Disparities in Psychiatric Care

CLINICAL AND CROSS-CULTURAL
PERSPECTIVES

Disparities in Psychiatric Care

CLINICAL AND CROSS-CULTURAL PERSPECTIVES

PEDRO RUIZ, MD

Professor and Interim Chair
Department of Psychiatry and Behavioral Sciences
University of Texas Medical School at Houston
Houston, Texas

Past President (2006–2007)
American Psychiatric Association

ANNELLE B. PRIMM, MD, MPH

Deputy Medical Director
Director of the Division of Minority and National Affairs
American Psychiatric Association
Arlington, Virginia

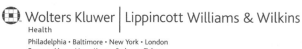
 Wolters Kluwer | Lippincott Williams & Wilkins
Health
Philadelphia · Baltimore · New York · London
Buenos Aires · Hong Kong · Sydney · Tokyo

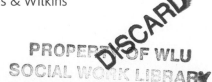

Acquisitions Editor: Charley Mitchell
Managing Editor: Sirkka Howes
Marketing Manager: Kimberly Schonberger
Designer: Holly Reid McLaughlin
Compositor: Maryland Composition/ASI

9 8 7 6 5 4 3 2 1

Library of Congress Cataloging-in-Publication Data

Disparities in psychiatric care : clinical and cross-cultural perspectives / [edited by] Pedro Ruiz, Annelle Primm.
     p. ; cm.
  Includes bibliographical references and index.
  ISBN 978-0-7817-9639-2 (alk. paper)
1. Mental health services—United States—Cross-cultural studies. 2. Minorities—Mental health services—United States. I. Ruiz, Pedro, 1936– II. Primm, Annelle.
  [DNLM: 1. Mental Health Services—United States. 2. Cross-Cultural Comparison—United States.
3. Healthcare Disparities—United States. 4. Socioeconomic Factors—United States. WM 30 D612 2010]
  RA790.6.D575 2010
  616.890089—dc22

2009002512

DEDICATION

Dr. Pedro Ruiz wishes to dedicate this book to his grandchildren Francisco A. Ruiz, Pedro P. Ruiz, Jr., Omar J. Holguin, III, and Pablo A. Holguin, who hopefully will one day live in a society that will be more sensitive and generous vis-à-vis persons with mental illness.

Dr. Annelle B. Primm wishes to dedicate this book to her daughter, India Delphine Primm-Spencer, who from a very young age, has shown extraordinary sensitivity to the needs of people with mental illness.

Dr. Pedro Ruiz and Dr. Annelle B. Primm also wish to dedicate this book to all people with mental illness worldwide. They suffer from real medical illnesses and, thus, deserve the highest quality of care together with universal access, comprehensive parity, and an environment where humane care will always prevail. We sincerely believe that health and mental health care should be a human right all over the world, not a privilege for those who can afford to pay for their care.

LIST OF CONTRIBUTORS

Sergio Aguilar-Gaxiola, MD, PhD Professor of Internal Medicine, University of California Davis School of Medicine; Director, Center for Reducing Health Disparities, Sacramento, California

Evaristo Akerele, MD Clinical Associate Professor, Department of Psychiatry, New York State Psychiatric Institute/Columbia University, New York, New York

Renato D. Alarcón, MD, MPH Professor, Department of Psychiatry and Psychology, Mayo Clinic College of Medicine; Medical Director, Mood Disorders Unit, Mayo Psychiatry & Psychology Treatment Center, Mayo Clinic, Rochester, Minnesota

Margarita Alegría, PhD Professor of Psychiatry, Department of Psychiatry, Harvard Medical School, Boston, Massachusetts; Director, Center for Multicultural Mental Health Research, Cambridge Health Alliance, Somerville, Massachusetts

David Baron, MSEd, DO Professor and Chair, Department of Psychiatry, Temple University; Psychiatrist-in-Chief, Temple-Episcopal Hospital, Philadelphia, Pennsylvania

Charles T. Barron, MD Clinical Assistant Professor, Department of Psychiatry, Mount Sinai School of Medicine, New York, New York; Director of Psychiatry, Elmhurst Hospital Center, Elmhurst, New York

Benedicto Borja, MD Clinical Assistant Professor, Department of Psychiatry, University of Maryland; Associate Director, Department of Residency Training, Sheppard Pratt Health System, Baltimore, Maryland

Douglas R. Bransfield, MBA, Esq. Red Bank, New Jersey

Robert C. Bransfield, MD Associate Director, Department of Psychiatry, Riverview Medical Center, Red Bank, New Jersey

José M. Cañive, MD Professor of Psychiatry and Neurosciences, University of New Mexico; Staff Psychiatrist & Director, Psychiatry Research, Behavioral Health Care Line & Research Service, New Mexico BA Health Care System, Albuquerque, New Mexico

Carlyle H. Chan, MD Professor and Vice Chair for Professional Development and Educational Outreach, Department of Psychiatry and Behavioral Medicine, Medical College of Wisconsin, Milwaukee, Wisconsin

Jack Drescher, MD Clinical Assistant Professor, Department of Psychiatry, New York Medical College, Valhalla, New York; Training and Supervising Analyst, Division of Psychoanalysis, William Alanson White Institute, New York, New York

Harold Eist, MD Psychiatrist, Bethesda, Maryland

Katherine Elliott, PhD Assistant Clinical Professor, Department of Pediatrics, University of California Davis, Psychologist, CAARE Diagnostic and Treatment Center, Sacramento, California

Anita Everett, MD, DFAPA Assistant Professor of Psychiatry, Johns Hopkins University; Section Chief, Community and General Psychiatry, Johns Hopkins Bayview, Baltimore, Maryland

Jacqueline Maus Feldman, MD Patrick H. Linton Professor; Director, Division of Public Psychiatry, Department of Psychiatry and Behavioral Neurobiology, University of Alabama at Birmingham, Birmingham, Alabama

Caroline E. Fisher, MD, PhD Assistant Professor, Department of Psychiatry, University of Massachusetts Medical School, Worcester, Massachusetts

Nimisha Gokaldas, MD Assistant Professor, Department of Psychiatry, School of Medicine, Oregon Health and Science University; Staff Psychiatrist, Mental Health, Portland VA Medical Center, Portland, Oregon

Marisela B. Gomez, MS, MPH, PhD, MD Social Health Concepts, Metairie, Louisiana

Warren W. Hewitt, Jr., MS Doctoral Candidate, School of Public Health and Policy, Morgan State University, Baltimore, Maryland; Center for Substance Abuse Treatment, Substance Abuse and Mental Health Services Administration, Rockville, Maryland

Michael Hollifield, MD Research Scientist, Pacific Institute of Research and Evaluation, Albuquerque, New Mexico

Ada Ikeako, MD Fellow in Psychoanalysis, Department of Psychiatry, New York University, Bellevue Hospital Center; Resident, Department of Psychiatry, Columbia University at Harlem Hospital Center, New York, New York

James Jackson, PhD Director and Research Professor, Institute for Social Research, University of Michigan, Ann Arbor, Michigan

Alex Kopelowicz, MD Associate Professor and Vice Chair, Department of Psychiatry and Behavioral Sciences, Geffen School of Medicine at UCLA, Los Angeles, California; Chief of Psychiatry, Olive View UCLA Medical Center, Sylmar, California

William B. Lawson, MD, PhD, DFAPA Professor and Chair, Department of Psychiatry and Behavioral Sciences, Howard University; Howard University Hospital, Washington, District of Columbia

Joseph B. Layde, MD, JD Associate Professor and Vice Chair for Education, Department of Psychiatry and Behavioral Medicine, Medical College of Wisconsin, Milwaukee, Wisconsin

Russell F. Lim, MD Associate Clinical Professor of Psychiatry and Behavioral Sciences, UC Davis School of Medicine, Sacramento, California

Maria D. Llorente, MD Professor of Psychiatry and Behavioral Sciences, Miller School of Medicine at the University of Miami; Chief, Psychiatry Service, Miami Veterans Administration Healthcare System, Miami, Florida

Steven R. Lopez, PhD Professor, Departments of Psychology and Social Work, University of Southern California, Los Angeles, California

Francis G. Lu, MD Clinical Professor, Department of Psychiatry, University of California, San Francisco; Director, Cultural Competence and Diversity, San Francisco General Hospital, San Francisco, California

Mario Maj, MD, PhD Professor and Chair, Department of Psychiatry; Head Physician, University of Naples, Naples, Italy; President, World Psychiatric Association

Spero M. Manson, PhD Professor and Head, American Indian and Alaska Native Programs, School of Medicine, University of Colorado Denver, Aurora, Colorado

Shunda McGahee, MD Clinical Fellow in Psychiatry, Harvard Medical School; Psychiatry Resident, Massachusetts General Hospital, Boston, Massachusetts

John S. McIntyre, MD Clinical Professor of Psychiatry, University of Rochester; Past Chair, Department of Psychiatry and Behavioral Health, Unity Health System, Rochester, New York

Rodrigo A. Muñoz, MD Clinical Professor of Psychiatry, University of California, San Diego, San Diego, California

Niru Nahar, MD, MPH Attending Psychiatrist, St. Joseph's Medical Center, Yonkers, New York

Ora Nakash, PhD Instructor of Psychology, Department of Psychiatry, Harvard Medical School, Boston, Massachusetts; Research Associate, Center for Multicultural Mental Health Research, Cambridge Health Alliance, Somerville, Massachusetts

Vernon I. Nathaniel, MD Chief Resident, Department of Psychiatry, Department of Psychiatry and Behavioral Sciences, Howard University Hospital, Washington, District of Columbia

John M. Oldham, MD, MS Professor and Executive Vice Chair, Menninger Department of Psychiatry and Behavioral Sciences, Baylor College of Medicine; Senior Vice President and Chief of Staff, The Menninger Clinic, Houston, Texas

Richard R. Pleak, MD Associate Professor of Clinical Psychiatry and Behavioral Sciences, Albert Einstein College of Medicine, Bronx, New York; Director of Education and Training, Child and Adolescent Psychiatry, Long Island Jewish Medical Center, New Hyde Park, New York

Annelle B. Primm, MD, MPH Deputy Medical Director, Director of the Division of Minority and National Affairs, American Psychiatric Association, Arlington, Virginia

Beny J. Primm, MD Executive Director, Addiction Research and Treatment Corporation, Brooklyn, New York

Andres J. Pumariega, MD Professor of Psychiatry and Behavioral Sciences, Temple University School of Medicine, Philadelphia, Pennsylvania; Chair of Psychiatry, The Reading Hospital and Medical Center, Reading, Pennsylvania

Daniel Rosen, PhD Assistant Professor, Counseling and Health Psychology, Bastyr University, Kenmore, Washington

Pedro Ruiz, MD Professor and Interim Chair, Department of Psychiatry and Behavioral Services, University of Texas Medical School at Houston, Houston, Texas

Roslyn Seligman, MD Professor of Psychiatry, University of Cincinnati College of Medicine; Faculty, Department of Psychiatry, University Hospital, Cincinnati, Ohio

Steven S. Sharfstein, MD, MPA Clinical Professor and Vice Chair of Psychiatry, University of Maryland School of Medicine; President and CEO, Sheppard Pratt Health System, Baltimore, Maryland

Jay H. Shore, MD, MPH Assistant Professor of Psychiatry, University of Colorado, Denver, Aurora, Colorado

William Sribney, MS Third Way Statistics, White Lake, New York

Altha J. Stewart, MD Executive Director, National Leadership Council on African American Behavioral Health

Ann Marie Sullivan, MD Clinical Professor of Psychiatry, Mount Sinai School of Medicine, New York, New York; Senior Vice President, Queens Health Network, Elmhurst Hospital Center, Elmhurst, New York

David Takeuchi, PhD Professor, Department of Sociology and School of Social Work, University of Washington, Seattle, Washington

Hendry Ton, MD, MS Assistant Clinical Professor, Department of Psychiatry and Behavioral Sciences, University of California Davis, Director of Education, Center for Reducing Health Disparities, University of California, Davis Health System, Sacramento, California

William A. Vega, PhD Professor of Family Medicine, University of California at Los Angeles, Los Angeles, California

Suzanne Vogel-Scibilia, MD Psychiatrist, Beaver County Psychiatric Services, Beaver, Pennsylvania

Serena Yuan Volpp, MD, MPH Clinical Assistant Professor of Psychiatry, New York University School of Medicine; Unit Chief, Residency Training Unit, Department of Psychiatry, Bellevue Hospital, New York, New York

Khakasa Wapenyi, MD Attending, Department of Psychiatry, Weill Cornell Medical College; New York Presbyterian Hospital, New York, New York

Henry C. Weinstein, MD Clinical Professor of Psychiatry; Director, Program in Psychiatry and the Law, New York University School of Medicine, New York, New York

Joseph J. Westermeyer, MD, MPH, PhD Professor of Psychiatry, University of Minnesota; Medical Director, Mental Health Department, Minneapolis VAMC, Minneapolis, Minnesota

Meghan Woo, ScM Research Assistant, Center for Multicultural Mental Health Research, Cambridge Health Alliance, Cambridge, Massachusetts

PREFACE

This book was conceived by Dr. Pedro Ruiz during his tenure as President of the American Psychiatric Association (APA) (2006–2007). The idea evolved from Dr. Ruiz's efforts to address all major obstacles faced by people with mental illness in the United States in their quest to secure access, parity, quality, and humane care. Dr. Ruiz's overall theme for his APA Presidential year was "Addressing Patient Needs: Access, Parity and Humane Care," and he decided to produce a book focusing on "psychiatric/mental health disparities" as his major Presidential project. A related initiative taken by Dr. Ruiz during his APA Presidential year was to build a strong and ongoing relationship with some of the most prominent mental health advocacy organizations. He achieved this goal with the National Alliance on Mental Illness (NAMI) and Mental Health America (MHA); this book, then, represents one of his core advocacy efforts as President of the APA.

Disparities in mental healthcare have existed for centuries, going as far back as when the world civilization began. We have seen many examples of attempts to improve and/or eliminate the negative impact of psychiatric/mental health disparities on people with mental illness all over the world. The initiatives introduced by William Tuke at the Retreat in York, England, in 1796, were directed to improve the treatment received by people with mental illness during this period. The book "Malleus Maleficarum" by the German Dominican fathers Sprenger and Kramer at Cologne University in 1846 also clearly depicts the negative perception of mental illness and people with mental illness at the end of the 15th century. The "moral treatment" efforts advanced by Dr. Philippe Pinel and other humanitarian figures at the end of the 18th century additionally demonstrate the desires to eliminate discriminatory practices and disparities within the mental healthcare system in Europe during this period. It may seem inconceivable that discriminatory practices and psychiatric/mental health disparities still exist in the 21st century and, in particular, in the United States, which is the most economically developed and powerful country in the entire world. In this context, Dr. Ruiz felt that a book addressing "psychiatric/mental health disparities" would constitute an ideal tool to address these discriminatory practices, not only in the United States but all over the world as well. Early in this project, Dr. Ruiz asked Dr. Annelle B. Primm, Director of the Office of Minority and National Affairs of the APA, to join him as a Co-Editor of this book.

This book is composed of six sections and a total of 33 chapters. Each section focuses on a set of relevant topics pertaining to "psychiatric/mental health disparities." Also, each chapter addresses the most important and significant issues pertaining to the section theme.

Section I focuses on the foundations of psychiatric disparities, and consists of two chapters. In Chapter 1, Anita Everett, MD, addresses the historical roots of psychiatric disparities. The role of the government, its impact on the mental healthcare system, and its implications for today's multiethnic and multicultural population are discussed. The historical perspectives related to the ideological aspects of the mental healthcare system over the last several centuries are also addressed in this chapter. In Chapter 2, Altha J. Stewart, MD, discusses the determinants of psychiatric/mental health disparities. Dr. Stewart identifies the following key factors that influence psychiatric disparities: (1) economic status, (2) cultural and ethnocentric issues, (3) racism, discrimination and prejudice, (4) lack of trust between patients and health care providers, and (5) lack of cultural competence within the healthcare system and the workforce.

Section II concentrates on psychiatric disparities among ethnic groups, and encompasses four chapters. In Chapter 3, William B. Lawson, MD, and Annelle B. Primm, MD, write about African Americans within the context of psychiatric disparities. The authors focus on diagnostic considerations, treatment, and prevention efforts. In Chapter 4, Renato D. Alarcon, MD, and Pedro Ruiz, MD, report on the Hispanic population who reside in the United States. The current demographics of this population, its cultural characteristics, and the mental healthcare system of this population subgroup, including access to care, diagnostic features, and potential solutions are all well addressed in this chapter. In Chapter 5, Francis G. Lu, MD, focuses on psychiatric disparities among Asian Americans and Pacific Islanders. Areas of focus include health insurance status, the mental healthcare system, stigma associated with mental healthcare, and future research perspectives. In Chapter 6, Jay H. Shore, MD, and Spero M. Manson, PhD, focus on American Indians and Alaska Natives. In this chapter, the authors address historical perspectives; the significance of the doctor-patient relationship; and promising practices, challenges, and future directions.

Section III, "Psychiatric Disparities Among Gender and Sexual Minorities," is composed of five chapters. In Chapter 7, Caroline Fisher, MD, and Roslyn Seligman, MD, report on psychiatric disparities among women. Specific issues such as diagnostic issues, treatment strategies, preventive measures, as well as relevant key issues, such as ethnicity and religion, are covered. In Chapter 8, Jack Drescher, MD, discusses psychiatric disparities among gay men. Dr. Drescher addresses factors that hinder research in this population subgroup; also, subgroup differences and definition challenges are discussed. Finally, the author discusses stigma-related issues and research challenges and makes recommendations for the DSM-V. In Chapter 9, Nimisha Gokaldas, MD, and Khakasa Wapengi, MD, delineate the psychiatric disparities among lesbians. They define this patient population subgroup and address "coming out" issues, suicide, diagnostic considerations, and treatment options. In Chapter 10, Serena Y. Volpp, MD, focuses on psychiatric disparities among the bisexual population subgroup. Dr. Volpp concentrates on epidemiological trends and methodological problems in defining bisexual population subgroups, as well as diagnostic considerations, suicide, and behaviors such as violence, addiction, eating habits, mental healthcare utilization, and understanding of disparities within this population. In Chapter 11, Richard R. Pleak, MD, covers psychiatric disparities among transgender persons. In this chapter, definitional issues and childhood and adolescent developmental, and adulthood issues are discussed.

Section IV focuses on psychiatric disparities among age groups, and is comprised of three chapters. In Chapter 12, Andres J. Pumariega, MD, discusses psychiatric disparities among children and adolescents. Topics include financial and cultural barriers, prevalence, and mental healthcare utilization. Ways of addressing and resolving psychiatric disparities are also discussed. In Chapter 13, Ann M. Sullivan, MD, and Charles T. Barron, MD, concentrate on key issues pertaining to psychiatric disparities in adulthood. An overview of racial and ethnic mental health disparities and their impact on caregivers and work roles is also presented in this chapter, as well as related diagnostic considerations. In Chapter 14, Maria D. Llorente, MD, Vernon I.

Nathaniel, MD, and Shunda McGahee, MD, focus on psychiatric disparities among older adults. Demographic changes are discussed, as well as epidemiological trends, workforce constraints, and diagnostic and treatment considerations.

Section V relates to psychiatric disparities among special populations, and includes seven chapters. In Chapter 15, Joseph J. Westermeyer, MD, Michael Hollifield, MD, and Jose M. Canive, MD, discuss psychiatric disparities among migrants and refugees. The authors discuss factors contributing to disparities, including patient-centered characteristics, stigma, lack of education, somatization, distrust, lack of knowledge about healthcare regulations, lack of resources, clinician/provider issues, and system factors, as well as family and community-based factors and natural disasters. In Chapter 16, Suzanne Vogel Scibilia, MD, covers issues pertaining to psychiatric disparities among rural populations. Additionally, she discusses key issues including marked infrastructure deficits and lack of key services such as crisis intervention and inpatient services, avoiding criminal justice interventions and transportation challenges. Other issues such as manpower recruitment and retention, available housing and supportive employment capabilities are also discussed in this chapter. Finally, recommendations to resolve disparities are made. In Chapter 17, Beny J. Primm, MD, Warren W. Mewitt, Jr., MS, Annelle B. Primm, MD, and Marisela B. Gomez, MD, focus on psychiatric disparities among addicted population subgroups, especially among African Americans. In this chapter, the most current epidemiological trends are described, utilization factors and quality of care factors are addressed; causes and consequence issues and prevention practices are presented. In Chapter 18, Henry C. Weinstein, MD, describes issues pertaining to psychiatric disparities among incarcerated populations. In this chapter, a flow chart depicting the steps of incarcerated persons within the criminal justice system is discussed; also addressed are overcrowding barriers within this system, as well as "bias" and language barriers. In Chapter 19, Jacqueline M. Feldman, MD, discusses psychiatric disparities among chronic mentally ill populations. In this chapter, the demographic trends of this population are depicted, as well as historical perspectives and unique barriers to care such as stigma, financial constraints, unresponsive care systems, impact of mental illness on the individual. In Chapter 20, Alex Kopelowicz, MD, Steven R. Lopez, MD, and William A. Vega, MD, report psychiatric disparities among disabled populations. In this chapter, the role of psychiatric rehabilitation is extensively discussed, as well as the need to integrate cultural aspects in the treatment of families. Additionally, the role of case management and access to care are fully addressed. In Chapter 21, Suzanne Vogel-Scibilia, MD, focuses on psychiatric disparities among mentally ill populations. In this chapter, the role of disability determinations is addressed, as well as the role of managed-care plans and the understaffing of outpatient care programs. Additionally, the extensive cost of specialized psychiatric care and the difficulties in accessing care are discussed. The importance of having good knowledge of how the mental healthcare system operates is also underlined in this chapter, as well as the vulnerabilities of the mentally ill homeless population.

Section VI defines how best to address psychiatric disparities, and it includes 12 chapters. In Chapter 22, Ora Nakash, PhD, David Rosen, PhD, and Margarita Alegria, PhD, address the culturally-sensitive evaluation vis-à-vis psychiatric disparities. In this chapter, the challenges and barriers in conducting mental health intakes with multicultural populations are described, as well as the impact of stereotyping and biases when processing minority patients' clinical information. Recommendations to overcome these challenges and barriers are presented, as well as ways of improving the system of care and the therapeutic alliance. In Chapter 23, Russell F. Lim, MD, focuses on the role of cultural competence. The author describes current federal policies, state policies, and the influence of the national accrediting agencies, professional organizations, and foundations. In Chapter 24, Benedicto Borja, MD, and Steven S. Sharfstein, MD, discuss the role of emergency care. The authors note the decline of state hospital beds and the current levels of mental healthcare utilization. They also discuss the role of psychiatric services provided by primary care providers and managed care; finally, future options directed to improve the healthcare system are covered. In Chapter 25, Rodrigo A. Munoz, MD, and Harold Eist, MD, write about the interrelation between providers and psychiatric disparities. In this chapter, health disparities are assessed, the role of disparities vis-à-vis systems of care are discussed, and historical perspectives, as well as payments challenges are defined; finally, potential solutions are considered. In Chapter 26, John M. Oldham, MD, and John S. McIntyre, MD, focus on the role of quality of care. In this chapter, a historic perspective of quality of care models is presented, including "pay-for-performance" and "maintenance of certification." In Chapter 27, William Sribney MS, Katherine Elliott, PhD, Sergio Aguilar-Gaxiola, MD, and Hendry Ton, MD, discuss the role of nonmedical interventions for mental health, non-MD, clinicians, and other human service providers for mental health; also, the use of complementary and alternative medicine for mental health are discussed extensively. Additionally, the implications for training and education with respect to the use of these models of mental healthcare are presented. In Chapter 28, Evaristo Akerele, MD, Niru Nahar, MD, and Ada Ikeake, MD, focus on the topic of psychiatric disparities in education and discuss issues pertaining to undergraduate, graduate, and postgraduate education in psychiatry. In Chapter 29, Carlyle H. Chan, MD, and Joseph B. Layde, MD, JD, consider the role of continuing medical education. They describe the structure of the continuing medical education system in the United States and address the challenges for continuing education in the care for depression. In Chapter 30, Margarita Alegría PhD, Meghan Woo, ScM, David Takeuchi, PhD, and James S. Jackson, MD, focus on ethnic and racial group-specific considerations. Coverage focuses on diagnostic and treatment considerations, preventive considerations, and areas for future research. In Chapter 31, Robert C. Bransfield, MD, and Douglas R. Bransfield, MBA, Esq, discuss the role of parity. The authors address the current burden of mental illness and its financial costs as well as the current technical capability of the mental healthcare system. Finally, the chapter discusses the consequences of not having mental health parity and the current cost of cost-containment practices. In Chapter 32, Mario Maj, MD, and David Baron, MD, present the current status of global perspectives with respect to psychiatric disparities. Key topics include the prevalence of mental disorders worldwide, with attention given to treatment gaps and treatment effectiveness; the current worldwide resources availability for mental healthcare, worldwide trends in mental healthcare, and the existing worldwide barriers to change the current mental health system of care. In Chapter 33, Pedro Ruiz, MD, and Annelle B. Primm, MD, focus on the need for universal access to care as a way of dealing with psychiatric disparities. In this chapter, the current situation vis-à-vis access to care in the United States is discussed. Attention is also given to the current mental healthcare needs of minority populations in the U.S., as well as to the role of managed care. Finally, solutions to the current crisis in the mental healthcare system of the United States are fully addressed and discussed.

We hope that this book will be useful in addressing the much needed changes facing the current mental healthcare system of the United States, and also the models for positive changes in mental healthcare systems worldwide. People with mental illness will hopefully benefit from this book and, thus, we should all unite: mental health professionals, governmental officials, advocacy organizations, consumer organizations, and society at large to ensure that all people with mental illness in this country and abroad have their mental healthcare needs addressed. Our patients deserve universal access to care, full and comprehensive parity of care, high quality of care, and humane care.

We also want to take this opportunity to deeply thank the tireless efforts of our contributing authors. Because of their hard work and full commitment to the goals and objectives of this book, we hope and expect that people with mental illness all over the world will have a more promising and bright future with respect to their mental healthcare needs; likewise, we also wish to recognize two sensitive and caring professionals in the staff of Lippincott Williams & Wilkins: Charles W. Mitchell, Executive Editor, and Sirkka Howes, Associate Managing Editor. Without their editorial guidance and professional commitment, as well as their ongoing support, this book would not have been produced. Additionally, we wish to thank the members of the American Psychiatric Association's Board-of-Trustees and the APA Medical Director and Chief Executive Officer, James H. Scully, MD, who fully supported this Presidential Project, and also had faith in the goals and objectives of this book. We additionally wish to recognize the excellent support that we received during this entire project from Alison Bondurant, MA, from the APA's Office of Minority and National Affairs, and Marie O. Gonzales-Arms, from U.T. Houston's Department of Psychiatry and Behavioral Sciences; they both worked very hard to make this project a reality. Finally, we remain indebted to people with mental illness in this country and abroad. We hope that they will be the true beneficiaries of this much needed collaborative effort.

Pedro Ruiz, MD
Houston, Texas

Annelle B. Primm, MD, MPH
Arlington, Virginia

FOREWORD

For generations the topic and stigma of mental health has been swept under the rug. We chose not to see it, to hear of it or to speak of it. It has been and continues to be an immediate negative label on the human race, which we must work collaboratively to change through education, understanding and partnerships. Mental illness does not discriminate. It touches all, regardless of race, gender, class or religion.

The impact of mental illness is very real and very scary to many. For more than one in four of our men and women returning from war who suffer or have suffered from traumatic brain injury or post-traumatic stress disorder, suicide has been a chilling choice. It is also the third leading cause of death for children under age 24, and statistics reveal that more than half of all prison and jail inmates suffer from mental illness. Increasingly the economic impact of mental illness, in addition to the personal impact, is being quantified, with lost productivity and absenteeism costing the United States economy upward of $200 billion a year.

According to the U.S. Surgeon General, 57 million Americans suffer from mental illness. Despite findings that most mental illnesses are highly treatable, only one in three individuals suffering from a mental illness seek and/or receive any treatment. Such low treatment rates can be attributed to the strong stigma associated with mental illness that persists. Yet we know that those who seek treatment can lead healthy and productive lives.

Additionally, individuals who do seek help are far too frequently facing difficulty accessing needed services, especially help that is linguistically and culturally appropriate. To meet the demand for mental health services, which is growing in every corner of our country, we must recognize, accept and dialogue using effective vernacular. It is critical for our country to provide help through access to trained professionals who can provide culturally competent services. We must also forge partnerships throughout our diverse communities to address the disparities in mental health care.

We must continue to educate ourselves, our friends, our families, and government and elected officials to work to remove the stigma associated with the idea of mental illness. By increasing awareness of mental health disparities, we can remove the first obstacle for those suffering from mental illness to receive assistance.

Disparities in Psychiatric Care is unrivaled in its extensive examination of disparities in the provision of multiple areas of mental health services. This valuable work utilizes evidence-based clinical approaches to establish a framework for mental health practitioners to prevent, reduce and eliminate disparities within mental health care. The comprehensive discussion that follows should be regarded as a leading guide for all who have an interest in the mental health and the wellbeing of those living with serious mental illness, as well as serve to educate the non-mental health community.

Thank you, Dr. Pedro Ruiz, for being a champion and a strong, dedicated partner during your tenure as President of the American Psychiatric Association and for your continued efforts in this important endeavor to bring awareness to the impact mental illness has on society and improve the mental health of all. By working together, we truly can make a difference and begin a new era for mental health.

Grace F. Napolitano
Member of Congress

TABLE OF CONTENTS

Foundations

1 Historical Perspectives

Anita Everett

INTRODUCTION

Celebrate diversity. These two familiar words are commonly paired in contemporary American culture. These words might be seen in community promotions, health systems, and other public places. *Celebrate* connotes a happy, positive, and joyous welcoming. *Diversity* implies difference within a group and commonly in this context is interpreted to mean differences in race and/or ethnicity. The word *diversity* itself today has a generally neutral connotation but often is associated with programs that promote inclusion of individuals from different and minority cultural and racial backgrounds. In our culture today, most Americans conceptually endorse the value of diversity; however, this is not universal and has not always been the case. We want to live and raise our children in communities that are diverse. We want our children to go to colleges that include diverse student bodies. A diverse community is thriving and vibrant in comparison to a homogenous community which may conjure images of economic and social stagnation. While we may have arrived at an ideological tipping point with regard to valuing the inclusion of racial and ethnic groups, we are a long way from achieving actual equal opportunity for all within contemporary American culture. Nowhere is disparity or disadvantage more critical than in healthcare. Persons who are unwell cannot participate fully in their lives or in the development of our country and culture. Addressing the needs of individuals from different racial and ethnic backgrounds is a situation every nation and group of people has had to address; it is a universal issue throughout time.

This chapter is designed to provide context and historical antecedents that have shaped contemporary United States policy and thought regarding diversity and disparity in our culture and in our healthcare system. Initially there are several concepts and definitions that will be reviewed. Examples of significant points in history with

1

particular focus on the strategies and/or policies that governments or ruling classes developed to address cultural diversity will be highlighted. The goal of this chapter is to provide a framework that will equip and inspire clinicians and other readers to develop and maintain a lifelong curiosity about and interest in providing excellent clinical care to individuals from different cultures, including those that in the United States are at a health disadvantage due to their ethnicity, race, culture, or origin. An additional goal would be to encourage all healthcare providers to advocate for these members of our culture so that we might all participate fully in the "life, liberty, and the pursuit of happiness" that was outlined as an inalienable or human right by our founding fathers.

CORE GOVERNMENT FUNCTIONS: DEFENSE AND JUSTICE

In framing a discussion on cultural diversity and disparity, it is necessary for clinicians to have a basic understanding of the powerful role government has in shaping attitude and practice toward individuals and groups from diverse cultures. Governments are formed when groups of people have a need for a common defense and some form of order or justice. Without government, people would be in anarchy. A recent example of near anarchy would be the situation in the nation of Iraq immediately following the deposition of Saddam Hussein.

Defense and justice are universally observed functions of all forms of government including monarchies, dictatorships, and democracies. A tribe in rural Africa might manifest these functions less formally with a council of elders that make determinations regarding justice within the tribe and create defensive strategies against natural (e.g., floods) and unnatural (e.g., rival tribe) external forces. Highly structured societies manifest the governmental functions of defense and justice much more formally through written laws, ordinances, precedents, and other deliberated and detailed documents. Although the word defense connotes protection from an external aggressor, for this chapter, it will also be understood more broadly to include military action against an external culture or enemy as in the case of one nation conquering another. Justice in this context of basic government functions includes a wide range of activities. Core functions of basic justice include: (a) the development and articulation of an ethical framework upon which justice is based; (b) a mechanism through which deliberation of potential breeches in the framework can be resolved; (c) decisions about common resource accrual and distribution (taxation); and (d) application of the framework (do these rights and rules apply to persons of all race, gender, and ethnicity, or only to certain subgroups within the jurisdiction of the government?).

In addition to the core functions of defense and justice, government often supports social programs deemed to be advantageous for the common good. These include programs such as education, civil infrastructure (roads, water, and electricity), public healthcare, welfare, disability, etc. The scale and scope of these sociocultural functions varies greatly and is generally associated with the stage of economic development of a nation. In times of peace, and once a nation has an established government that is recognized by its people, needs related to social and cultural function can be addressed. A familiar paradigm that we might consider here would be Maslow's Hierarchy of Needs. As clinicians, we are accustomed to the application of this hierarchy of needs on an individual level. Individuals must have certain basic survival needs met, such as food and shelter, before they can progress to work on other more sophisticated issues. Governments or nations in early development generally cannot begin to work on social and cultural functions until basic security and justice are developed. The extent to which government should provide benefits broader than defense and justice have been debated throughout U.S. history. Today, what is sometimes referred to as liberal ideology generally promotes a broader government role in providing human services that support a civil society, whereas conservative ideology generally advocates for individual choice, and a government role that is more limited and does not expect government to provide broader social welfare programs. This division in thought becomes critical when applied to the issue of U.S. healthcare policy. Is healthcare and mental healthcare for all citizens a universal human right that falls within the justice duty of government, or is government-sponsored healthcare an optional social program? If healthcare is viewed as a human right, all individuals within a government's domain, irrespective of culture of origin, gender, or race should have equal access to it. If government-sponsored healthcare is an optional social program, then it is logical that government resources would be used for certain parts of the population that are in accord with the priorities in the ethical framework for resource distribution of a nation. An example of this is our Medicaid program. The provision of healthcare to poor children, who are at a health disadvantage through no fault of their own, provides justice by giving an equal start in life to all potential good citizens. In the recent years, there have been efforts to contain Medicaid costs and one strategy has been the institution of a requirement of proof of citizenship as a condition for eligibility. This is an example of one of many ways in which the U.S. healthcare system is difficult for individuals from other cultures to access and understand.

ONE NATION, MANY CULTURES: MELTING POTS AND MOSAICS

Several terms are often used to shape policy toward the inclusion or exclusion of diverse groups within a community, society, and a nation. All nations, governments, and societies need to determine how they are going to address individuals that represent different cultures or are minority components. *Assimilate* is a term used to describe the integration of a person or group of people into a larger group so that the original differences are minimized or eliminated. If a person is assimilated successfully into an alien culture, he or she becomes part of that culture and loses attributes of his or her native culture.

The term *melting pot* has historically been used to describe U.S. policy toward the inclusion of persons immigrating to the United States. Melting pot is a term used to describe a society consisting of individuals from different cultures and ethnic groups that are brought together to create one emergent culture. Inherent in the idea of melting pot are themes of assimilation and a single emergent blended culture such that the characteristics of the culture of origin are minimized.

In contrast to a melting pot, some governments have envisioned or promoted a *mosaic* as a framework. With a mosaic policy orientation, there is acceptance and recognition of individual cultures that remain intact and at the same time exists within a nation or country. Canadian immigration policy has been described as promoting a cultural mosaic. While a cultural mosaic policy may be useful to encourage immigration and settlement in a country with great land mass and low population such as Canada, this policy orientation could result in a weaker national government with less sense of national cohesion and less national identity.

Tolerance is a policy or approach that includes the recognition of different cultures or groups without attempting to suppress the native qualities of that culture. In a tolerance policy, immigrants may have limited opportunities to participate in national development and leadership; rather their existence would be tolerated. Early Jim Crow laws in some U.S. southern states codified the separation of whites from blacks. These laws conceptually codified tolerance. African Americans were expected to obey these laws which outlined the details of segregation in public spaces. Later in this process, because of the inability or unwillingness of communities to provide separate and equal services, schools and public spaces became a foundation for the American Civil Rights movement. The concept in the U.S. Declaration of Independence that men are created equal and have inalienable rights to pursue life, liberty, and happiness has been clear from the outset. Exactly to whom these rights apply has been clarified and refined over time.

A policy of *intolerance* would generally include mechanisms to actively eliminate diversity and may range from the narrow immigration policy to aggressive racial and/or ethnic cleansing. A contemporary example of intolerance would be in Rwanda in 1994, wherein the Hutu tribe by policy and military action attempted to eliminate members of the Tutsi tribe. Current attempts to heal the animosity and anarchy created by this civil war include the development of a strong emergent national identity with virtually no recognition of tribal identity. Thus the goal is a kind of melting pot or blending of two native cultures.

THREE ERAS IN TIME: ALEXANDER OF MACEDONIA, THE RENAISSANCE, AND U.S. HISTORY

The remainder of this chapter includes a discussion of three eras in history that have been influential in the development of current policy and attitude toward cultural diversity in the United States. All governments and the people within them must develop a policy toward individuals and groups from other cultures. It is hoped that examples from each of these highly influential eras would provide stimulating new insight into the foundations of cultural diversity in the United States. Three eras will be reviewed: Alexander the Great and Hellenistic Alexandria, the Renaissance, and mid-20th century history of the United States. In each section, a brief review of the cultural aspect of the era will be addressed. Additionally, highlights regarding the scientific and medical developments in each era will be discussed.

Alexander the Great and International Tolerance

Alexander the Great (356–323 BC) was a remarkable figure in the Classic or Hellenistic era. He is known as a highly ambitious warrior and was from Macedonia. In his quest to rule the world, he captured not only Greece but also the powerful kingdom of Persia (now Iran). Greece itself had many cultural similarities with his native Macedonia; Persia, however, was a very different culture. Herodotus, an ancient historian in the 5th century BC delineated four elements that comprise a culture: genealogy, language, religion, and custom. Genealogy in this context refers to the family and place of origin. Being able to establish oneself as Greek was important as one had to be Greek to compete in the Olympic games. Kings and leaders in the Persian Empire were generally direct descendants of other kings and were considered to have a divine right to rule. A familiar example of this is the role of pharaoh in

Egyptian culture which for much of this era was under Persian rule. In contrast, Greek and Macedonian rulers were considered to be the first among peers. They were individual citizens with leadership qualities that made them worthy for the ruling class. There was an easy merging of language, religion, and custom when Alexander captured and subsequently ruled Greece. The capture of Persia, however, resulted in Alexander becoming the ruler of a multinational, conglomerated empire. Rather than demand assimilation as was the custom of the era, in ruling Persia he supported a policy of tolerance. He openly encouraged his leaders to marry into Persian families. This style of openness to diverse cultures supported the development of one of the most influential cities of this era—Alexandria, Egypt. Alexandria was a vibrant city where individuals from a variety of cultures and races lived. Alexandria was a well-known international trading port as well as an intellectual mecca where the first museum and the first school of mathematics were developed. Scientific leaders of the day were beginning to be able to provide explanations for natural events that were previously believed to be the will of the gods. Medical science was influenced by the work of the Greek physician, Hippocrates. Hippocrates sought explanations for the causes and treatments of illnesses that were based on reason and physical observation. This was in contrast to the prevailing belief that sickness represented the will or punishment of a god. The oath developed by Hippocrates (1) serves as a cornerstone of contemporary professional ethics and includes the principle of equity in treatment for all individuals that seek medical attention (2). Not much is described about mental illness in accounts of history of this era. Some individuals with mental illness were likely to have been perceived to have had special prophetic powers given by a god. In conclusion, Alexander the Great serves as an example of a global superpower who ruled the multinational empire he developed with a policy of cultural tolerance and diversity. It is widely recognized that the cultural diversity of Alexandria served as a critical foundation for the great accomplishments that were developed in the world in this era. This era is the foundation of Western civilization and is an important underpinning of U.S. culture.

The Renaissance and Humanism

The second historical era that has fundamental influence on contemporary society, culture, and ultimately health disparity, is the Renaissance. This is an era that directly impacted the ideology of our forefathers as they formulated the guiding principles that the United States was founded on. The intellectual background for what constitutes a human right was developed from the humanistic ideology of the Renaissance.

The term Renaissance comes from the Latin for *rebirth* and is believed to stem from a renewed interest in the study of ancient Greek, Egyptian, and Persian culture in this period. This period roughly extends from 1400 to 1700. Several ancient texts had been found and translated from Greek and Arabic into Italian, French, and English. The recent development of the printing press enabled widespread dissemination of information and ideology. It is in this period that *Humanism*, or the formal study of man, his history, and culture flourished (3). Humanism provided a foundation for the questioning of the divine right to rule. Generations of monarchs and ruling elite had asserted that they had the authority to wage war, to impose taxes, to govern, and to live lavish lives based on a divine right. The ruling class was above reproach due to this divine right to rule. Reacquaintance with Greek ideology stimulated consideration that great leaders such as Alexander the Great might earn the privilege of rule through an affirmation by peers. This resulted in cracks to the divine right entitlement of monarchs and served as a foundation for the development of democratic governments such as the United States and later in France.

Scientific developments of the era included a formalization of the scientific method of observation and recording reproducible results. This time was the primordial soup from which the industrial era, or a drive for the practical application of science was born. While some medical science discoveries were made in this era, medicine was not seen as a profession or science that held many answers. Much of the entire world was at ongoing risk of massive deaths due to the plague and other infectious diseases which medical science of the time had no reliable treatments for. With regard to mental health, this was an era that saw some hope for management of mental illness through the application of humanistic approaches. Although the *moral treatment* method did not become standard approach until later in the 1800s, it had its foundation in humanism of the Renaissance. The idea behind moral treatment is that the provision of a dignified environment that is clean and orderly together with attention to human cultural, educational, and social needs would result in cure for mental afflictions.

The Declaration of Independence was written primarily by Thomas Jefferson who was highly influenced by late Renaissance humanism. This document is the pivotal document that articulated the rationale for independence from the tyrannies of the British monarchy. The first sentence of this document reads as follows: "We hold these truths to be self-evident, that all men are created equal, that they are endowed by their Creator with certain unalienable Rights, that among these are Life, Liberty and the pursuit of Happiness." In this single powerful sentence, Jefferson clearly asserts that all men are created as equal. He does not limit the fundamental right to life, liberty, and the pursuit of happiness just to citizens, to property holders, to whites, to the educated, to native-born persons, or to the nobility, rather he broadens this to all persons. Much of this ideology is influenced by the writings of John Locke. A second critical point in this opening statement is the assertion that this equality is an inalienable or undeniable right that is based on natural law and is not bestowed by a monarch, government, or ruling class. He asserts that equality is a human right that supersedes the policy of a government and in fact can be legitimately used as a reason individuals might secede from a particular government to form their own government that does not violate these natural or human rights.

The United States Pledge of Allegiance, with more efficient wording, affirms the expectation of equality for all. These words are: "I pledge allegiance to the flag of the United States of America . . . one nation under God, indivisible, with liberty and justice for all." The idea that individuals could come to the United Stated to escape the tyranny of other governments and live a life that is relatively unencumbered by the tyrannies of government resonates to this day throughout the world. In these thoughts there is a kind of inherent expectation for assimilation: the idea that one culture will emerge from the assimilation of many—the melting pot. As we will explore in the final section of this chapter, it is the actual enforcement of the details of these well grounded principles of equality for all that have been the cause of intense political, social, and cultural debate in recent years. The very idea on which we were founded, that individuals from tyrannical governments can come to the United States, assimilate, and then be able to participate fully in U.S. society has not truly manifested itself. The lack of ability to resolve these issues has resulted in our current situation of cultural, social, and health disparities.

The Great Society

In this third and final section, we will review several historical developments that have played a role in shaping current cultural disparity in the United States. Our founding fathers built our nation on the concept that persons are created equal and that all people have certain unalienable rights. Working out the details as to who was included and the role of government in enforcing those rights was the challenge of the next several generations of Americans.

In the years following the Revolutionary War, the United States grew in terms of population and land mass. It is beyond the scope of this chapter to review the many details of the circumstances that led to the Civil War in the United States. There were competing interests in keeping the states united as a single government versus allowing the practice of slavery with its associated human rights violations that were inconsistent with the ideology of equality as established in the Declaration of Independence. From the very beginning of the United States until after the Civil War, this was among the most contentious issues that the United States as a young government was forced to address. Within the army itself, colored units served in the war but were kept separate from other units. Following the Civil War there was a policy of tolerance toward African Americans. This resulted in separate schools, medical and professional services, etc. A need for teachers and other professionals in African American communities resulted in the development of several colleges and professional schools which are still in existence today and are often referred to as historically black colleges and universities. Many of these schools are very active in advocating for the elimination of disparities for traditionally underserved racial and ethnic groups.

There are some parallels to the experience of African Americans in cities that were the destiny of immigrants mostly on the East Coast from European countries such as Ireland and Italy and on the West Coast from countries such as China and Mexico. Often these new arrivals to the United States chose to live in segregated areas. These areas, known as "Little Italy," "Little Poland," or "Chinatown," within these cities were usually not legally segregated. A significant difference in these populations was that the individuals who were mostly white came of their own choice and many times were voluntarily seeking a better life free from human rights violations and extreme poverty. Americans of African descent, however, usually were brought to the United States forcefully to work as slaves. Residents of all of these communities have often experienced stigma.

There are numerous examples of intense containment or profiling of individuals based on culture in recent U.S. history. Specific examples of this include the use of Japanese Internment camps in the 1940s as well as various neo-Nazi movements and the profiling of individuals who practice Islam.

It was by executive order of President Truman in September 1954 that the U.S. Armed Forces first became desegregated. This order specifically directed that all soldiers would be treated equally and would no longer be segregated in terms of active duty, pay, or benefits as veterans. The large scale and far reaching scope of the U.S. Armed Forces as an employer made this policy a very significant milestone in American history.

The post-World War II era was a very exciting time. The dawn of the space era was associated with an almost unbridled hope that through science, humankind would be able to develop solutions to our greatest challenges. It was a time of great hope for many. It was also a time of increasing racial tensions within the United States. Historically, tolerance had been supported by policies of racial segregation, and these polices were increasingly challenged in the courts and by public protests in the first several decades following WWII.

Medicine in particular shared in the successes of science of this time. Through the successes of public health coupled with research and health promotion, many deadly infectious diseases were contained and irradiated. With technology, many incurable diseases were able to be diagnosed and treated; many cancers can be successfully treated. Mental health in mid-20th-century U.S. history was very institution based. It was in 1963 that then President Kennedy enacted the Community Mental Health Act. This act promised to support the development of community mental health centers that could treat individuals in outpatient settings.

Having started with equality for all men, U.S. policy purported opportunity for all on one hand, but progressively supported a policy of cultural tolerance throughout much of the first 200 years. This was clearly demonstrated less than a century ago in public county school systems and by trends in the development of separate state-operated asylums for colored insane patients. States and local governments tried to support separate institutions but virtually none were able to support the institutions provided to Americans of African descent at the same level of support that schools and institutions designed for other persons received. The idea that services and communities could be equal but separate was progressively challenged legally and ultimately was deemed unconstitutional by the U.S. Supreme Court with the assertion that different but equal is inherently unequal (4) and thereby unconstitutional. With this opinion, states and local governments were given great latitude in the timeliness with which they desegregated their public facilities which was yet another source of ongoing tension.

Thus, for more than 200 years since the inception of U.S. democracy, there have been many significant refinements in the details of policy and law about the ability of individuals from other cultures and races to participate fully in United States culture. As a nation, we have worked through many difficult times yet there remain many individuals who are disadvantaged and are unable to participate fully in American culture based on their culture of origin and/or race.

CONCLUSION

The United States is a relatively young country, however, our democratic government itself is among the most mature democracies in the world. We have a very solid foundation and have made many advances in working out details that define our nation as being one that respects human rights individually as well as through a government that supports the rights of all individuals to pursue life, liberty, and happiness. One of the most outstanding issues that face us today is our approach to cultural disparity at the local community, state, and national levels. We as a nation need to be able to respect and celebrate the cultural diversity that makes our communities and nation great while working toward and maintaining a society that provides truly equal opportunity for all who want to engage fully in our culture. Equal opportunity for all is an entrenched component of our society and we are still working to achieve this.

This chapter began with a brief exploration of the phrase *celebrate diversity*. Addressing the needs of individuals from different racial and ethnic backgrounds is a situation every nation and group of people has had to address; it is a universal issue throughout time. U.S. policy in general supports a melting pot or assimilation policy with growing recognition of the value that diversity adds to thriving communities in the United States. The United States is a strong nation because of the diversity within it. Disparities based on racial and ethnic origin must be eliminated.

References

1. Greek Medicine. Hippocrates and the rise of rational medicine. NIH medical history Web site. Available at: http://www.nlm.nih.gov/hmd/greek/greek_rationality.html. Accessed January 8, 2009.
2. National Library of Medicine Web site. Available at: http://0-www.nlm.nih.gov.catalog. llu.edu/hmd/greek/greek_timeline.html. Accessed August 1, 2008.
3. Garraty JA, Gay P. *The Columbia History of the World*. New York: Harper and Row; 1972:504.
4. Barnes R. Divided court limits use of race by school districts.Washington Post article on the Supreme Court decision to support desegregation. Available at: http://www. washingtonpost.com/wp-dyn/content/article/2007/06/28/AR2007062800896. html. Accessed January 8, 2008.

2 Determinants of Disparities

Altha J. Stewart

"Of all forms of inequality, injustice in health is the most shocking and the most inhuman."–The Rev. Martin Luther King, at the Second National Convention of the Medical Committee for Human Rights, Chicago, March 25, 1966.

The first Report on Mental Health issued by the Surgeon General acknowledged that despite an understanding of the debilitating nature of mental illness, the strong science on which effective treatments are based, and the importance of early recognition and treatment to achieve recovery, racial and ethnic minority groups tended to receive lesser quality of mental health services (1). The Surgeon General's Supplemental Mental Health Report, as well as subsequent studies, reported that racial and ethnic minority patients present later and with more disabling conditions, greater impairment in functioning, and greater levels of psychosocial problems. Some studies suggest that other factors related to racial and ethnic differences in diagnosis are that clinicians may not accurately perceive and evaluate the symptoms of emotional distress in individuals from these groups or that these groups may exhibit different tolerance thresholds for symptoms of mental illness and different help-seeking behaviors (2–4). The emerging literature regarding treatment outcomes for racial and ethnic minorities suggests that other contributing factors include uncertainty in clinical decision making and difficulty in the communication between patients and physicians. In addition, patient surveys commissioned by the Kaiser Family Foundation and the Commonwealth Fund described adverse experiences with health professionals, with more African Americans and Hispanic Americans feeling unfairly treated or disrespected because of their racial or ethnic background. Such experiences certainly influence the level of comfort in seeking and participating in treatment.

The term *disparity* appeared in the 1985 *Report of the Secretary's Task Force on Black and Minority Health*, and it is noteworthy that the social and cultural determinants of overall poorer minority health status identified in that report continue to play a significant role in the disparities in healthcare for racial and ethnic minorities seen today. These factors include:

- socioeconomic status
- cultural and ethnocentric issues
- racism, discrimination, and prejudice (individual and institutional)
- lack of trust between patients and healthcare providers
- lack of cultural competence in healthcare system and workforce

The literature related to disparities includes various definitions for the term. The National Institutes of Health (NIH) workgroup provided the federal government's first definition of disparity as "differences in the incidence, prevalence, mortality and burden of diseases, and other adverse health conditions that exist among specific population groups in the United States"; the *Healthy People 2010* report regarded disparities as "differences that occur by gender, race or ethnicity, education or income, disability, living in rural localities or sexual orientation"; and the Institute of Medicine (IOM) report defined disparities as "racial or ethnic differences in the quality of healthcare that are not due to access-related factors or clinical needs, preferences, and appropriateness of intervention."

Notable dissenters in the health disparities debate, such as Klick and Satel (5), described the evolution of the definition of "disparity" as moving from a cause-neutral imbalance to an unfair and pernicious difference. They believe that groups studying disparities discounted more benign explanations, attributed racial bias to data never designed to study discrimination, and then erroneously concluded that the cause of the disparities must be bias. They proposed that the race-based disparity theories and suggested remedies, diverted energy, and resources and led policy makers away from a true public health solution to the problem of improving care for all Americans, irrespective of minority group membership. Carpenter-Song et al (6), in an anthropological critique of cultural competence models, observed that culture is not a "static variable" and that "narratives of culture" in the health services and disparity discussion fail to account for cultural variation and ignore other important sources of health disparities.

Concern about racism and its effects on psychiatric practice have been discussed in the psychiatric literature since the 1970s. It is well documented that misdiagnosis and more serious clinical diagnoses occur more often in ethnic minority patients (7). There is also substantial evidence that these patients more often received medication rather than psychotherapy, received care in more restrictive settings (2), and minority children and adults were more likely to be placed in custodial settings than treatment settings compared to their white counterparts (8).

Although the science base on racial and ethnic minority mental health remains inadequate, available research concludes that these groups also have less access to availability of care. They face greater exposure to racism, discrimination, violence, and poverty. Living in poverty has the most measurable effect on the rates of mental illness, with individuals in the lowest socioeconomic status about two to three times more likely to have a mental disorder. Racism and discrimination are stressful events that may also adversely affect mental health, placing minorities at increased risk for mental illnesses, such as depression and anxiety. In general, depression is underdiagnosed and inadequately managed in racial and ethnic minorities, compared with whites. Depression is associated with a high social burden and substantial reduction in quality of life (9). It is also associated with an increased prevalence of chronic diseases for which racial and ethnic minorities are at high risk, and may significantly affect the course of comorbid medical illnesses (10). These disparities have resulted in a greater disability burden from unmet mental health needs, and efforts to increase utilization and improve overall mental health have been hindered by shame, stigma, discrimination, and mistrust.

Over the last four decades, numerous books and journal articles have been published, which expands the literature that attempts to describe, analyze, and explain disorders, whose etiology and management are related to the psychological consequences of racism, discrimination, societal inequities, and economic inequality. In 1970, Sabshin et al (8) reported that substantial evidence indicated that psychiatry has a structuralized pattern of racism, influencing treatment accessibility, mental health treatment and practices, research, and the professional functioning of psychiatrists. This was expanded to include all of medicine when the *2002 IOM Report* placed heavy emphasis on the failure of the medical profession to purge its ranks of prejudice, a shortcoming that was "rooted in historic and contemporary inequities."

Trierweiler et al (11) reported that even when standardized diagnostic criteria are used, clinical judgment and clinician characteristics play a differential role in how symptoms are attributed to African American and white patients. When compared to available epidemiologic community research studies which find no differences in schizophrenia diagnoses by ethnicity, it suggests that racial biases exist in the diagnostic process (12).

Much more work needs to be done to determine the effects of whether to address the factors noted above with regard to treatment, cost effectiveness, and consumer satisfaction. Bell and Williamson (13) reviewed articles on special populations published in *Psychiatric Services* between 1950 and 1999. They reported that in the 50-year period studied, 36 articles addressed issues in African American mental health (including the 1994 special issue on psychiatric services for African American patients), 15 addressed issues related to the mental health of Native Americans and Alaska Natives, 15 articles were published on issues related to the mental health of Asian Americans and Pacific Islanders, and a total of 21 articles on Hispanic American issues were published.

Scientists, biological and social, have endeavored to study the questions, problems, and issues related to these factors and their impact on psychological development in racial and ethnic minorities. Numerous conferences, meetings, and public forums of all sorts have encouraged dialogue between the professionals and the people they study to frame the issues and work on solutions. Research on effective psychotherapeutic interventions and innovative treatment models, psychopharmacological practices, and consumer-directed community support services has resulted in the development of culturally appropriate services for patients from racial and ethnic minority groups based on evidence from actual clinical treatment practices. The field of cross-cultural psychiatry has evolved from the study of unusual, exotic, or isolated clinical syndromes in non-Western countries to a continuum that includes cultural competence in clinical practice and the application of the Outline for Cultural Formulation in *Diagnostic and Statistical Manual of Mental Disorders Fourth Edition* (DSM-IV; and DSM-V once completed). With all the knowledge available to the field that recognizes the relevance of social, cultural, and ethnic influences on mental illness, why is it that we are still facing disparities in mental healthcare for racial and ethnic minorities?

The answer to this question begins with a review of the various aspects of cultural identity that influence awareness and understanding of mental illness, symptom manifestation, and treatment adherence. This is essential to obtain the historical information needed to better understand the individual's perspective on health, mental illness, help-seeking, and acceptable treatments. Approaching the patient by starting a conversation to assess his or her cultural identity allows the clinician to:

1. Identify potential strengths and natural supports, improving likelihood of successful treatment outcome
2. Identify potential cultural conflict that may impede treatment adherence and success
3. Be better informed about the patient's understanding of his or her illness and treatment and dispel myths and misconceptions
4. Attempt to demonstrate understanding of the individual as a whole person rather than only as an ill person

Clinicians may also find information obtained in the cultural identity assessment useful in the analysis of the mental health of individuals from each of the racial and ethnic minority groups (14). This is also important for a full understanding of the appreciation of culturally defined "normalcy" within the historical context of the influence of the discrimination experienced by each culture on mental health within the larger society.

Lu et al (15) listed the following common aspects of cultural identity:

- ethnicity
- race
- country of origin
- language
- gender
- age
- marital status
- sexual orientation
- religious/spiritual beliefs
- socioeconomic status
- education
- other identified groups
- migration history
- level of acculturation
- degree of affiliation with above

In addition to understanding factors that contribute to an individual's cultural identity, it is important to understand the history of the primary racial and ethnic minority groups in the United States, their historical relationship with the majority white population, and the likely psychological impact of their experiences of racism, discrimination, societal inequities, and economic inequality.

America has a history of legalized discrimination with each of the four federally recognized racial and ethnic minority groups—enslavement of early Africans followed by a century of segregation for their descendants, discrimination of early Chinese immigrants and the internment of Americans of Japanese descent during the 1940s, the forced relocation of Native Americans to reservations in remote locations and forfeiture of their land to whites, and the historically detrimental policies toward people of Hispanic heritage which continues today. The role of this societal legacy is a significant factor in the development of mental health disparities that exist today. Racist and discriminatory experiences are associated with psychological and physical stress for both minority groups and whites. Poorer overall health status with increased chronic medical illnesses and self-reports of ill health has been observed in several studies over the last decade.

John Hope Franklin wrote in 1969 that "color and race are at once among the most important and the most enigmatic factors at work in our society." Understanding the history of sociocultural factors related to experiences of racial and ethnic minorities will help clinicians and other mental health professionals navigate through the impediments, stereotypes, and assumptions that lead to substandard, disparate care, because preventing disparities is the only way to eliminate them.

From the early days of American psychiatry, it was clear that the mental health field was not immune from societal assumptions regarding racist attitudes and behaviors and their influence on therapeutic encounters. The history of mental health practices illustrates how the social environment has often incorporated and distorted the "science" underlying psychiatric interventions and treatment.

It is well documented that ethnic minority populations do not receive the same quality of healthcare as whites do. From the early days of the healthcare system in the United States, many factors have affected access to care, as well as type and quality of care available, including socioeconomic status, environment, gender, and race. Racial and ethnic minorities are disproportionately represented in high-need populations, e.g., foster cares, jails, prisons, homeless shelters, and refugee resettlement programs. Recent studies have also suggested evidence of provider behaviors and practice patterns as contributors to these disparities, with clinical provider-patient communication representing a significant barrier.

In addition, fundamental system issues have been identified, including:

- limited entry points into the treatment system, especially for specialty care such as psychiatric services, and
- lack of insurance, especially for racial and ethnic minorities.

The origins of the disparities acknowledged today have their roots in the early days of this country. Like the rest of the evolving medical system, psychiatry and the social service professions were nurtured by the race and class-based systems of the day. While all racial and ethnic minority groups have experienced, in general, poorer outcomes than whites, the experience of African Americans is perhaps most illustrative of the influence of racism, class bias, prejudice, and resultant disparities in mental health.

Early 19th-century theorists proposed that the "uncivilized races" (i.e., slaves and Indians) had much less or almost no mental illness. Benjamin Rush, the "father of American psychiatry," wrote several articles and medical treatises dealing with blacks including "an account of the diseases peculiar to the Negroes in the West Indies, and which are produced by their slavery," where he expressed concern for both the mental and physical effects of slavery. In *Medical Inquiries and Observations upon the Diseases of the Mind*, published in 1812 and considered the first textbook in American psychiatry, Rush described a variant of madness or insanity induced by grief that had been observed among slaves in the Caribbean soon after they entered into perpetual slavery in the West Indies.

White physicians during this time frequently promoted alternate mechanisms of disease based on race, resulting in the development of a lexicon of "Negro diseases." Rush's contribution included his theory of the Negro's blackness stemming from a leprous-like disease. He believed that finding a cure and removing the blackness would promote racial harmony and lead to white's greater acceptance of African Americans, suggesting that he understood well the impact of physical differences on the mental health of blacks and whites. This position was further supported by some of his abolitionist writings where he emphasized the "detrimental effects of slavery on the mind or mental health of the Negro."

The issue of psychiatric "scientific evidence" in support of the institution of slavery was revisited with the 1840 census report of increasing mental illness in African Americans the farther north they lived. Dr. Samuel Cartwright reported "discovery" of a new disease, *drapetomania*, with the sole symptom of causing the desire in African Americans to run away. The cure was to "whip the devil out of the patient and in extreme cases to cut off toes."

Segregation was the rule for most asylums, when they accepted blacks at all. When no state hospital was available, blacks were often confined to jail. In the south, there was little state provision, as slaves were generally taken care of by their masters. Eastern State Hospital at Williamsburg, Virginia, believed to be the first state hospital in the United States, accepted blacks from its founding in 1774, but after the Civil War in 1869 a separate hospital was built for blacks, Central State Hospital in Petersburg, Virginia. In the north, Worcester State Hospital in Massachusetts, established in 1833, remodeled a brick shop on the grounds to create separate quarters for blacks when it opened. (16) Lim's *Clinical Manual of Cultural Psychiatry* and the Surgeon General's Supplemental Report on Mental Health provide more detail on the historical influence of the early experiences and documented disparities in clinical care for each of the four federally recognized racial and ethnic groups in the United States. (2,17)

Individuals from racial and ethnic minority groups also experienced racist and discriminatory behaviors as they attempted to join the ranks of psychiatric professionals. African Americans and other minorities were not accepted into US medical schools until the mid-19th century. As the first African American to obtain a formal medical education, James McCune Smith (1811–1865) was the first African American to make a submission to a U.S. medical journal (*The Annalist* in 1874). He also has the distinction of refuting the use of the fraudulent 1840 U.S. census data by then Secretary of State John Calhoun who attempted to use the data to rally congressional support for continuing slavery to protect the slaves from the "insanity of freedom."

Dr. Solomon Carter Fuller (1872–1953) was the first African American psychiatrist in the United States, completing his psychiatric training with Emil Kraeplin, and then going on to work with Alois Alzheimer. He completed his training in Europe because of the difficulties he experienced when he attempted to enter private practice or receive an appointment in clinical neurology and psychiatry in the Massachusetts State Hospital system. Fuller went on to teach Karl Menninger at Harvard Medical School and was an invited participant at the 20th anniversary of Clark University in 1909 on the occasion of Sigmund Freud's visit to America.

Charles Prudhomme, distinguished African American psychiatrist and member of the American Psychiatric Association (APA), reported his disappointment when the APA leadership in 1952 resisted his request to support *Brown v. Board of Education* by submitting a brief *amicus curiae* regarding the negative psychological consequences of "separate but unequal" facilities, stating his request was an example of his "continuing acting out" (16).

The American health and mental health systems were founded on principles of Western medicine, emphasizing objective evidence based on scientific inquiry. This method, however, did not take into account the cultural and social context of individuals from minority groups, which are significant determinants for behavior of clinicians and patients as they encounter each other in clinical therapeutic situations. Along with the larger social issues of poverty, discrimination, and racism, these cultural factors often lead to misunderstandings that result in mistrust, bias, and poor outcomes for those who seek mental health services.

The Surgeon General's Supplemental Mental Health Report and its core message of "culture counts," the development and use of the DSM-IV Outline for Cultural Formulation, and publications such as the *Clinical Manual of Cultural Psychiatry* all provided strategies for bringing cultural issues into the clinical encounter, enriching our understanding of patients and improving outcomes. Ruiz (18) offered useful definitions of culture, race, and ethnicity to assist the busy psychiatrist understand the difference between the three terms. He also noted the availability of good resources in the psychiatric literature to address important issues for racial and ethnic minority groups pertaining to racial identity, applications of culturally sensitive psychotherapy approaches, empirical issues pertaining to psychodynamic processes, transference and countertransference situations, and other clinically relevant topics within the context of cross-cultural psychiatry. And, while we continue to use the term "minority," the rate of growth for racial and ethnic groups in the United States signals that by 2025, populations of color will represent the majority of citizens and might be more appropriately called *emerging majorities* (19). These changing racial and cultural demographics are making this country more pluralistic and multiethnic than ever before in our history. This increasing diversity will increase interracial therapeutic encounters and clinicians must develop a better understanding of the impact of these racial differences on help-seeking, diagnosis, treatment, and outcomes. Psychiatry must also improve participation by members of racial and ethnic minority groups in clinical care and research, especially related to factors affecting treatment seeking, treatment preference, and response to psychotropic medication and psychotherapy.

RECOMMENDATIONS

Any recommendation for eliminating disparities and improving mental health services to racial and ethnic minorities must acknowledge the influence of culture at every level of the service delivery system. The use of available practices that are appropriate and effective with racial and ethnic minority populations will do much to improve access to and quality of care provided.

This is especially important at the level of individual clinicians. Physician recognition of disparities has remained relatively low despite the wealth of information regarding the pervasiveness of disparities in healthcare. Vanderbilt et al (20) conducted interviews with physicians actively engaged in reducing healthcare disparities, especially regarding what life experiences led them to become engaged in addressing disparities and what specific strategies they were using to improve quality of care and to reduce disparities for racial and ethnic minority patients. They concluded that factors that are important in reducing disparities include: treating all patients with respect and understanding, active listening, maintaining eye contact, understanding the patient's background and needs, and being accountable for ensuring patient understanding. More work should be done in this area to improve clinician-patient communication and the interactions that result in adverse treatment outcomes, greater burden of illness, and poorer quality of life.

Psychiatric researchers have historically been reluctant to study mental health issues in nonwhite populations. This is, in part, related to the tensions that exist when dealing with racial and ethnic issues because discussion of disparities is a reminder that large segments of the population do not have adequate healthcare and implicates the healthcare system and practitioners as part of the problem. While the methodology may be complex, making studies about nonwhite populations difficult, the entire mental health community (patients and clinicians) will benefit from a better understanding of how factors such as acculturation, help-seeking behaviors, stigma, ethnic identity, racism, and spirituality provide protection from or risk for mental illness in racial and ethnic minority populations (13).

More research is encouraged to determine effective methods to reduce the impact of social problems such as community violence, racism, and discrimination. The results of such studies will assist in efforts to build on community strengths, foster recovery and resilience, and educate families and communities about mental health, mental illness, and treatment effectiveness. Although education alone is not the answer, training for patients as well as clinicians must be implemented to improve identification and acknowledgement of mental illness in racial and ethnic minority populations. Additional research is needed to determine the efficacy of culturally oriented interventions that have proven more effective than "traditional" practices in reducing dropout rates for ethnic minority patients. Research is also needed to determine the best methods to change attitudes and behaviors that will improve utilization of mental health services by racial and ethnic minority communities. Messages to reduce stigma, increase awareness, and promote principles of recovery must be tailored to the cultural context of each community.

Finally, addressing disparities in mental health will require building capacity in the system for improving research, training, and clinical treatment in an effort to create culturally competent services with treatment guidelines based on rigorous empirical study. Capacity building must include community health centers where many racial and ethnic minority patients and families prefer to receive mental health services. Other nontraditional service settings such as churches, foster care programs, correctional systems, homeless shelters, and refugee programs must be able to provide some level of care for the high-need, at-risk populations they serve. The language barriers facing many racial and ethnic minority populations must be overcome to ensure that persons with limited English proficiency (LEP) have meaningful access to services.

As the United States becomes a more multiethnic society, we must develop a better understanding of the meaning of race, culture, and ethnicity within the context of psychiatric care. This is crucial if we are to reduce the disparities in the current health and mental healthcare systems. In this way, we move closer to achieving our goal of improving the diagnosis and treatment of psychiatric disorders among the racial and ethnic minority groups who reside in the United States.

References

1. U.S. Department of Health and Human Services. *Mental Health: A Report of the Surgeon General.* Rockville, Md: U.S. Department of Health and Human Services, Substance Abuse and Mental Health Services Administration, Center for Mental Health Services; 1999.
2. U.S. Department of Health and Human Services. *Mental Health: Culture, Race, and Ethnicity—A Supplement to Mental Health: A Report of the Surgeon General.* Rockville, Md: U.S. Department of Health and Human Services, Substance Abuse and Mental Health Services Administration, Center for Mental Health Services; 2001.
3. Smedley BD, Stith AY, Nelson AR. *Unequal Treatment: Confronting Racial and Ethnic Disparities in Health Care.* Washington, DC: The National Academies Press; 2002.
4. West JC, Herbeck DM, Bell CC, et al. Race/ethnicity among psychiatric patients: variations in diagnostic and clinical characteristics reported by practicing clinicians. *FOCUS* 2006;4;48–56.
5. Klick J, Satel S. *The Health Disparities Myth: Diagnosing the Treatment Gap.* Washington, DC: American Enterprise Institute Press, 2006.
6. Carpenter-Song EA, Schwallie MN, Longhofer J. Cultural competence reexamined. *Psychiatr Serv* 2007;58:1362–1365.
7. Adebimpe VR. Overview: White norms and psychiatric diagnosis of black patients. *Am J Psychiatry* 1981;138:279–285.
8. Sabshin M, Diesenhaus H, Wilkerson R. Dimensions of institutional racism in psychiatry. *Am J Psychiatry* 1970;127:787–793.
9. Druss BG, Rosenheck RA, Sledge WH. Health and disability costs of depressive illness in a major U.S. corporation. *Am J Psychiatry* 2000;157:1274–1278.

10. Kristofco RE, Stewart AJ, Vega W. Perspectives on disparities in depression care. *J Contin Educ Health Prof* 2007;27:S18–S25.
11. Trierweiler SJ, Neighbors HW, Munday C, et al. Differences in patterns of symptom attribution in diagnosing schizophrenia between African American and non–African American clinicians. *Am J Orthopsychiatry* 2006;76:154–160.
12. Whaley AL. Cultural mistrust and clinical diagnosis of paranoid schizophrenia in African American patients. *J Psychopath Behav Assess* 2001;23:93–100.
13. Bell CC, Williamson J. Articles on special populations published in psychiatric services between 1950 and 1999. *Psychiatr Serv* 2002;53:419–424.
14. Ton H, Lim RF. The assessment of culturally diverse individuals. In: Lim RF, ed. *Clinical Manual of Cultural Psychiatry*. Washington, DC: American Psychiatric Publishing, Inc., 2006;3–31.
15. Lu FG, Lim RF, Mezzich JE. Issues in the assessment and diagnosis of culturally diverse individuals. In: Oldham JM, Riba MB, eds. *American Psychiatric Press Review of Psychiatry, Vol 14*. Washington, DC: American Psychiatric Press, Inc., 1995:477–510.
16. Prudhomme C, Musto DF. Historical perspectives on mental health and racism in the United States. In: Willie CV, Kramer AM, Brown BS, eds. *Racism and Mental Health*. Pittsburgh: University of Pittsburgh Press, 1973;25–57.
17. Lim RF, ed. *Clinical Manual of Cultural Psychiatry*. Washington, DC: American Psychiatric Publishing, Inc.; 2006.
18. Ruiz P. Addressing culture, race, and ethnicity in psychiatric practice. *Psychiatr Annals* 2004;34:527–532.
19. Primm AB. Understanding the significance of race in the psychiatric clinical setting. *FOCUS* 2006;4:6–8.
20. Vanderbilt SK, Wynia MK, Gadon M, et al. A qualitative study of physicians' engagement in reducing healthcare disparities. *J Natl Med Assoc* 2007;99:1315–1322.

Disparities Among Ethnic Groups

3   African Americans

Annelle B. Primm and William B. Lawson

INTRODUCTION

People of African descent in the United States represent a heterogeneous group of cultures and origins that is becoming increasingly diverse (1). As a group, however, they experience disparities in access to and quality of general healthcare and mental healthcare. Their mental health and experiences in the psychiatric clinical setting are complicated by a multiplicity of historical and contemporary factors that will be addressed in this chapter. Our hope is that this analysis will provide direction for future efforts to improve the mental health status and clinical psychiatric outcomes of people of African heritage.

DEFINITION OF THE POPULATION

In this chapter, the term *African American* will refer to the broad spectrum of individuals of African heritage who reside in the United States, approximately 12% of the population. The majority of these persons were born in the United States and are descendants of slaves with origins primarily in West Africa (2). However, other groups included among African Americans are immigrants and refugees seeking asylum in the United States in recent decades from nations in the Caribbean, Central America, South America, and East, Central, West, and South Africa, and their descendants. The people in these groups represent a wide variety of cultures, languages, and mores. It is important to note that immigration is increasing the diversity of individuals referred to as African Americans (1). In many major cities as many as one third of African Americans are Caribbean immigrants or they are first- or second-generation offspring. Despite their diversity, all individuals of African ancestry must deal with the specter of racism, which may be a more important contributor to disparities in treatment than such factors as socioeconomic status (1).

DIAGNOSTIC CONSIDERATIONS

According to large-scale national studies using validated structured interviews, African Americans experience the full range of psychiatric disorders (3). For the most part, prevalence rates are similar to or lower than their counterparts in other racial and ethnic groups. However, smaller clinical studies show that African Americans are overrepresented in certain diagnostic groups, including dysthymic disorder, isolated sleep paralysis, and cognitive disorders (2). Moreover, clinicians continue to overdiagnose such disorders as schizophrenia at the expense of mood and anxiety disorders at rates that cannot be accounted for by studies using the more valid structured interviews (4,5). Underrecognition of some mental disorders and excessive misdiagnosis of others may contribute to some of the treatment disparities. In this section, we will examine the African American experience and disparities with regard to the epidemiology and clinical diagnosis of four major disease categories: anxiety disorders, depressive disorder, bipolar disorder, and schizophrenia.

ANXIETY DISORDERS

Some anxiety disorders may show a higher prevalence among African Americans. The Epidemiologic Catchment Area study (ECA), a household survey using structured interviews found higher rates of anxiety disorders among African Americans than other populations (6). In contrast, the National Comorbidity Survey (NCS) replication also used structured interviews and found lower rates of anxiety disorders in racial and ethnic minorities (3). Methodological differences may partially explain the difference. The ECA study was conducted in five cities and oversampled minorities, whereas the NCS was conducted nationally and did not oversample people of color or include persons from institutional settings where people of color are overrepresented. However, prevalence rates based on diagnoses by clinicians invariably find lower rates of anxiety disorders in African Americans (4,7). Misdiagnosis is clearly a factor.

Socioeconomic factors can play a role in the higher prevalence of some anxiety disorders. Posttraumatic stress disorder in particular has been found more often in African Americans, possibly because African Americans are overrepresented in inner cities, which have higher crime rates and poverty, and in combat situations in the military (4,8). Yet, this disorder often is either underdiagnosed or misdiagnosed as other disorders such as schizophrenia. Hence, the evidence is inconclusive at this point about the actual prevalence of anxiety disorders among people of color, and specifically African Americans (7).

What are some of the underlying causes of patient and/or clinical disregard or misinterpretation of anxiety disorder symptoms in African Americans? The lack of use of structured, reliable, and cross-culturally validated assessment instruments could be a factor, although the *Diagnostic and Statistical Manual of Mental Disorders* (DSM) IV is considered to be an important improvement over older diagnostic systems (4). Another potential contributor to underdiagnosis of anxiety disorders is the lack of recognition of subsyndromal symptoms, which may be deemed culturally acceptable responses to environmental stress. The frequent co-occurrence of psychotic symptoms and paranoid ideation among African Americans with anxiety disorders is another possible explanation for the misdiagnosis of anxiety subtypes (4). Moreover, African Americans are more likely to seek help in primary care settings, where general medical conditions top the list of differentials (8).

SCHIZOPHRENIA

For many years, African Americans have been regarded as having an increased risk of schizophrenia, and they still are at nearly a 10-fold risk of being diagnosed with schizophrenia compared with other populations of color (4,5,9). However, the ECA study found no difference in the prevalence of schizophrenia among African Americans when socioeconomic status was controlled, and the NCS Replication found that African Americans were less likely than European Americans to have nonaffective psychosis, primarily schizophrenia (3,6). Higher rates of schizophrenia in clinical settings have been consistently reported for African Americans compared with other ethnicities in inpatient and outpatient settings, often associated with correspondingly lower rates of affective disorders (9). It has been presumed that affective disorders were being misdiagnosed in favor of schizophrenia. Yet, even with the use of the DSM IV, this pattern of overdiagnosis of schizophrenia in African Americans persists, occurring in a variety of settings, including the Veterans Administration, facilities for juveniles, and public and private facilities (9).

The persistence of this diagnostic disparity is not caused by variance in criteria but rather by failure on the part of the clinician to obtain adequate information and overinterpretation of Schneiderian first-rank symptoms as being exclusively associated with schizophrenia (5). It is not uncommon for African Americans to present with these types of symptoms when experiencing a mood disorder. Additional possible explanations are clinician bias regarding the presence of mood disorders in African Americans and lack of knowledge about idioms of distress among African Americans, such as anger, irritability, and somatic complaints (9). Patient factors include suspiciousness and mistrust, often characterized as "healthy paranoia," and delays in seeking treatment until the crisis point is reached, which may further complicate the diagnostic process (9).

To prevent misdiagnosis, it is necessary to consult family and others in the patient's life so that culturally accepted idioms of distress are not misconstrued. Furthermore, it is essential to consider schizophrenia as a diagnosis of exclusion only after ruling out mood, anxiety, and other disorders from the differential diagnosis.

DEPRESSION

Although schizophrenia has been overdiagnosed among people of African descent, mood disorders, including major depression and bipolar disorder, have been underdiagnosed (5). Depression is a significant problem among African Americans. Williams and colleagues (10) found in the National Survey of American Life (NASL) that rates of depression among African Americans (10.4%) and Afro-Caribbeans (12.9%) were lower than that of white Americans (17.9%). However, rates of subsyndromal depression and dysthymic disorder are higher among people of African descent (11). As a result, higher rates of depression in general are found in African Americans when compared with their Caucasian counterparts.

Both the NCS and NASL found that major depressive disorder in African Americans including those of Caribbean origin is typically overlooked, undiagnosed, untreated, inadequately treated, more severe, and/or associated with greater disability. It is disturbing to note that only 45% of African Americans and 24% of Caribbean Americans with major depression received any treatment (10). Among the underlying reasons for unmet need for depression care among people of African descent is the presentation of depressive symptoms, other then sadness, that still meet the usual depressive criteria. These include the alternate symptoms of irritability, hostility, and somatic symptoms that the clinician may interpret as another psychiatric disorder or even a general medical condition. The problem is further enhanced by the failure of many African Americans to recognize depression when they are suffering from it. This phenomenon is graphically demonstrated in the book "Black Pain" by Terrie Williams (12).

Suicide is an important consequence of depression and is a reminder that depression can be a mortal illness. In the past, suicide was thought to be rare in African Americans. Recent studies, however, have shown that young men of African descent do not differ in rates from their white counterparts in suicide rate (13).

BIPOLAR DISORDER

African Americans are often diagnosed as having schizophrenia or depression when they have bipolar disorder. Although the ECA and NCS studies found little racial difference in prevalence, bipolar disorder was thought to be nonexistent among African Americans until recently (4,5). Misdiagnosis of bipolar disorder when it first presents itself is common in any population. African Americans, however, are much more likely to be underdiagnosed or misdiagnosed at rates of 90% with first presentation (14). A high likelihood of symptom presentations that include irritability, anxiety, or psychosis often lead to the misdiagnosis of schizophrenia. Moreover, many patients often first present with depressive symptoms. Cultural factors that may color the presentation, cultural ignorance, and stereotypical beliefs contribute to the misdiagnosis and missed diagnosis. The preference for service by primary care providers is also a factor because primary care providers often are not familiar with the many ways that bipolar disorder may present and believe it is rare outside of psychiatric settings. Yet, recent studies show that bipolar disorder may make up 10% to 20% of patients in primary care settings (15).

TREATMENT CONSIDERATIONS

The scientific literature is replete with examples of psychiatric treatment disparities experienced by African Americans (1,4). As noted above, the large depression survey amply described the undertreatment of depression and subsequent poorer outcome, even when income was controlled. Other studies have shown that less than a quarter of African Americans receive evidence-based treatment for most mental disorders (16). When African Americans receive psychiatric care, they tend to receive more invasive and potentially detrimental care and they receive less of the more benign forms of treatment. They are more likely to be involuntarily committed, placed in seclusion and restraint, or given higher doses of medication (7). These differences are probably a result of delay in treatment caused by lack of availability, stereotypical beliefs about African

Americans being more hostile, and unwillingness by the provider to be therapeutically engaged. The location and circumstances surrounding psychiatric care for African Americans is also problematic, with high rates of use in emergency rooms, inpatient settings, correctional settings, and primary care settings (2,17). African Americans continue to receive inadequate or no treatment in primary care settings (18).

Among children and youth with mental health needs, African Americans are more likely to be found in the juvenile justice system than are white youth with identical presentations (4). Few African American children and youth receive treatment in private hospitals, day treatment, or case management services. Most receive care, if at all, in publicly funded hospitals and residential treatment centers. Those who are in the juvenile justice system are underreferred for mental health services (1).

Socioeconomic (S-E) factors are important. The direct cost of providing service to someone with schizophrenia, for example, exceeds the median family income of African Americans (9); however, even when S-E is controlled, significant disparities remain (1).

Attitudes of the provider clearly contribute to some of the disparity. African Americans are less likely to be offered either evidence-based pharmacotherapy or psychotherapy (16). They are also less likely to get different types of psychotherapy (19). African Americans are less likely than other groups to get evidence-based or optimal treatment in both the primary care and the VA system as well as in public or private mental health settings (18,20). African Americans are less likely to be prescribed newer antipsychotics or antidepressants (7,9). They are less likely to be given electroconvulsive therapy. It is an important treatment modality for depression especially when the depression is intractable, in emergency situations where the risk of suicide is high, or in elderly populations or others who have a low tolerance for antidepressant medication. Electroconvulsive therapy is offered less often to African Americans than to whites even when several factors including S-E are controlled (21).

Attitudes among African Americans can interfere with treatment acceptance. A recent qualitative study queried low-income African Americans who were receiving psychotherapy for the treatment of depression about reasons that African Americans with emotional or psychological problems underuse mental health services. The most frequent response was stigma, followed by dysfunctional coping behavior, shame, and denial (22). A study from the New York State Psychiatric Institute found that although African Americans were more likely than whites to believe that mental health professionals could help people with depression and schizophrenia, they were more likely to believe that treatment was unnecessary (23). In addition, African Americans were more likely to believe that prayer and faith alone was all that was necessary to treat depression.

ETHNOPSYCHOPHARMACOLOGY

Many clinicians are unaware of potential racial/ethnic differences in pharmacological response. For example, many anticipate that people of African descent will respond to medication similar to the way other racial and ethnic groups do because there is considerable genetic similarity across racial and ethnic groups. Unfortunately, many also believe that African Americans require more medication, based on the misconception that African American males are more hostile (4). However, the evidence suggests that African Americans may require, if anything, less medication because of differential pharmacological response.

The importance of ethnic factors in pharmacotherapy gained clinical importance with the medication marketed as BiDil. This agent was tested as a treatment for congestive heart failure and was found to be consistently effective only in African Americans. It subsequently was the first agent receiving FDA approval for a specific racial/ethnic group (17). Racial differences in treatment response and side effect profiles have also been reported with psychotropic agents.

African Americans may require lower doses of antipsychotic and antidepressant medications than do Caucasians. Cytochrome P 450 enzymes metabolize greater than 90% of drugs in clinical use, including antipsychotic and antidepressant medications. Individuals with relatively inactive CYP2D6 alleles (which account for 25% of metabolism of commonly used drugs) tend to have higher plasma levels of antipsychotics and antidepressants (24). Fifty percent of people of African ancestry have reduced functioning or nonfunctioning alleles. This leads to slower metabolism of older antipsychotics or tricyclic antidepressants and higher plasma levels. Chronically higher plasma levels may be associated with an increased risk of side effect intolerance of the medication, which in turn can lead to poorer adherence to treatment and should be compensated for with lower doses in African Americans than in Caucasians to achieve a therapeutic response.

Clinically, African Americans tend to be more likely to discontinue medication (4). African Americans are also more likely to develop tardive dyskinesia when receiving first-generation antipsychotics (25).

In the treatment of schizophrenia and other psychotic disorders, African Americans are less likely to receive newer-generation antipsychotic medications, which are associated with fewer extrapyramidal symptoms, amelioration of negative symptoms of schizophrenia, and a lower risk of tardive dyskinesia. This presents a challenge of choice to the clinician because the newer-generation antipsychotics pose higher risks of type 2 diabetes and significant weight gain, for which African Americans and other populations of color are at greater risk than are Caucasians (7,26). In any case, African Americans are more likely to receive antipsychotic medications when other agents may be as effective and to receive excessively higher doses when ethnopharmacological research would suggest that lower doses are needed.

African Americans may also have a different response to antidepressants at a receptor level. The STAR*D study, the first large-scale naturalistic study of current antidepressant treatment, presented sequentially, showed that African Americans had poorer responses and longer periods to remission with initial treatment with citalopram and poorer outcomes generally (27). African Americans appear to be less likely to have an allele or type of serotonin receptor that is associated with antidepressive response (28).

African Americans may have less access to some psychotropic medications because of their side effect profile. African Americans have preexisting low leukocyte counts at baseline, also known as benign leucopenia, which is not associated with increased pathology. This is a barrier to prescribing of agents with agranulocytosis as a side effect to otherwise healthy African Americans (7). Such agents include clozapine, which is shown to be more effective than other antipsychotic agents in treating treatment-refractory schizophrenia despite metabolic side effects. Also, carbamazepine is used to treat bipolar disorder, but it has agranulocytosis as a side effect as well.

African Americans are known to show a higher red blood cell–to–plasma ratio of lithium concentration when compared with Asians and Caucasians, and this finding was consistent even when the lithium levels were in therapeutic range (17). This difference is significant because of diminished lithium tolerability in African Americans and more side effects with high red blood cell/plasma ratios. As a consequence, African Americans with mood disorders are less likely to have lithium treatment prescribed as a single agent or as adjunctive therapy, even though it is effective and relatively inexpensive.

Pharmacokinetic and pharmacogenetic factors may explain why African Americans discontinue psychotropic medication more frequently than other groups (4,29). However, sociocultural factors are also important. Medication adherence is particularly an issue among African Americans, given their mistrust of physicians and psychiatrists, stigma associated with mental illness, and concerns about addictiveness of medication (19). Numerous other factors such as homelessness, substance abuse, support systems, affordability, cultural norms, and medication side effects can affect initiation and maintenance of pharmacologic treatment. To acquire information in these areas, the clinician should get a comprehensive personal and social history and, if given permission, talk to the family to identify potential barriers to successful treatment.

Psychotherapy is effective in the treatment of African Americans and is more acceptable than medication to many, especially in depression treatment (30). Taking into consideration patients' and the therapists' racial identities and worldviews, transference and countertransference are important. The psychotherapeutic relationship is vulnerable to bias and stereotyping which are sometimes unintentional and subconscious; yet, reside at the crux of disparities (31). These factors have considerable impact on care and clinical decision-making (2).

CLINICIAN–PATIENT COMMUNICATION, PATIENT CENTEREDNESS, AND CULTURAL COMPETENCE

Physician communication is a key factor in improving the quality of care and outcomes of patients of African descent. Collins and colleagues (32) found in a national telephone survey that African Americans and other people of color do not fare as well as whites with regard to patient-physician communication. Also, physicians were 23% more verbally dominant and engaged in 33% less patient-centered communication with African American patients than with white patients (33). African Americans and other people of color report being treated with disrespect or looked down on in their therapeutic relationships (34).

A recent study of African American and white patients in primary care with depressive symptoms revealed racial disparities in communication between primary care physicians and their patients. The study found that although there were no racial differences in the level of symptoms, physicians made fewer depression-related statements to African American patients than to white patients. Even when depression discussion occurred, physicians determined that fewer African American than white patients were experiencing significant emotional distress. This situation makes evident the need for improvements in communication to help reduce racial disparities in depression care (35).

The false notion that African Americans are more hostile is made worse by dysfunctional communication between patients and providers and by distance on social, economic, and ethnic levels. When patients become suspicious and hostile toward the mental health system, they often choose alternative sources of care or become noncompliant.

Language is an important aspect of cultural identity as well as communication, as spelled out in the DSM-IV-TR Cultural Formulation (DSM IV TR). Among the broad spectrum of people of African descent in the United States, the primary language spoken is standard English, with some speaking in nonstandard English dialects. Among immigrant and refugee populations of African descent, languages including Haitian, Creole, French, Portuguese, and Spanish are commonly spoken. It is important to provide mental health services in the language that the patient speaks at home by making available bilingual psychiatric clinicians or at least trained translators or interpreters. The National Standards for Culturally and Linguistically Appropriate Services (CLAS), promulgated by the Office of Minority Health, also urge the provision of signage and written materials in the languages spoken by patient populations. Patients who speak English as a second language are more likely to be misdiagnosed as having schizophrenia when they have depression (4). Limited English-proficient individuals may be turned away, may be forced to find their own interpreter (often a family member or friend), may not come back to a second appointment, may not adhere to treatment, or may not receive appropriate and necessary treatment. A growing number of people of African descent are facing this potential barrier to treatment (36).

The important correlated concept of cultural competence entails engagement of patients as partners in problem solving and decision-making, holistic consideration of social and cultural context, and the consequences of patients' experiences with illnesses. Social and cultural barriers between healthcare providers and patients may affect the quality of healthcare. Some African Americans harbor distrust of healthcare providers and institutions on the basis of historical or ongoing experiences of discrimination (4). Providers may harbor overt or subconscious biases about people of color that influence their interactions and decision-making (2,4).

Spirituality plays an important role in African American life, promoting mental health and prevention and serving as a key source of support (1). Collins and colleagues (32) report that 12% of African Americans use alternative care for religious or cultural reasons compared with 4% of whites. Many African Americans rely solely on spiritual support in lieu of professional treatment.

The religious diversity among people of African descent in the United States is considerable. Although Christianity, and its various denominations including Catholicism and Protestant denominations, is the predominant religion, African Americans belong to a wide range of faiths including Islam, Judaism, Buddhism, Yoruba, and other belief systems. Religion has been recognized as a source of strength for African-descendent populations, contributing to mental health promotion and resilience. However, religious beliefs and fervent expression, especially among fundamentalist Christian worshippers, have been misconstrued as signs of psychopathology. Many fundamentalists believe that mental health treatment may be inconsistent with their faith. This underscores the importance of psychiatrists and other mental health professionals in understanding the normative manifestations of the religious beliefs and practices of the African American subpopulations they serve.

Patient centeredness is an approach to the patient as a unique individual with his or her own story; one that requires the physician to understand the patient as well as the disease. It involves exploring the illness experience, understanding the whole person, finding common ground regarding management, incorporating prevention and health promotion, and being realistic about personal limitations. The physician tries to enter the patient's world and to see the illness through the patient's eyes (9).

Part of understanding the whole person involves understanding the family role. Family involvement can influence outcomes in people with schizophrenia, and African Americans are no exception. African Americans tend to be supportive in their family involvement with a loved one with schizophrenia. Yet, they also are more likely to believe that the mentally ill individual may be dangerous (9). Nevertheless, behavior that may be toxic in other cultures, such as high emotionality, intrusiveness, and critical comments, does not predict poor outcomes in African Americans (9). These findings underscore the importance of culture in determining how the family interacts with a member who is severely mentally ill.

PREVENTIVE CONSIDERATIONS

Taking a public health approach to mental health and psychiatric illness, one should consider primary prevention. Much of recent psychiatric research has focused on identifying the genetic basis of mental disorders (9). Identifying risk genes for mental disorders does not preclude extragenetic factors. For example, Caspi and associates (37) showed that a serotonin receptor allele was indeed a risk gene for depression. However, it was associated with depression only in individuals with a history of childhood abuse. Thus, genetic factors probably interact with environmental stressors such as physical abuse, substance abuse, or other physical or social insults to cause a mental disorder. Identifying and addressing these stress factors may prevent the development of some disorders.

Primary prevention involves taking proactive steps to prevent illness, such as intervening with support after loss, trauma, or disaster to protect against depression or anxiety disorders in vulnerable people or providing prophylactic treatment for depression or schizophrenia in African Americans with a strong family history. Such actions are infrequently attempted. Nevertheless, despite a strong focus on the genetics of mental illness, factors such as substance abuse, family rearing, and stress seem to interact with risk genes to determine if a mental disorder is expressed or has a poor outcome.

"Risk factors are not predictive factors due to protective factors" is an important concept, particularly in mental health. It dictates that mental health professionals invest resources in protective factors, such as social support and social fabric, which can serve as a buffer against inevitable stressors and negative environmental conditions that many African Americans encounter. Such investment can foster resilience in populations that might otherwise fall prey to significant challenges to mental health or outright expression of psychiatric illness in the face of overwhelming stressors or negative life events.

CONCLUSION

Dove and colleagues (38) provide a series of corrective measures for mental health disparities, including:

- Decreasing the discriminatory attitudes associated with psychiatric illness through education
- Improving communications and providing training in social skills for people with mental illness
- Increasing access and availability of psychiatric care in communities with significant levels of unmet need
- Increasing the number of providers serving African American populations
- Increasing educational efforts to enhance adherence to treatment

The mental health system and its providers must become more patient-centered and receptive to the needs of African Americans and their families. A system based on compassion may explain the superior outcomes seen in third-world countries and recovery-based provider systems.

References

1. U.S. Department of Health and Human Services: *Mental Health: Culture, Race, and Ethnicity—A Supplement to Mental Health: A Report of The Surgeon General.* Rockville, MD: U.S. Department of Health and Human Services, Substance Abuse and Mental Health Services Administration; 2001.
2. Primm A. Cultural issues in assessment and treatment: African American patients. In: Lim RF, ed. *Clinical Manual of Cultural Psychiatry.* Washington, DC: American Psychiatric Publishing, Inc.; 2006.
3. Kessler RC, Berglund P, Demler O, et al. Lifetime prevalence and age-of-onset distributions of DSM-IV disorders in the National Comorbidity Survey Replication. *Arch Gen Psychiatry* 2005;62(6):593–602.
4. Lawson WB. Mental health issues for African Americans. In: Guillermo B, Trimble JE, Burlow AK, eds. *Handbook of Racial and Ethnic Minority Psychology.* Thousand Oaks, CA: Sage Publications, Inc.; 2002.
5. Strakowski SM, Keck PE Jr, Arnold LM, et al. Ethnicity and diagnosis in patients with affective disorders. *J Clin Psychiatry* 2003;64:747–754.
6. Robins LN, Locke B, Regier DA. An overview of psychiatric disorders in America. In Robins LN, Regier DA, eds. *Psychiatric Disorders in America: The Epidemiologic Catchment Area Study.* New York: The Free Press; 1991:328–366.
7. Lawson WB. Identifying interethnic variations in psychotropic response in African-Americans and other ethnic minorities. In: Ng CH, Lin KM, Singh BS, eds. *Ethno-Psychopharmacology Advances in Current Practice.* Melbourne, Australia: Cambridge University Press Australia and New Zealand; 2007.
8. Alim TN, Graves E, Mellman TA, et al. Trauma exposure, posttraumatic stress disorder and depression in an African American primary care population. *J Natl Med Assoc* 2006;98:1630–1636.
9. Lawson WB. Clinical issues in the pharmacotherapy of African Americans. *Psychopharmacology Bull* 1996;36:278–281.
10. Williams DR, Gonzalez HM, Neighbors H, et al. Prevalence and distribution of major depressive disorder in African Americans, Caribbean blacks, and non-Hispanic whites: Results from the National Survey of American Life. *Arch Gen Psychiatry* 2007;64(3):305–315.
11. Brown D, Keith V, eds. *In and Out of Our Right Minds: The Mental Health of African American Women.* New York: Columbia University Press; 2003.
12. Williams T. Black Pain. *It Just Looks Like We're Not Hurting.* New York: Scribner; 2008.
13. Joe S, Baser RE, Breeden G, et al. Prevalence of and risk factors for lifetime suicide attempts among blacks in the United States. *JAMA* 2006;296(17):2112–2123.
14. Lawson WB. Bipolar Disorder in African Americans. In: Georgiopoulos AM, Rosenbaum JM, eds. *Perspectives in Cross-Cultural Psychiatry.* Philadelphia: Lippincott Williams & Wilkins, 2005:135–142.
15. Graves RE, Alim TA, Aigbogun N, et al. Diagnosing bipolar disorder in primary care clinics. *Bipolar Disord* 2007;9(4):318–323.
16. Wang PS, Berglund P, Kessler RC. Recent care of common mental disorders in the United States: Prevalence and conformance with evidence-based recommendations. *J Gen Intern Med* 2000;15(5);284–292.
17. Lawson WB. Schizophrenia in African Americans. In: Mueser KT, Jeste DV, eds. *Clinical Handbook of Schizophrenia.* New York: The Guilford Press; 2008.
18. Stockdale SE, Lagomasino IT, Siddique J, et al. Racial and ethnic disparities in detection and treatment of depression and anxiety among psychiatric and primary health care visits, 1995–2005. *Med Care* 2008;46(7):668–677.

19. Atdjian S, Vega WA. Disparities in mental health treatment in U.S. racial and ethnic minority groups: Implications for psychiatrists. *Psychiatric Services* 2005;56:1600–1602.

20. Chermack ST, Zivin K, Valenstein M, et al. The prevalence and predictors of mental health treatment services in a national sample of depressed veterans. *Med Care* 2008;46(8):813–820.

21. Breakey WR, Dunn GJ. Racial disparity in the use of ECT for affective disorders. *Am J Psychiatry* 2004;161(9):1635–1641.

22. Cruz M, Pincus HA, Harman JS, et al. Barriers to care-seeking for depressed African Americans. *Int J Psychiatry Med* 2008;38(1):71–80.

23. Anglin DM, Alberti PM, Link BG, et al. Racial differences in beliefs about the effectiveness and necessity of mental health treatment. *Am J Community Psychol* 2008;42(1–2):17–24.

24. Bradford LD. CYP2D6 allele frequency in European Caucasians, Asians, Africans and their descendants. *Pharmacogenomics* 2002:3:229–243.

25. Glazer WM, Morgenstern H, Doucette J. Race and tardive dyskinesia among outpatients at a CMHC. *Hosp Comm Psychiatry* 1994;45:38–42.

26. Bailey RK. Atypical psychotropic medications and their adverse effects: A review for the African American primary care physician. *J Natl Med Assoc* 2003;95(2):137–144.

27. Lesser IM, Castro DB, Gaynes BN, et al. Ethnicity/race and outcome in the treatment of depression: results from STAR*D. *Med Care* 2007;45(11):1043–1051.

28. McMahon FJ, Buervenich S, Charney D, et al. Variation in the gene encoding the serotonin 2A receptor is associated with outcome of antidepressant treatment. *Am J Hum Genet* 2006;78:804–814.

29. Olfson M, Marcus SC, Tedeschi M, et al. Continuity of antidepressant treatment for adults with depression in the United States. *Am J Psychiatry* 2006;163:101–108.

30. Cooper LA, Gonzales JJ, Galio JJ, et al. The acceptability of treatment for depression among African American, Hispanic, and White primary care patients. *Med Care* 2003; 41(4):479–489.

31. Smedley BD, Stith AY, Nelson AR, eds. Institute of Medicine of the National Academies. *Unequal Treatment: Confronting Racial and Ethnic Disparities in Health Care.* Committee on Understanding and Eliminating Racial and Ethnic Disparities in Health Care. National Academies Press, 2004. Available at http://www.iom.edu/?id=16740.

32. Collins TC, Clark JA, Petersen LA, et al. Racial difference in how patients perceive physician communication regarding cardiac testing. *Med Care* 2002;40(1 Suppl):127–134.

33. Johnson RL, Roter D, Powe NR, et al. Patient race/ethnicity and quality of patient-physician communication during medical visits. *Am J Public Health* 2004;94(12):2084–2090.

34. Blanchard J, Lurie N. R-E-S-P-E-C-T: Patient reports of disrespect in the health care setting and its impact on care. *J Fam Pract* 2004;53(9):721–730.

35. Ghods BK, Roter DL, Ford DE, et al. Patient-physician communication in the primary care visits of African Americans and whites with depression. *J Gen Intern Med* 2008; 23(5):600–606.

36. Summit Health Institute for Research and Education, Inc. *Giving Voice to the Voiceless: Language Barriers and Health Access Issues of Black Immigrants of African Descent.* Supported by The California Endowment. Los Angeles, CA; 2005.

37. Caspi A, Sugden K, Moffitt TE, et al. Influence of life stress on depression: Moderation by a polymorphism in the 5-HTT gene. *Science* 2003:18;301(5631):386–389.

38. Dove HW, Anderson TR, Bell CC. Mental Health. In Satcher D, Pamies R, eds. *Mental Health in Multicultural Medicine and Health Disparities.* New York: McGraw Hill; 2006:295–304.

4 | Hispanic Americans

Renato D. Alarcón and Pedro Ruiz

INTRODUCTION

This chapter will initially present a brief history and demographic data related to the Hispanic (or Latino) population in the United States. An overview of the mental health picture of this group will be followed by diagnostic and treatment considerations and by the examination of potential preventive factors. Beyond similarities with other racial and ethnic minorities, Hispanics in the United States experience significant disparities in the provision of appropriately designed services, characteristics of the mental health workforce, and the plight of the special subpopulations: children and adolescents, the elderly, women, gays, lesbians and bisexuals, and other emerging groups. The conclusions will focus on needs and priorities and on possible approaches to solve or improve the existing realities.

HISPANICS IN THE UNITED STATES

For centuries before the arrival of the Spanish colonizers, indigenous groups, particularly of Mayan and Aztec origin, populated areas of what is now the Western portion of the United States. Spain conquered Mexico during the 16th century and founded a powerful vice royalty in that territory. American pioneers of the "March Toward the East" during the 18th century found well-established native *pueblos*, mixed-population villages, and Spanish-speaking communities in what are now California, Arizona, and Texas. The foundation of the Republic of Texas and the U.S.-Mexican war fostered the expansion of the growing United States, driven by historical developments, ideological forces ("the Manifest Destiny"), and economic factors exemplified by the purchase of the Louisiana Territory.

On the East, the expeditions of Ponce de León looking for the "Fountain of Eternal Youth" in what is now Florida, Hernando de Soto crossing the Mississippi River, and the establishment of advance posts of Spanish explorers and adventurers along the southern and southwestern borders of the current United States reflect, unquestionably, a significant presence of Spanish-speaking populations long before the emergence of the country as a world political and economic power.

The 20th century witnessed a significant growth of the U.S. population as a whole, the pervasive, systematically increasing presence of immigrants and their descendants being one of its most salient features. Hispanics from Mexico, Central and South America, Puerto Ricans migrating from the island to the continent, and other immigrants, legal and undocumented, have lived through, at times, a stormy assimilation process for the last six to eight decades. The contribution of Hispanics to the population growth, economic progress, cultural pluralism, and demographic diversity of today's United States is an irrefutable reality.

CURRENT DEMOGRAPHICS

It is well known that Hispanics constitute, at this point in history, the largest and fastest-growing minority group in the United States. Recently released figures from the U.S. Census Bureau (1) show that by July 2007, the Hispanic population reached a total of 45.5 million (out of a minority population of 100.7 million), 15.1% of the estimated total U.S. population of 301.6 million. Census projections indicate that the Latino population will double from 15% of today to 30% by 2060. Mexican-Americans constitute 55.2% of all Hispanics, followed by Central and South Americans (14.3%), Puerto Ricans (9.6%), Cubans (4.3%), and other Hispanics (6.6%).

The state of California has the largest Hispanic population (13.2 million), followed by Texas (8.6 million) and Florida (3.8 million). Texas had the largest numerical increase between 2006 and 2007 (308,000), followed by California (258,000) and Florida (131,000). In the state of New Mexico, Hispanics comprise the highest portion of the total population (44%), with California and Texas (36% each) next in line. Furthermore, Hispanics as a whole are younger than the average age of the overall American population: 27.6 vs. 36.6 years. Almost 34% of the Hispanic population was younger than 18 years, compared with 25% among the total population. In 10 years, a quarter of the 10- to 14-year-olds will be Hispanic.

Two more demographic factors are important to consider. First, the surge in the U.S. Hispanic population appears to be primarily driven by birth and not immigration, the result of Hispanic women's high fertility rate (84 births per 1000 women, compared with 63 per 1000 non-Hispanic women) (2,3). Between 2003 and 2007, about 62% of the increase in Hispanics came from births, a significant difference with the 1980s and 1990s when the flood of Hispanic immigrants (particularly from Mexico and Central America) sustained most of the group's population rise. Furthermore, Hispanic women give birth on average to 2.8 children, compared with 1.8 children for white women (a rate of 2.1 is necessary to maintain a stable population).

The second observation is that the Hispanic population is moving from its traditional centers of settlement to other areas in the country. Rather than staying on the West Coast (primarily California) or in the Southwest area (primarily Texas), Hispanics, particularly Mexicans and Mexican-Americans, are moving to the Southeast and the Midwest. Puerto Ricans are concentrated in the New York metropolitan area, and Cubans live primarily in Southern Florida. However, "nontraditional" states such as Georgia, the Carolinas, Minnesota (which had an increase of 166% of its Hispanic population in a period of 5 years), Nebraska, and Iowa are seeing continuous growth. The search for better opportunities and lower costs of living are the main reasons for this internal migration.

EDUCATIONAL AND SOCIOECONOMIC SITUATIONS

Although there has been some improvement in the number of Hispanics achieving a high school diploma (currently, less than 50 %), almost 35% of those 25 years or older have less than a ninth grade education, and less than 12% have graduated from college. This has, of course, economic implications because Hispanic people are 3 times as likely as non-Hispanic whites to live below the poverty level (about 25% vs. 8%). The unemployment rate also hits hardest on the Hispanic population (close to 7% in the year 2000). Beyond large urban centers, a new trend in Hispanic settlements seems to be moving toward small communities to take jobs in industries such as meat packing, textiles, and construction. Somewhat paradoxically, there is marked growth in spending by Hispanics (1). It is said that Hispanics control more disposable income than any other minority group, a figure that has been placed at $860 billion a year and is expected to reach $1.3 trillion by 2012.

CULTURAL CHARACTERISTICS

Although some regional variations and local or indigenous dialects are used, by and large Spanish is the language spoken by the vast majority of Hispanic persons. Sixty percent to 65% of Hispanics are Catholic, and 25% are Protestant—a phenomenon that has been confirmed in numerous studies, breaking a tradition of centuries. From a strictly cultural point of view, Hispanics profess a significant "personalization" of religion, emphasize issues of guilt and shame, and a great deal of spirituality permeates their perceptions of both health and illness.

Compared with Caucasians, Hispanics are more likely to never marry (40% vs. 24.4%), more likely to be single parents (23.7% vs. 13% among women), and less likely to be widowed or divorced. *Familismo*, the deep identification with and attachment to the nuclear and extended family, is one of the strongest cultural features of the Hispanic population. It emphasizes the values of interdependence, connectedness, and sharing, together with the acceptance of a hierarchical authority structure. Hispanics have a significant concern about privacy, and their strong religious and spiritual background make them more prone to attribute significant benign or malignant power to external forces (4).

Gender roles in Hispanic families seem to follow (although this may be declining) the same hierarchal structure. This characteristic includes *machismo*, the ideal of the strong, powerful, active man, and *marianismo*, the ideal of the submissive, docile, and yet resilient woman. In many cases, however, both features have been exaggerated by popular culture myths or stereotypes. Sociocentrism or collectivism, the emphasis on needs, objectives, and goals of the group prevailing over those of individual members, is another important cultural feature. *Simpatia*, the avoidance of direct anger and confrontation between people to make relationships flow smoothly and nicely, interacts with other features such as fatalism (mix of pessimism, acceptance, and resilience), dependency (born out of respect for age and authority figures), and hypersuggestibility (relevant in transactions with healthcare providers) (4,5).

MENTAL HEALTH IN THE U.S. HISPANIC POPULATIONS

Clinical epidemiological investigations have provided a general yet changing picture of mental health among Hispanics in the United States. There is a small but selected group of studies dating back to the early 1980s and 1990s (6). The National Latino and Asian American Study (NLAAS) (7) used methodology similar to the National Comorbidity Survey (NCS) and has produced cogently relevant information from a representative sample (8). The information below summarizes findings from some of these studies.

GENERAL FINDINGS

Confirming previous results, the NLAAS (which used the World Mental Health Composite International Diagnostic Interview [CIDI] as its main tool) found that immigrants appear to have lower rates of psychiatric disorders than second- and third-generation Latinos in the United States. For disorders such as depression, anxiety, and substance abuse disorders, the lifetime prevalence estimate shows a rate of 36.8% for U.S.-born Latinos compared with 23.8% for foreign-born Latinos; past-year prevalence was 18.6% for U.S.-born and 13% for those foreign-born.

Whereas prevalence estimates are similar for men and women, in comparisons among the different Latino subgroups, Puerto Ricans tended to show higher figures in some disorders (anxiety, particularly post-traumatic stress disorder) than Cubans, Mexicans, or other groups. Comparatively, Mexican men and women are less likely to have a history of depressive disorders, and Cuban men are less likely to have anxiety or substance abuse disorders (7).

ACCESS AND UTILIZATION OF HEALTH SERVICES

There are well-demonstrated culturally based patterns of help-seeking among Hispanics. Because of the emphasis on privacy and the strong family ties and connections with and respect for authority figures, the health services as such may be the last resort in many physical and mental health cases among Hispanics. Before seeing a physician or a health professional, Hispanics may resort to relatives, friends, priests, community leaders, neighbors, teachers, and the like. In the case of mental problems, it is even more evident that they would rather be seen by a non–health professional (including folk healers, *curanderos*, and similar figures) than by psychiatrists, psychologists, or other mental health professionals.

On the other hand, data are consistent regarding the role of factors such as legal status, financial means, insurance coverage, and related areas contributing to a delay in the search for and access to mental health services (9). Actually, African Americans and Hispanics had no or less care or access to care when needed, or delayed care compared with whites for specific conditions such as alcoholism and drug abuse (10). Significant portions of Latino populations in the United States are uninsured for medical expenditures compared with blacks and non Hispanic whites. Nevertheless, among the Hispanic subpopulations, Puerto Ricans were 5.5 times more likely to receive Medicaid coverage than Mexican-Americans and Cuban Americans (11).

Cultural beliefs and habits, language barriers, insufficient numbers of Hispanic manpower in the healthcare professions, low educational and socioeconomic levels, differences in the recognition of mental health problems, the high number of uninsured Hispanics, and ethnic and racial prejudices and discrimination are factors that limit the access to services. Analyses from the 1990 to 1992 NCS indicated that poor Latinos (with a family income of less than $15,000 per year) have lower access to specialty care than poor nonLatino whites. Latinos were likely to have two or more previous-year psychiatric disorders than nonLatino whites and African Americans (9,10). The combined effect of poverty and minority status places particular population groups at a higher risk of reduced access to mental health services. Vega et al. (12) show that immigrants are unlikely to use mental health services even when they have a recent disorder but may use general practitioners, which raises questions about the appropriateness, accessibility, and cost-effectiveness of mental healthcare for this population.

SPECIFIC CLINICAL ENTITIES

A general premise in the overall assessment of specific clinical conditions should be that nonbiological, environmental, or sociocultural factors play an etiopathogenic role. Some of the demographic and cultural characteristics mentioned above, in connection with factors such as migration status or reception by the host culture, contribute to what some clinicians would call predisposing personalities or psychological make-ups of vulnerability, resilience, or a combination of both. Hispanics may show specific forms of experiencing symptoms that, in turn, have some impact on their help-seeking behaviors, approach to treatment, levels of compliance, clinical outcomes, and overall quality of life.

Depression and Other Mood Disorders

It has been demonstrated that depression may be more severe among Latino patients, perhaps because many of them fail to recognize the symptoms; on the other hand, suicidality is less marked in adults but appears to be on the rise among Mexican-American youth (7,10). Symptoms such as social isolation, apathy, and/or excessive use of alcohol as a self-medicating attempt are well-known clinical characteristics among Hispanics. Irritability has been observed, but not to the point of physical violence because factors such as sociocentrism, *familism*, religious faith, respect, and other cultural features may play a preventive role. Poor compliance with medication intake is an important observation, perhaps related to both cultural and financial factors.

Anxiety Disorders

The clinical picture of anxiety among Latinos tends to be more overt in expression of emotional lability, restlessness, or verbal and nonverbal manifestations. Generalized anxiety disorder with concomitant panic attacks may be seen more frequently among Hispanics, a cultural twist of which may be a relatively high incidence of *susto* or *ataque de nervios*, considered characteristically Hispanic culture-bound syndromes (13). Similarly, agoraphobia and social phobia are seen frequently and have been ascribed to social isolation, differences in relational styles, and fear of being judged or humiliated by others. Finally, higher exposure to traumatic events (14), higher rates of unemployment and underemployment with financial consequences, overrepresentation of households headed by single women experiencing both gender role stresses, and separation from family members may contribute to posttraumatic stress disorder–like symptoms among Hispanics (7).

Psychoses

The dominant clinical perception is that psychotic conditions among Hispanics tend to show more overt delusions or hallucinations. The religious content of both of these psychopathological manifestations responds to cultural conditions. Pharmacologically, the need of lower doses of antipsychotics has been confirmed in different studies in Latino populations, with possible pharmacogenomic explanatory substrates (15).

Substance Use Disorders

Alcohol abuse seemed to be predominant among Hispanic patients but, in recent years, there is a significant increase of polysubstance abuse, particularly marijuana, cocaine, heroin, narcotic and hallucinogenic agents, methamphetamine, and other stimulants. Although the clinical pictures may be similar, the issue of frequency of abuse and modalities of combination of drugs is noteworthy (16). The legal and judicial implications of these behaviors are evident.

Personality Disorders

Although it is very difficult to say which of the DSM-IV TR personality disorder clusters is most frequent among Hispanics, there may be a trend toward cluster C, particularly the dependent and avoidant types. The former may be related to family structures and culturally inspired hierarchal principles; the latter is related to difficulties in social interactions (language, living quarters, neighborhoods, interactions with the host culture) or to sheer financial factors. It has been said that antisocial and related cluster B personality features are less frequently seen among Hispanics compared with others, but there is a dearth of epidemiological data (17). Cultural distinctions about cluster A disorders may be difficult to ascertain because of the possible neurobiological or neurocognitive roots of these categories; paradoxically, the mistaken assignments of these diagnoses to Latino adolescents and young adults is fairly frequent.

Eating Disorders

There seems to be less frequency of eating disorders (particularly, anorexia nervosa) among Latino patients, particularly girls. This may have to do, again, with culturally determined features, parental influence, and concepts about an ideal body image. Nevertheless, like in many other groups, the tendency toward more Westernized notions of body image may contribute to a small but steady increase of these disorders.

Dementia and Other Geriatric Disorders

As in other conditions, there seems to be an upward trend in the frequency of these disorders among Hispanics (7–9). Nevertheless, the role of concomitant medical problems cannot be underestimated because aging, socioeconomic factors, and biological predispositions can make them worse. In turn, the impact of these conditions on mental performance, particularly higher functions, may be noticeable.

Chronic Medical Conditions and Mental Health

Among Hispanics, conditions such as diabetes mellitus, arthritis, hypertension, urinary/bowel incontinence, kidney disease, ulcers, and stroke with residual speech problems predict high levels of depressive symptoms. Hispanic populations seek large amounts of care for sexually transmitted diseases and obstetrical problems and smaller amounts for specific entities such as AIDS and adverse fetal outcomes. The mental health impact of all these conditions is self-evident and is aggravated by the limited access to care (5,18). Among Hispanic cancer patients, the roles of family and religious faith are important components of quality of life. Among cardiovascular female patients, functional impairment has a stronger association with depressive symptoms than angina or physical inactivity. Similarly, among patients with systemic lupus erythematosus, attitudes toward the disease, fatigue, and pain have greater impact on self-perceived functional levels than more objective measures of disease activity (19). Last but not least, the physical and emotional well-being of custodial grandparents in Latino families, the health status of partners of patients with chronic diseases, and the presence of chronic diseases among children and adolescents appear to be growing problems in this population group (9).

Acculturative Stress

Focused more on immigrants, this condition has an unsteady nosological status (20). Nevertheless, it is clear that it does not belong to the traditional post-traumatic stress disorder category, even though it shares some symptoms with it. The characteristics of onset, duration, severity, and management styles of acculturative stress are different among Hispanic populations. The clinical manifestations are a mix of anxiety, depression, dysphoria, agitation, confusion, and subsequent interpersonal difficulties. It may start later, about 6 months after the patient's arrival in the country, and the social and occupational interferences due to the disorder are evident. On the other hand, Hispanic individuals with these manifestations seem to respond well to opportune interventions.

MENTAL HEALTHCARE FOR HISPANICS

Many authors agree that there is a de facto racial and ethnic segregation in U.S. healthcare. Health facilities, nursing homes, access to community health services, private care, and other statistics show consistent patterns of segregation. The link between health and poverty needs to be addressed (21). Living in a disadvantaged community militates not only against access to amenities but also to healthful food, opportunities for physical activity, and medical and other services. In addition, insecurity, fear of crime, implications of low socioeconomic status, and lack of social support are all features of disadvantaged communities that result in obvious inequalities in healthcare and concomitant mental health repercussions. The Hispanic population is prominently situated in the "firing line" of these pervasive realities.

Attempts to assimilate to an economic and cultural ideal in the United States, while retaining an identity now clouded by a minority status, exert particular pressure on Latino men and women. It is important to be aware in both general practice and psychiatric settings of the risk factors for depressive and other disorders affecting Latinos at even higher levels of acculturation.

POSSIBLE APPROACHES AND SOLUTIONS

A better understanding of these deep-seated social inequalities will be a first step toward the correction of the problems. It is important to set a good catalogue of needs as well as priorities; nevertheless, the approach should be global, frontal, and determined. In the context of coronary heart disease (a chronic condition, like many mental illnesses), Diez Roux et al. (22) suggested two potential targets of public health interventions: enhancing the social and psychological resources of individual people and improving the quality of neighborhood and communal life. From the policy-making vantage point, together with a legislative push toward equity (steps such as the recent approval of Medicare parity are encouraging), the health system should dovetail performance incentives with enhancement of racial and ethnic equity in access and provision of services (23). Targeted infusions of expertise and technology in deprived areas, by providing funding for investment in needed infrastructure, should be pursued.

Attention should be paid to the role of cultural factors in the different phases of the Hispanic patients' contact with the mental health system. This includes language use, the management of diverse explanatory models, attitudes toward therapies, family interactions, and further treatment of those whose response may be ineffective or inappropriate (24). The dearth of Spanish-speaking mental healthcare providers cannot be faced with the expectation that a sufficient number of native-language Hispanics will join the workforce anytime soon. On the other hand, resilience among Hispanics is a matter of continuous debate but is still lacking in consistent research evidence. Generally speaking, it may be a compositum of psychological, ethical, moral, behavioral, and neurobiological factors. No one should rely only on the latter to explain a set of attributes that reflect essential principles of the human condition.

Improving mental healthcare for Hispanics is a challenge. Several authors and organizations have outlined steps and strategies aimed at a reasonably paced improvement of the situation (25,26). In summary, the following areas should be examined, prioritized, and implemented:

1. Community advocacy for the outreach and expansion of science-based approaches, evidence-based research efforts, support of education, training, and career-development initiatives.
2. Promotion of culturally competent health and mental health services, including a linguistically competent workforce, and a parallel development of community-based options for Hispanics to learn English. This applies also to professionals such as translators, social workers, and physician assistants.
3. Professional competence that implies protection of the patient's confidentiality, honesty and ethical behavior, fair distribution of resources, absence of conflicts of interest, and commitment to the continuous improvement of scientific knowledge.
4. Promote an appropriate representation of Hispanic professionals in pertinent Federal, state, and local agencies, as well as in board memberships and leadership positions in major mental health organizations.

The Hispanic population, as does the great majority of the U.S. population, would support the rational development and implementation of a comprehensive health insurance plan directed to cover all sectors of the population currently uninsured. This should include mandatory provision of basic health insurance coverage for all workers in the labor sector. The implementation of a health and mental healthcare system that integrates different disciplines (primary care practitioners and psychiatrists, for example) would enhance an efficient use of human and technological resources. The promotion of appropriate professional representation from ethnic minority groups would strengthen the potential of public and private educational and research institutions. Advocating appropriate allocation of research funds geared to the unique health and mental healthcare needs of the U.S. Hispanic population and other minorities in this country is another well-delineated objective.

CONCLUSION

Hispanics in the United States are a human group in the most powerful country of the world, striving to reach a level of identity, presence, recognition, and achievement that may appropriately reflect their increasing demographic growth. At the same time, their health and mental health needs have peculiar and unique characteristics related to social, political, and economic factors, as much as to a strong and well-established historical and cultural legacy. In such context, the clinical picture of different conditions may have unique facets that need to be considered in diagnostic systems and in the identification of therapeutic targets, treatment strategies, and outcome assessments. Priority needs in the public, community, educational, and research areas must be met. Advocacy, a culturally competent workforce, leadership, and organizational visibility are items of significant value for Hispanic patients, their families, and health professionals. Well-planned, comprehensive approaches aimed at erasing mental health and healthcare disparities in general should, therefore, be meaningfully addressed.

The authors wish to express their deep appreciation to Juan Ramos, PhD, for his valuable assistance in the preparation of this chapter.

References

1. U.S. Census Bureau Press Release. U.S. Hispanic population surpasses 45 million—Now 15 percent of total. Washington, DC, May 1, 2008.
2. Gonzales F. Hispanic Women in the United States, 2007. Available at http://www.pewhispanic.org. Washington, DC, May 8, 2008:1–28.
3. Dougherty C, Jordan M. Surge in U.S. Hispanic population driven by births, not immigration. *Wall Street Journal,* May 1, 2008:A3.
4. López AG, Katz I. An introduction. In: López AG, Carrillo E, eds. *The Latino Psychiatric Patient. Assessment and Treatment.* Washington, DC: American Psychiatric Publishing, Inc, 2001:3–18.
5. Pérez-Stable EJ, Nápoles-Springer AM. Physical health states of Latinos in the U.S. In: López AG, Carrillo E, eds. *The Latino Psychiatric Patient. Assessment and Treatment.* Washington, DC: American Psychiatric Publishing, Inc, 2001:19–36.
6. Alarcón RD. Culture, mental health and chronic medical illnesses: The Hispanic perspective. *Workshop on Depression and Medical Diseases. Bridging a Cultural and Clinical Divide.* National Hispanic Medical Association Meeting. San Francisco, CA, May 5, 2003.
7. Alegría M, Mulvaney-Day N, Torres M, et al. Prevalence of psychiatric disorders across Latino subgroups in the United States. *Am J Public Health* 2007;97:68–75.
8. Alegría M, Mulvaney-Day N, Woo M, et al. Correlates of past-year mental health service use among Latinos: Results from the National Latino and Asian American Study. *Am J Public Health* 2007;97:76–83.
9. Alegría M, Canino G, Ríos R, et al. Inequalities in use of specialty mental health services among Latinos, African Americans, and non-Latino Whites. *Psychiatr Serv* 2002;53:1547–1555.
10. Wells K, Klap R, Koike A, et al. Ethnic disparities in unmet need for alcoholism, drug abuse and mental health care. *Am J Psychiatry* 2001;158:2027–2032.
11. Treviño FM, Moyer E, Burciaga-Valdez R, et al. Health insurance coverage and utilization of health services by Mexican Americans, mainland Puerto Ricans, and Cuban Americans. *JAMA* 1991;265:233–238.
12. Vega WA, Kolody B, Aguilar-Gaxiola S, et al. Gaps in service utilization by Mexican Americans with mental health problems. *Am J Psychiatry* 1999;156:928–934.
13. Guarnaccia PJ. Ataques de Nervios in Puerto Rico: Culture-bound syndrome or population illness? *Med Anthropol* 1992;15:1–14.
14. Galea S, Ahern J, Resnick H, et al. Psychological sequelae of the September 11 terrorist attacks in New York City. *N Engl J Med* 2002;346:982–987.
15. Smith M. Etnopsicofarmacología Psiquiátrica en América Latina. In: Alarcón RD, Mazzotti G, Nicolini H, eds. *Psiquiatría,* 2ª. ed. México D.F.: El Manual Moderno 2005:994–1002.
16. Ruiz P, Langrod JG: Hispanic Americans. In: Lowinson JH, Ruiz P, Millman RB, et al, eds. *Substance Abuse: A Comprehensive Textbook,* 4th ed. Philadelphia: Lippincott Williams & Wilkins, 2005:1103–1112.

17. Alarcón RD, Foulks EF, Vakkur M. *Personality Disorders and Culture. Clinical and Conceptual Interactions.* New York: Wiley & Sons, 1998:133–171.
18. Taningco MTV. *Revisiting the Latino Health Paradox.* Tomás Rivera Policy Institute, August 2007:14.
19. Fernández M, Alarcón GS, Calvo-Alén J, et al. A multiethnic, multicenter cohort of patients with systemic lupus erythematosus (SLE) as a model for the study of ethnic disparities in SLE. *Arthritis Rheum* 2007;57:576–584.
20. Lara M, Gamboa C, Kahramanian MI, et al. Acculturation and Latino Health in the United States: A review of the literature and its sociopolitical context. *Ann Rev Public Health* 2005;26:367–397.
21. Krugman P. Poverty is poison. Op-Ed, *New York Times,* February 18, 2008.
22. Diez Roux AV, Stein MS, Arnett D, et al. Neighborhood of residence and incidence of coronary heart disease. *N Engl J Med* 2001;345:99–106.
23. Blustein J. Who is accountable for racial equity in health care? *JAMA* 2008;299:814–816.
24. Folsom DP, Gilmer T, Barrio C, et al. A longitudinal study of the use of mental health services by persons with serious mental illness: Do Spanish-speaking Latinos differ from English-speaking Latinos and Caucasians? *Am J Psychiatry* 2007;164:1173–1180.
25. Ruiz P. Hispanics' mental health plight. Available at http://www.behavioral.net. November/December, 2005:17–20.
26. National Alliance of Multi-Ethnic Behavioral Health Associations (NAMBAH). *Blueprint for the National Network to Eliminate Disparities in Behavioral Health.* Working draft. Washington, DC, 2008.

5 Asian Americans and Pacific Islanders

Francis G. Lu

INTRODUCTION

This chapter will begin with a description of the population of Asian Americans and Pacific Islanders (AAPIs), their health status, health insurance coverage, and access to healthcare to provide a foundation of important information to contextualize the other studies discussed. Mental health disparities for AAPIs were brought into the forefront by the landmark 2001 *Mental Health: Culture, Race, and Ethnicity: A Supplement to Mental Health: A Report to the Surgeon General* (1) and this chapter will review the key findings of Chapter 5, "Mental Health Care for Asian Americans and Pacific Islanders." Recent studies of mental health and psychiatric care disparities involving AAPIs will then be discussed, which reveal the complexity of cultural identity and sociocultural environmental variables that must be considered both to understand the origin of these disparities and to design interventions to reduce these disparities. Finally, future directions in research on AAPI disparities will be discussed.

DEFINITION OF THE POPULATION

As of 2006, there were more than 14.9 million Asian Americans and 1 million Native Hawaiian and Pacific Islanders in the United States (2). Although Native Hawaiians are an important ethnic group, they will be designated in this chapter under the rubric of "Pacific Islanders." The significant heterogeneity between Asian Americans and Pacific Islanders can be seen in this startling reality: "Asian Americans, as a whole, have higher educational attainment rates, higher median household incomes, and lower rates of poverty compared with non-Hispanic whites. However, the exact opposite is true of Native Hawaiians and Pacific Islanders" (3).

AAPIs are a fast-growing racial group in the United States. The population grew 3.2% (either alone or in combination with one or more other races) between 2005 and 2006, the highest of any race group during that time period. The projected number of U.S. residents in 2050 who will identify themselves as single-race Asians is 33.4 million. They would comprise 8% of the total population by that year, in contrast to 5.3% now (2).

The term AAPI must always be decontextualized in assessing an individual patient to understand the complexity of the cultural identity variables to avoid at the clinical encounter level stereotyping and overgeneralizations, which can contribute to health and mental healthcare disparities. For example, there are as many as 43 distinct ethnic groups. In 2004 to 2006 pooled data (3), the rank order by percentage of the largest ethnic groups were: Chinese, 21%; Filipino, 15%; Asian Indian, 14%; Vietnamese, 11%; Korean, 9%; other Southeast Asian, 7%; and Native Hawaiian and Pacific Islander, 5%. The AAPI population is concentrated in the Western United States, with more than half of this group in the West. The states with the largest populations in 2004 are California (5 million), New York (1.4 million), and Texas (882,000).

A second key cultural identity variable is country of birth and immigration versus native-born status. The majority of AAPIs were born outside of the United States and immigrated; the specific waves of immigration vary by ethnic group and historical circumstances of U.S immigration/exclusion laws, war, and economic promise, among other factors (1). More than two-thirds of AAPIs are U.S. citizens (about 33% by birth, 37% by naturalization). The Japanese had the highest proportion of natives (about 58%) and Koreans the lowest (about 24%), and Asian Indians had the highest proportion of foreign-born, non-U.S. citizens (about 41%) (5).

The linguistic diversity within the AAPI population comprises more than 100 languages and dialects. Two and one-half million people in the United States age 5 years and older speak a Chinese dialect at home. After Spanish, Chinese is the most widely spoken non-English language in the country. Tagalog, Vietnamese, and Korean are each spoken at home by more than 1 million people (2). In addition, some AAPI populations have high rates of limited English proficiency, which can contribute to health and mental health disparities. For example, these percentages of AAPIs live in linguistically isolated households, where no one age 14 years or older speaks English "very well": Hmong, 61%; Cambodian, 56%; Laotian, 52%; Vietnamese, 44%; Korean, 41%; and Chinese, 40% (1).

Other significant cultural identity variables of AAPIs that bear on mental health disparities that will be discussed later include age, socioeconomic status, gender, and sexual orientation, among others.

HEALTH STATUS, HEALTH INSURANCE COVERAGE, AND ACCESS TO HEALTHCARE

In general, the health status of AAPIs is rated by self-report to be better than that of non-Hispanic whites and members of other racial and ethnic groups. Eleven percent of AAPI adults rated their health as fair or poor compared with 23% of American Indians/Alaska Natives, 22% of African Americans, 18% of Hispanics, and 13% of non-Hispanic whites (3). Within the AAPI group, there are variations. For example, 15% of Vietnamese rated their health status as fair or poor compared with 8% of Japanese.

Health insurance status is well known to cause health and mental health differences in access to care, quality of care, and outcomes, so it was factored out of the definition of healthcare disparities in the landmark 2002 Institute of Medicine's *Unequal Treatment: Confronting Racial and Ethnic Disparities in Health Care* (6). Native Hawaiians and PIs are more likely to be uninsured and more likely to be on Medicaid than both Asians and nonwhite Hispanics. Employer-sponsored coverage ranges from as low as 49% among Koreans to a high of 77% among Asian Indians. Reliance on Medicaid and other public coverage ranges from 4% in Asian Indians to 19% among other Southeast Asians. Koreans have the highest rate of uninsured (31%), followed by Native Hawaiians and PIs (24%) (3).

Alegría and colleagues (7) examined the role that population vulnerabilities play in insurance coverage for a representative sample of Latinos and Asians in the United States. Using data from the National Latino and Asian American Study (NLAAS), these analyses compared coverage differences among and within ethnic subgroups, across states and regions, among types of occupations, and among those with or without English language proficiency. Extensive differences exist in coverage between Latinos and Asians, with Latinos more likely to be uninsured. Potential explanations included the type of occupations available to Latinos and Asians, reforms in immigration laws, length of time in the United States, and regional differences in safety-net coverage.

Health insurance status greatly affects access to health and mental healthcare. Individuals without insurance are more likely to lack a usual source of healthcare; for example, 11% of insured AAPIs lack a usual source of care compared with 52% of uninsured AAPIs. This approximately 1-to-4 ratio is also seen among Chinese, Filipino, Asian Indian, and non-Hispanic white groups.

MENTAL HEALTHCARE FOR ASIAN AMERICANS AND PACIFIC ISLANDERS

The 2001 *Mental Health: Culture, Race, and Ethnicity: A Supplement to Mental Health: A Report to the Surgeon General* (1) described the mental health disparities of the four major racial and ethnic groups in the United States (AAPI, African American, Hispanic, American Indian/Alaska Native) compared with the non-Hispanic white population in the following ways: (i) less access to services, (ii) less likely to receive needed services, (iii) more likely to receive poor quality of care when treated, and (iv) underrepresented in mental health research. Taken as a whole, these mental health disparities exerted a disproportionately greater disability burden on these four racial and ethnic minority populations and became an imperative for them to be reduced and eventually eliminated. Separate chapters were devoted to each of the four racial and ethnic minority populations, and the report ended with "A Vision of the Future," a chapter that made six broad recommendations: (i) continue to expand the science base, (ii) improve access to treatment, (iii) reduce barriers to treatment, (iv) improve quality of care, (v) support capacity development, and (vi) promote mental health. In 2001, as a follow-up to the Surgeon General's Report, the American Psychiatric Association (APA) Board of Trustees, led by President Richard Harding, convened a steering committee to reduce disparities in access to psychiatric care, which created the APA's strategic plan to eliminate mental health disparities. It was approved by the Board of Trustees in December 2004 (8).

Chapter 5 ("Mental Health Care for Asian Americans and Pacific Islanders") of the 2001 *Mental Health: Culture, Race, and Ethnicity: A Supplement to Mental Health: A Report to the Surgeon General* (1) focused on the topic of mental healthcare disparities for AAPIs. After a description of the historical and demographic characteristics of AAPIs (including ethnicity, language, immigration, geographic distribution, family structure, education, income, and physical health status), the chapter described the limited knowledge about the following topics related to AAPI mental health disparities, for which the Surgeon General recommended further research to expand the science base.

Need for Mental Healthcare

Our knowledge of the mental health needs of AAPIs is limited. National epidemiological studies have included few AAPIs or people whose English is limited. The largest study to focus on AAPIs (i.e., the CAPES study) examined the prevalence of mood disorders in a predominantly immigrant Chinese American sample. This study found lifetime and 1-year prevalence rates for depression of about 7% and 3%, respectively. These rates are roughly equal to general rates found in the same urban area.

Although overall prevalence rates of diagnosable mental illnesses among AAPIs appear similar to those of the white population, when symptom scales are used, AAPIs show higher levels of depressive symptoms than do white Americans. Furthermore, Chinese Americans are more likely to exhibit somatic complaints of depression than are African Americans or non-Hispanic whites. Small studies of symptoms of emotional distress have found few differences between AAPI youth and white youth.

AAPIs may experience culture-bound syndromes such as neurasthenia and hwa-byung. Neurasthenia is characterized by fatigue, weakness, poor concentration, memory loss, irritability, aches and pains, and sleep disturbances. Hwa-byung, or "suppressed anger syndrome," is characterized by symptoms such as constriction in the chest, palpitations, flushing, headache, dysphoria, anxiety, and poor concentration.

Compared with the suicide rate of white Americans (12.8 per 100,000 per year), the rates for Filipino (3.5), Chinese (8.3), and Japanese (9.1) Americans are substantially lower. However, Native Hawaiian adolescents have a higher risk of suicide than other adolescents in Hawaii, and older Asian American women have the highest suicide rate of all women over age 65 years in the United States. There is also a growing concern about increasing suicide rates in the Pacific Basin.

High-Need Populations

AAPIs are not overrepresented among high-need, vulnerable populations such as people who are homeless, incarcerated, or have substance abuse problems. However, they are heavily represented among refugees. Many Southeast Asian refugees are at risk for posttraumatic stress disorder (PTSD) associated with trauma experienced before and after immigration to the United States. One study found that 70% of Southeast Asian refugees receiving mental healthcare met diagnostic criteria for PTSD. In a study of Cambodian adolescents who survived Pol Pot's concentration camps, nearly half experienced PTSD and 41% suffered from depression 10 years after leaving Cambodia.

Availability of Mental Health Services

Nearly 1 of 2 AAPIs will have difficulty accessing mental health treatment because they do not speak English or cannot find services that meet their language needs. Approximately 70 AAPI providers are available for every 100,000 AAPIs in the United States compared with 173 per 100,000 whites. No reliable information is available regarding the Asian language capabilities of mental health providers in the United States.

Access to Mental Health Services

Overall, about 21% of AAPIs lack health insurance, compared with 16% of all Americans. The rate of Medicaid coverage for eligible AAPI families is well below that of whites. For example, among families with incomes below 200% of the federal poverty level, whites are twice as likely as Chinese Americans to enroll in Medicaid. It has been suggested that lower Medicaid participation rates are, in part, due to widespread but mistaken concerns among immigrants that enrolling in Medicaid jeopardizes applications for citizenship.

Use of Mental Health Services

AAPIs appear to have the extremely low utilization of mental health services relative to other U.S. populations. For example, in the CAPES study, only 17% of those experiencing problems sought care. Among AAPIs who use services, severity of disturbance tends to be high, perhaps because AAPIs tend to delay seeking treatment until symptoms reach crisis proportions. Although more research is needed, shame and stigma are believed to figure prominently in the lower utilization rates of AAPI communities. AAPIs tend to use complementary therapies at rates equal to or higher than white Americans.

Appropriateness and Outcomes of Mental Health Services

Few studies examine the response of minorities to mental health treatment. One study found that AAPI clients had poorer short-term outcomes and less satisfaction with individual psychotherapy than did white Americans. Another study found that older Chinese Americans with symptoms of depression responded to cognitive behavior therapy as did other multiethnic populations. AAPI clients matched with therapists of the same ethnicity are less likely to drop out of treatment than those without an ethnic match. Preliminary studies suggest that AAPIs respond clinically to psychotropic medicines in a manner similar to white Americans but at lower average dosages. Research is needed to identify key components of culturally appropriate services for AAPIs (9).

NEED FOR MENTAL HEALTH CARE AND USE OF MENTAL HEALTH SERVICES: RECENT STUDIES

As noted in the previous section, a major need in our understanding of mental health disparities was comprehensive epidemiological information about mental disorders and service utilization in AAPIs correlated with some of the cultural identity and socioenvironmental variables discussed in the above section on the Definition of the Population. Margarita Alegría and her colleagues (10) have embarked on a most important study, which includes the first national epidemiological survey of Asian Americans in the United States, to accomplish this goal.

The National Latino and Asian American Study (NLAAS) provides national information on the similarities and differences in mental illness and service use of Latinos and Asian Americans. The NLAAS is one of the most comprehensive studies of Latinos and Asian Americans ever conducted using up-to-date scientific strategies in the design, sampling procedures, psychiatric assessments, and analytic techniques. The final NLAAS sample consisted of 2554 Latino respondents and 2095 Asian American respondents. To allow for important subgroup analysis, respondents were further stratified into the following ethnic subgroup categories: Puerto Rican, Cuban, Mexican, other Latinos, Chinese, Vietnamese, Filipino, and other Asians. Data collection took place between May 2002 and November 2003. To be eligible to complete the NLAAS, respondents were required to be 18 years of age or older, living in the noninstitutionalized population of the coterminous United States or Hawaii, and of Latino, Hispanic, Spanish, or Asian descent. The NLAAS instrument was administered in the respondent's choice of the following languages: English, Spanish, Chinese, Vietnamese, or Tagalog by fully bilingual lay interviewers.

NLAAS data analyses will provide important baseline information about Latinos and Asians that will be critical when assessing whether there are diminished mental health disparities by the year 2010 (Healthy People 2010). NLAAS publications and papers in preparation address a wide range of different topics of importance for Asian and Latino mental health, including the prevalence of disorders across Latino and Asian subgroups, issues regarding language and measurement of disorder, sociocultural influences on mental disorder, and health and mental health service patterns for Latinos and Asian Americans (11).

Two articles (12,13) utilizing data from NLAAS looked at the role of nativity and immigration among other factors on prevalence of mental disorders and service utilization. Takeuchi and colleagues (12) examined lifetime and 12-month rates of any depressive, anxiety, and substance abuse disorders in a national sample of Asian Americans. The relationships between immigration-related factors and mental disorders were different for men and women. Among women, nativity was strongly associated with lifetime disorders, with immigrant women having lower rates of most disorders compared with U.S.-born women. Conversely, English proficiency was associated with mental disorders for Asian men. Asian men who spoke English proficiently generally had lower rates of lifetime and 12-month disorders compared with nonproficient speakers. Abe-Kim and colleagues (13) examined rates of mental health–related service use (i.e., any, general medical, and specialty mental health services) as well as subjective satisfaction with and perceived helpfulness of care. About 8.6% of the total sample (n = 2095) sought any mental health–related services; 34.1% of individuals who had a probable diagnosis sought any services. Rates of mental health–related service use, subjective satisfaction, and perceived helpfulness varied by birthplace and by generation. U.S.-born Asian Americans demonstrated higher rates of service use than did their immigrant counterparts. Third-generation or later individuals who had a probable diagnosis had high (62.6%) rates of service use in the previous 12 months. They concluded that Asian Americans demonstrated lower rates of any type of mental health–related service use than did the general population, although there are important exceptions to this pattern according to nativity status and generation status.

Paralleling these studies, Breslau and Chang (14), using data from the National Epidemiological Survey of Alcohol and Related Conditions (NESAEC) of 1236 Asian Americans, discovered that foreign-born Asian Americans had a lower prevalence of all psychiatric and substance abuse disorders than did U.S.-born Asian Americans. These differences reached statistical significance for social phobia, agoraphobia/panic disorder, and all categories of substance use disorder. Furthermore, for all classes of disorder, after arrival in the United States, risk for first onset of disorder among the foreign born rises over time to a level equal to that of the U.S.-born Asian Americans, suggesting that the duration of experience in the United States contributes to risk.

Using the same NLAAS database, Cochran and colleagues (15) examined the hypothesis that lesbian, gay, and bisexual adults who are Latino or Asian American may be at elevated risk for mental health and substance use disorders, due to the experience of multiple sources of discrimination in addition to possible anti-gay stigma. About 4.8% of the sample identified themselves as lesbian, gay, bisexual, and/or reported recent same-gender sexual experiences. Although few sexual orientation–related differences were observed, among men, gay/bisexual men were more likely than heterosexual men to report a recent suicide attempt. Among women, lesbian/bisexual women were more likely than heterosexual women to evidence positive 1-year and lifetime histories of depressive disorders. These findings suggested a small elevation in psychiatric morbidity risk among Latino and Asian American individuals with a minority sexual orientation. However, the level of morbidity among sexual orientation minorities in the NLAAS appeared similar to or lower than that observed in population-based studies of lesbian, gay, and bisexual adults.

Investigating the underutilization of mental health services by high-risk racial/ethnic minority youth in San Diego, Garland and colleagues (16) controlled for confounding sociodemographic or clinical predictors of service use (e.g., family income, functional impairment, caregiver strain) that might account for disparities. Participants were 1256 youths ages 6 to 18 years who received a variety of outpatient, inpatient, and informal mental health services in a large, publicly funded system of care (including the child welfare, juvenile justice, special education, alcohol and drug abuse, and mental health service sectors). Youths and caregivers were interviewed with established measures of mental health service use, psychiatric diagnoses, functional impairment, caregiver strain, and parental depression. Significant racial/ethnic group differences in likelihood of receiving any mental health service and, specifically, formal outpatient services, were found after the effects of potentially confounding variables were controlled. Specifically, non-Hispanic whites had the highest rates of service use for any mental health service and for outpatient services, whereas AAPIs had the lowest utilization rates, which was about 50% lower. Race/ethnicity did not exert a significant effect on the use of informal or 24-hour care services.

The Barreto and Segal (17) study suggested that aggregating Asian subpopulations into a single group in services research is no longer appropriate. They explored the use of mental health services by Asian Americans and other ethnic populations (n = 104,773) in California to assess the role of ethnicity and diagnosis in predicting 6-month use of services. East Asians used more services than Southeast Asians, Filipinos, other Asians, Caucasians, African Americans, Latinos, and Native Americans, even when severity of illness was taken into account. They concluded that attention needed to be placed on the needs of Southeast Asians and other Asians, whose service use patterns approximated those of the traditionally most underserved groups, African Americans and Latinos. Although this study had significant limitations caused by the retrospective data collection process, it underscores the critical need to disaggregate AAPIs into ethnic groups in future research.

Sentell and colleagues (18) investigated the role of limited English proficiency (LEP) on mental health service utilization, using data from the 2001 California Health Interview Survey of adults aged 18 to 64 who provided language data (n = 41,984). Participants were categorized into three groups by self-reported English proficiency and language spoken at home: (i) English-speaking only, (ii) bilingual, and (iii) non-English speaking. Mental health treatment was measured by self-reported use of mental health services by those reporting a mental health need. Non–English-speaking individuals had lower odds of receiving needed services than those who only spoke English, when other factors were controlled. The relationship was even more dramatic within racial/ethnic groups: non–English-speaking AAPIs and non–English-speaking Latinos had significantly lower odds of receiving services compared with AAPIs and Latinos who spoke only English. The authors concluded that because LEP is concentrated among AAPIs and Latinos, it appeared to contribute to racial/ethnic disparities in mental healthcare.

Chow and colleagues (19) examined racial/ethnic disparities in mental health service access and use while living in neighborhoods at different poverty levels in New York City. They compared demographic, clinical characteristics, and service use patterns of whites, blacks, Hispanics, and Asians living in low-poverty and high-poverty areas. Logistic regression models were used to assess service use patterns of minority racial/ethnic groups compared with whites in different poverty areas. They found that residence in a poverty neighborhood moderates the relationship between race/ethnicity and mental health service access and use. Disparities in using emergency and inpatient services and having coercive referrals were more evident in low-poverty than in high-poverty areas. They concluded that neighborhood poverty was a key to understanding racial/ethnic disparities in the use of mental health services. For AAPIs living in high-poverty neighborhoods compared with whites, they found a twofold use of emergency services, less likelihood to have had prior mental health service use, and more likelihood of being diagnosed with schizophrenia. Furthermore, as compared with whites, they were less likely to have been referred by any recognized referral sources including self-referral, family, friends, social service agencies, and the criminal justice system. They surmised that "perhaps because of cultural factors of stigmatization and shame, Asian clients are largely isolated and have limited access and few contacts with the service system" (p. 796).

STIGMA OF MENTAL ILLNESS AND INTERVENTIONS: RECENT STUDIES

Stigma about mental illness in the AAPI population was recognized in the 2001 Surgeon General Report as one of the major reasons for mental health disparities, especially about utilization of mental health services. Five studies among others add to this literature.

Rao and colleagues (20) studied whether racial/ethnic differences existed in stigmatizing attitudes toward people with mental illness among community college students. Multiple regression models were used to investigate racial/ethnic differences in students' perceived dangerousness and desire for segregation from persons with mental illness both before and after participation in an anti-stigma intervention. At baseline, African Americans and Asians perceived people with mental illness as more dangerous and wanted more segregation than Caucasians, and Latinos perceived people with mental illness as less dangerous and wanted less segregation than Caucasians. Similar patterns emerged after the intervention, except that Asians' perceptions changed significantly such that they tended to perceive people with mental illness as least dangerous of all the racial/ethnic groups. These concluded that racial/ethnic background and socialization may help to shape explanatory models of mental illness and lead to mental illness stigma. Therefore, targeting antistigma interventions to racial/ethnic background of participants may be helpful.

Snowden (21) investigated the involvement of the family on service utilization in a large, representative sample of persons receiving public mental health treatment in California. They examined whether ethnic minority consumers were more likely than white consumers to live with their families and to receive family support and then evaluated whether differences observed in family involvement explained treatment disparities observed in outpatient and inpatient mental health services. Results indicated that Asian American and Latino consumers, especially, were considerably more likely than white consumers to live with family members and to receive family support. Ethnocultural differences in living with family did explain treatment intensity disparities whether or not consumers described themselves as dependent on family support. They believed the results supported the hypothesis that cultural differences in family involvement and support played a role in explaining mental health treatment disparities.

The review by Gary (22) summarized the literature on the stigma of mental illness as it is experienced by four ethnic minority groups in the United States. Concerns about prejudice and discrimination among individuals who suffer burdens related to mental illness were delineated: self-stigma, family stigma, and community and public stigma. He proposed that ethnic minority groups, who already confront prejudice and discrimination because of their group affiliation, suffer double stigma when faced with the burdens of mental illness. When combined with the possible lack of culturally and linguistically competent services, the double stigma in an ethnic minority group can impede accessing and continuing in services.

Shin and Lukens (23) showed how a culturally sensitive psychoeducational intervention with Korean Americans can reduce stigma. The study used data from an urban outpatient clinic in Queens, New York, to assess the effects of a 10-week psychoeducational intervention for Korean American adults with a diagnosis of schizophrenia who were randomly assigned to either an experimental group that provided a culturally sensitive psychoeducational group program in addition to individual supportive therapy or a control group that offered only individual supportive therapy. The two groups were compared on pretreatment and posttreatment measures of psychiatric symptoms, attitudes about and understanding of mental illness, and coping skills controlled for the effects of gender and education. Compared with the control group, the psychoeducational group showed significantly reduced symptom severity and perception of stigma and greater coping skills immediately after treatment.

After publication of the initial work by Chen and colleagues in New York City (24), Yeung and colleagues (25) investigated whether integrating psychiatry and primary healthcare improved referral to and treatment acceptability of mental health services among Chinese Americans. The "Bridge Project," a program to enhance collaboration between primary care and mental health services for low-income Chinese immigrants, was implemented at South Cove Community Health Center in Boston. The project consisted of conducting training seminars to primary care physicians to enhance recognition of common mental disorders, using a primary care nurse as the "bridge" to facilitate referrals to the Behavioral Health Department of the same facility and colocating a psychiatrist in the primary care clinic to provide onsite evaluation and treatment. The rates of mental health service referrals and successful treatment engagement before and during the project were compared. During the 12-month period of the Bridge Project, primary care physicians referred 64 (1.05% of all clinic patients) patients to mental health services, a 60% increase in the percentage of clinic patients referred in the previous 12 months. Eighty-eight percent of patients referred during the project showed up for psychiatric evaluation, compared with 53% in the previous 12 months. Integrating psychiatry and primary care was shown to be effective in improving access to mental health services and in increasing treatment engagement among low-income immigrant Chinese Americans.

RESEARCH ON DISPARITIES: FUTURE DIRECTIONS

One of the six recommendations of the Surgeon General in the last chapter of his report was to expand the science base to reduce disparities. One major challenge has been the underrepresentation of all racial and ethnic minorities in research studies as well as the need for community-engaged research. Chen and colleagues (26) described their experience of building research programs in a community-based healthcare facility in New York City. They learned: (i) mental health services research can be carried out in a community health center with minimal intrusion on usual patient flow; (ii) the effort must be shared between the health center and the community; (iii) barriers to participation in mental health research programs are multifactorial, ranging from conceptual, cultural, and attitudinal biases to practical concerns inherent in the ethnic minority population; and (iv) resistance can be overcome by working with participants' cultural and social needs and using their explanatory belief models when developing and pursuing studies. The science base has often come to be synonymous with evidence-based medicine and practice, which can be most challenging when applied to racial and ethnic minority populations, as discussed by Isaacs and colleagues (27). In addition to the underrepresentation of patients in the research studies, other challenges include: (i) lack of analyses on the impact of ethnic, linguistic, or cultural factors; (ii) limited resources devoted to the research of culturally specific practices; (iii) lack of theory development related to the relationships between culture, mental health disorders, and treatment; (iv) the absence of culturally relevant treatment outcomes; and (v) limited involvement of ethically and culturally diverse researchers. To deal with these challenges, Isaacs and colleagues advocate for the inclusion of practice-based evidence as "a range of treatment approaches and supports that are derived from, and supportive of, the positive cultural attributes of the local society and traditions. Practice-based evidence services are accepted as effective by the local community, through community consensus, and address the therapeutic and healing needs of individuals and families from a culturally-specific framework. . ." (p.16). Finally, research on disparities needs infrastructure support. In September 2007, the Asian American Center for Disparities Research opened at University of California, Davis, headed by Nolan Zane, PhD (28). This center has been funded by NIMH for 5 years at 3.9 million dollars. It is the only NIMH-funded, Asian-specific center on Asian American mental health disparities. Partnering with the National Asian American and Pacific Islander Mental Health Association and other community-based organizations, its objectives are:

- Conduct programmatic, problem-oriented research toward the empirical testing of effective clinical treatments for Asian American populations;
- Conduct research that has theoretical and policy significance for Asian Americans in particular and the mental health field in general;
- Promote and conduct research that addresses key methodological issues involved in the study of diversity and disparities;
- Serve as the focal point and stimulus for researchers conducting Asian American disparities research on a national level by maintaining and enhancing a network of researchers, service providers, and policy makers to facilitate theory and methodology development; and
- Bridge science into mental health practice, in particular, concerning cultural influences that affect critical problems of treatment and service delivery such as medical nonadherence and premature dropout.

The future of disparities research for AAPIs is bright indeed!

References

1. U.S. Department of Health and Human Services. *Mental Health: Culture, Race and Ethnicity: A Supplement to Mental Health: A Report to the Surgeon General.* Rockville, MD: U.S. Department of Health and Human Services, 2001.
2. U. S. Census Bureau: Accessed on October 15, 2008, available at http://www.census.gov/Press-Release/www/releases/archives/facts_for_features_special_editions/011602.html.
3. Henry J. Kaiser Family Foundation: Race, Ethnicity and Health Care Fact Sheet: Health Coverage and Access to Care Among Asian Americans, Native Hawaiians and Pacific Islanders. April 2008. Accessed on October 15, 2008, available at http://www.kff.org/minorityhealth/7745.cfm.
4. Du N. Issues in the treatment and assessment of Asian American patients. In: Lim R, ed. *Clinical Manual of Cultural Psychiatry.* Washington, DC: American Psychiatric Press, Inc, 2006.
5. U.S. Census Bureau. *The American Community–Asians: 2004.* 2007. Accessed on October 15, 2008, available at http://www.census.gov/prod/2007pubs/acs-05.pdf.
6. Institute of Medicine: *Unequal Treatment: Confronting Racial and Ethnic Disparities in Health Care.* Washington, DC: National Academy Press, 2002.
7. Alegría M, Cao Z, McGuire TG, et al. Health insurance coverage for vulnerable populations: Contrasting Asian Americans and Latinos in the United States. *Inquiry* 2006;43(3):231–254.
8. Ruiz P, Primm A. APA's efforts to eliminate disparities. *Psychiatr Serv* 2005;56(12):1603–1605.
9. Substance Abuse and Mental Health Services Administration (SAMHSA). Accessed October 15, 2008, available at http://mentalhealth.samhsa.gov/cre/fact2.asp.
10. Alegría M, Takeuchi D, Canino G, et al. Considering context, place, and culture: The National Latino and Asian American Study. *Int J Methods Psychiatr Res* 2004;13(4):208–220.
11. Center for Multicultural Mental Health Research. Accessed October 15, 2008, available at http://www.multiculturalmentalhealth.org/nlaas.asp.
12. Takeuchi D, Zane N, Hong S, et al. Immigration-related factors and mental disorders among Asian Americans. *Am J Public Health* 2007;97(1):84–90.
13. Abe-Kim J, Takeuchi D, Hong S, et al. Use of mental health related services among immigrants and U.S. born Asian Americans: Results from the National Latino and Asian American Study. *Am J Public Health* 2007;97(1):91–98.
14. Breslau J, Chang D. Psychiatric disorders among foreign-born and U.S.-born Asian-Americans in a U.S. national survey. *Soc Psychiatry Epidemiol* 2006;41:943–950.
15. Cochran S, Mays V, Alegría M, et al. Mental health and substance use disorders among Latino and Asian American lesbian, gay, and bisexual adults. *J Consult Clin Psychol* 2007;75(5):785–794.
16. Garland AF, Lau AS, Yeh M, et al. Racial and ethnic differences in utilization of mental health services among high-risk youths. *Am J Psychiatry* 2005;162(7):1336–1343.
17. Barreto RM, Segal SP. Use of mental health services by Asian Americans. *Psychiatr Serv* 2005;56(6):746–748.
18. Sentell T, Shumway M, Snowden L. Access to mental health treatment by English language proficiency and race/ethnicity. *J Gen Intern Med* 2007;22(Suppl 2):289–293.
19. Chow JC, Jaffee K, Snowden L. Racial/ethnic disparities in the use of mental health services in poverty areas. *Am J Public Health* 2003;93(5):792–797.
20. Rao D, Feinglass J, Corrigan P. Racial and ethnic disparities in mental illness stigma. *J Nerv Ment Dis* 2007;195(12):1020–1023.
21. Snowden L. Explaining mental health treatment disparities: Ethnic and cultural differences in family involvement. *Cult Med Psychiatry* 2007;31:389–402.
22. Gary FA. Stigma: Barrier to mental health care among ethnic minorities. *Issues Ment Health Nurs* 2005;26(10):979–999.

23. Shin SK, Lukens EP. Effects of psychoeducation for Korean Americans with chronic mental illness. *Psychiatr Serv* 2002;53(9):1125–1131.

24. Chen H, Kramer EJ, Chen T. The bridge program: A model for reaching Asian Americans. *Psychiatr Serv* 2003;54(10):1411–1412.

25. Yeung A, Kung WW, Chung H, et al. Integrating psychiatry and primary care improves acceptability to mental health services among Chinese Americans. *Gen Hosp Psychiatry* 2004;26(4):256–260.

26. Chen H, Kramer E, Chen T, et al. Engaging Asian Americans for mental health research: Challenges and solutions. *J Immigration Health* 2005;7(2):109–116.

27. Isaacs MR, Huang LN, Hernandez M, et al. *The Road to Evidence: The Intersection of Evidence-Based Practices and Cultural Competence in Children's Mental Health.* Washington, DC: The National Alliance of Multi-Ethnic Behavioral Health Associations; 2005.

28. Asian American Center for Disparities Research at University of California, Davis. Accessed October 15, 2008, available at http://psychology.ucdavis.edu/aacdr/.

6 American Indians and Alaska Natives

Jay H. Shore and Spero M. Manson

INTRODUCTION

As the original inhabitants of the lands that became the United States, mental health disparities for American Indian and Alaska Native populations are deeply rooted in the history of the country's development. This history has created dynamic and complex social, political, economic, and cultural contexts that affect the mental health of this population. This chapter begins with an overview of mental health disparities in American Indian and Alaska Natives with concentration on sociopolitical contexts, diversity of this population, and the current state of their mental health status and treatment. Attention is then focused on patient-provider interactions and the impact of the larger ecology in which these interactions are nested. A discussion of future challenges and directions for the mental health services for American Indians and Alaska Natives concludes the chapter, with an emphasis on the role of traditional treatments, the promise of technology, and issues raised by evidence-based practices.

MENTAL HEALTH OF AMERICAN INDIAN AND ALASKA NATIVES: HISTORY AND CONTEXT

Health disparities for minority populations are defined strongly by sociopolitical contexts. American Indians and Alaska Natives are unique among American minorities in their historical and current relationship with the U.S. government. From first contact, European settlers' interactions with the native groups were characterized by conquest, seizure of resources, compulsory relocation, and systemic campaigns of genocide. The new government of the United States continued these practices, developing policies of resettlement, attempted assimilation, and forced reservation relocation. By the 20th century, most American Indian tribes had been exterminated, dispersed, or driven onto federally created reservations. On the reservations, tribes continued to face threats to their identity from explicit governmental policies, for example, with federal laws banning traditional religious practices. The latter half of the 20th century for many American Indian and Alaska Native communities brought self-determination, self-governance, community and cultural rights, and greater awareness of the challenges facing American Indian communities.

Disparities in mental health for American Indians and Alaska Natives are inherently tied to the history and current sociopolitical landscapes experienced by this population. Present-day American Indians and Alaska Natives are characterized by incredible diversity in terms of their culture, environments, and socioeconomic circumstances. A detailed examination of this diversity is beyond the scope of this chapter, but there are currently 562 federally recognized tribes (1) representing a diverse array of distinct cultural groups and a wide range of acculturation. There are more than 200 different languages with more than a quarter million of the 4 million Americans (1.5% of the U.S. population) identifying themselves as having American Indian or Alaska Native heritage who speak a native language at home. Through the 1980s, most American Indians or Alaska Natives lived on reservations or trust land, but today only 20% live there, with greater than 50% of this population residing in urban and suburban areas. Because of the geographic isolation of many reservations, a substantial portion of this population continues to live in rural areas, with more American Indians living in rural areas compared with whites (42% vs. 23%) (2).

American Indian and Alaska Native communities have a unique relationship with the U.S. government as sovereign entities who retain all aspects of self-government not subsumed by the government, which continues to exercise significant control over these communities (3). Through its treaty obligations the U.S. government is required to provide healthcare services, including mental health, to federally recognized tribes, which the Indian Health Service (IHS) oversees. Only 20% of this population has direct access to IHS clinics, which are largely reservation based (2). The healthcare received by this population is delivered by a wide array of systems including the IHS, other federal organizations (e.g., SAMSHA, IIRSA), state agencies, private providers, and tribally run healthcare services.

American Indian and Alaska Native mental health disparities cannot be understood without understanding the healthcare resource gap that exists for this population. The IHS is the largest provider of care for this population. It has an estimated 59% of the resources required to provide the needed care and spends 50% of the national average per enrollee on health expenditures. Estimates for 2003 for the IHS were roughly $1900 per person annually versus $6000 for Medicaid recipients and $5200 for veterans (4). Only half of American Indians and Alaska Natives have employer-based healthcare coverage (72% for whites). Roughly one-quarter have Medicaid as a primary insurer, with another quarter having no healthcare coverage compared with 16% of the general population without coverage (2). This shortfall in healthcare resources for these communities plays a significant role in the ability to adequately address mental health problems.

The definitive work to date on American Indian and Alaska Native mental health disparities appears in the Surgeon General's Report on Mental Health Health's supplement on Culture, Race, and Ethnicity published in 2001 (5). It provides a detailed overview of historical contexts, current status, mental healthcare needs, service utilization, services outcomes, prevention, and mental health promotion for this population. The report also contains salient case studies, which add a clinical context to the material. This work arrives at several important conclusions:

• Compared with other populations, there is insufficient data on mental health problems and treatment for American Indians and Alaska Natives, but the existing data show that this population suffers significant mental health disparities compared with the general population. More data are required across the lifespan for this population.
• Native peoples are overrepresented in vulnerable populations (homeless, incarcerated, trauma victims) that are often in need of mental healthcare.

- Significant comorbidity exists in this population between mental health and substance use disorders. These are unlikely to be dealt with in conventional treatment settings.
- The availability of culturally appropriate treatment, accessible services (both financially and geographically), and accompanying medical care is critical in the provision of effective services for this population.
- A better understanding of the financing and organization of mental health service for American Indians and Alaska Natives is needed to characterize the rapidly changing service delivery environment.
- Mental health treatment guidelines have been developed on the basis of the majority population, with little specificity for minority groups despite evidence of the importance of ethnic and cultural differences. Research must focus on the applicability, outcomes, and modifications for treatment guidelines for American Indians and Alaska Natives.
- Improved methods are needed to better integrate traditional healing and spiritual practices that can complement mental healthcare for this population.
- A greater focus on prevention strategies and an exploration of individual and collective strengths and resiliencies of American Indians and Alaska Natives is warranted.

Over the ensuing 8 years, sustainable progress has been achieved regarding many of the recommended lines of inquiry. Worth briefly reviewing here is the American Indian Service Utilization, Psychiatric Epidemiology, Risk, and Protective Factors Project (AI-SUPERPFP) (6,7).

AI-SUPERPFP and its associated findings were not available at the time and therefore not addressed in the Surgeon General's Report. AI-SUPERPFP represents the largest psychiatric epidemiology project ever conducted on two well-defined samples of American Indians. Drawing on more than 3000 tribal Southwest and Northern Plains tribal members living on or near their home reservations, the lifetime and 12-month prevalence of nine psychiatric disorders were estimated together with patterns of service utilization. Its design allowed direct comparison with the National Comorbidity Survey, highlighting the contrast to the general U.S. population. Overall, AI-SUPERPFP demonstrated that this sample of American Indians had at least comparable or greater mental healthcare needs when compared with the general population. Substance- and trauma-related disorders were among the more prevalent problems (7). Additionally, as in other studies with this population, use of traditional healing services was common (6).

THE PROVIDER-PATIENT RELATIONSHIP AND CLINICAL DISPARITIES

Having briefly reviewed the general context of American Indian and Alaska Native mental health disparities, we now turn to clinical perspectives on these disparities. The relevant literature is scarce and generally descriptive in nature. As underscored in the Surgeon General's Report, the integration of general mental health treatment guidelines with best practices for American Indian and Alaska Native populations has not been systematic. The published literature is silent in respect to randomized controlled outcome trials with this population on either specific pharmacological or behavioral health interventions. Finally, although the majority of American Indians and Alaska Natives reside in urban areas, much of the work to date has focused on reservation or community residents, contributing to an important gap in knowledge about mental health disparities for urban Native populations. The clinical encounter between mental health providers and American Indian and Alaska Native patients underscores the most obvious disparities in mental healthcare. Using the lens of the Cultural Formulation for the *Diagnostic and Statistical Manual*, 4th edition (DSM-IV) (8), we draw on our experience of the University of Colorado Denver's American Indian and Alaska Native Programs (AIANP) to discuss challenges, pitfalls, and assets in clinical work with this special population.

The Cultural Formulation for DSM-IV, hereafter referenced as the Cultural Formulation, is the most widely known transcultural approach used in psychiatry. It encourages one to consider the cultural identity of the patient, the patient's cultural explanation of distress, cultural factors related to the psychosocial environment, and cultural factors in the treatment relationship, synthesizing these elements together in an overall cultural assessment for diagnosis and care. Of particular relevance are the backgrounds of both the patient and provider and the impact of culture on the patient-provider relationship (8). The background, past experiences, and cultural identities of both the patient and the provider set the stage for the clinical interactions, determining idioms of distress and cultural context that influence the treatment process.

American Indians and Alaska Natives represent an enormous array of cultural beliefs about healing, health, and illness. These beliefs affect a patient's expression, manifestation of, and communication about their distress. In addition to the diversity of cultural idioms of illness, one's degree of "acculturation" needs to be considered with respect to each patient and the extent to which each patient adheres to traditional tribal concepts of mental health and illness. This becomes more complicated in light of the multiple cultural systems that patients may identify with, which includes traditional beliefs, Western culture, and regional cultural and urban versus rural cultural perspectives. The interplay of these belief systems with each unique cultural background determines the patient's expression and communication of distress. For example, previous work on satisfaction of care among American Indian elders revealed that those with a higher self-report of Indian ethnic identify report lower levels of satisfaction with medical care and higher levels of frustration in communicating with providers (9).

Communication can be further complicated when working with patients whose primary language is their tribal language. In the AIANP clinical programs, it is rare to encounter an elder who does not speak English at least as a second language. Although clinical interactions may be carried out in English, our experience has demonstrated that often the meaning differs between patients and providers. For example, in the Northern Plains the term "lonely" is often used by bilingual patients to describe states similar to depression. The meaning of "lonely" for Native speakers goes beyond the feeling of being without company, often referring to a feeling or state of social disconnectedness from one's family and community. The concept of "lonely" often correlates clinically and approximates feelings of depression. Providers need to remain alert to patient's use of specific words and enquire further about context and meaning.

Despite diverse beliefs, there are common and shared aspects of American Indian and Alaska Native cultures. In partnership with the National Center for Posttraumatic Stress Disorder, we developed a program (*Wounded Spirit, Ailing Hearts)* to educate providers working with Native veterans (10). This program discusses general values of Native culture that may clash with dominant society values. Among these are (i) placing tribe and extended family before self; (ii) focusing on today rather than preparing for tomorrow; (iii) valuing age over youth; (iv) cooperative rather than a competitive stance in working with others, emphasizing patience and humility over aggression; (v) orientation toward the land and living in harmony with the environment versus conquering and controlling the environment; (vi) honoring the intuitive and mysterious rather than skepticism; (vii) having flexible rules rather than a rule for every contingency; (viii) judging for oneself rather than depending on external aides to perform the function of judging; and (ix) different ways of conceptualizing time. Dominant Western culture is time-driven, whereas many traditional tribal cultures believe things should happen at the "right time," unfolding as opposed to rigidly dictated by a schedule. Providers working with American Indian and Alaska Native patients must have a general knowledge about the diversity of this population, specific communication issues that may arise, and common shared values in Native cultures.

The providers' background also has a significant impact on the clinical process. The type of provider working with Native populations is directly influenced by the larger social and economic environments. There is a significant deficit of behavioral health providers who are American Indian and Alaska Native (11). Even if a provider is Native, unless practicing in his/her home community, he/she interacts with patients of different cultural backgrounds. Being Native may help to bridge cultural gaps, but it does not guarantee culturally appropriate care. Providers who are trained in cross-cultural settings with Native populations are critical to culturally appropriate care. Because of lower salaries, remote locations, complex cases, and limited resources, it is often difficult for the IHS and other health systems serving American Indians and Alaska Natives to recruit and retain mental health specialists (11).

Tension exists for providers between general versus explicit knowledge about the specific tribal group with whom they are working. General knowledge of American Indian and Alaska Native values and specific knowledge of a tribe's history, environment, and customs must be integrated by the provider during individual clinical encounters. Level of acculturation and individual group identity must be taken into account to facilitate this fit. This can be especially challenging for providers serving a patient population from multiple different tribal backgrounds (e.g., an urban clinic), where tribal origin may differ from one clinical encounter to the next.

Providers should familiarize themselves with the histories, environments, and cultures of the specific tribal groups from which their patients originate. This can be accomplished through an array of recourses including published materials, colleagues, meetings, trainings, patients, and community events. We recommend taking a detailed cultural history during the initial assessment that includes tribal background, first language spoken (tribal vs. English), current languages spoken and identity of patient's primary language, traditional practices in the home and developmental environments, current engagement in traditional practices, spiritual history, and past and current use of traditional healing. This part of the assessment also offers the provider an opportunity to learn more about the patient's culture of origin. This approach also facilitates rapport with the patient by allowing the provider to express interest and begin the dialogue around cultural issues at an early stage in the patient-provider relationship.

In addition to properly assessing their patients' background, mental health providers working with American Indian and Alaska Native patients must be adept at monitoring the clinical process. For example, our clinical experience has shown that for many American Indian and Alaska Native patients from more traditional backgrounds, direct confrontation, particularly with an authority figure such as a physician, is considered impolite. Such patients will verbally agree with their providers' recommendations and/or report to the provider what they think a provider wants to hear. Providers who have an overly paternalistic/confrontational style are at risk of misreading politeness for compliance. This type of interaction may lead to poor adherence with treatment, decreasing communication, and worsening clinical outcome.

Many American Indian and Alaska Native cultures have strong narrative traditions. American Indian and Alaska Native elderly patients with a traditional identity often have a narrative style of expressing themselves. This can lead to frustration from patient as well as the provider when the latter attempts to use a symptom checklist or follows a highly structured interview. Abruptly cutting off or redirecting patients during an initial interview not only inhibits the history gathering but can interfere with further communication and establishing the patient-provider relationship. Ideally, providers must respect the narrative structure and should be prepared to be flexible with their clinical time to do so, especially for initial assessments. If time is an issue, explaining this can prevent damaged rapport and communication. In our clinical experience, it is possible with careful attention to conduct highly structured interviews and at the same time honor the narrative flow of the patient, although this requires more time for the assessment process.

Family and community can be very important to American Indian and Alaska Native patients. Involving family early in the treatment process, when clinically feasible, can improve the process of care. It is important to educate family and community members about a patient's mental health problems and destigmatize mental illness for the patient.

Finally, in any negotiated treatment with the patient, providers should enquire about the role of traditional treatments. For those patients expressing interest or currently engaged in traditional treatments, providers may want to consider formal or informal collaboration with traditional healers (12). At the very least, providers should attempt to understand traditional treatments, the beliefs surrounding this treatment, and how such traditional treatment can affect the care offered by the provider.

So far, we have reviewed issues to improve clinical disparities with American Indians and Alaska Natives by addressing patient and provider factors that contribute to disparities, which are summarized in Table 6.1. However, major gains for patients can be accomplished through improvements in the systems of mental health treatment and delivery. An important priority should focus on knowledge, training, and availability of providers. Providers need information on cultural background, pertinent mental health problems (e.g., trauma, substance disorders), the clinical process, and knowledge of best practices. This area is clearly underdeveloped, and more research is required. We must look to training as an ongoing process throughout a provider's career. Methods to disseminate this knowledge especially must be developed to assist those working in rural areas. Increasing the availability of culturally competent mental health providers for American Indian and Alaska Native populations is critical to effectively address clinical disparities.

The next section examines several recent developments that have potential to address many aspects of clinical disparities. These include evidence regarding traditional treatments, technologies that have fostered new models of care delivery, information dissemination, and the growing movement of evidence-based and personalized medicine.

PROMISING PRACTICES, CHALLENGES, AND FUTURE DIRECTIONS

Undoubtedly, addressing funding and treatment challenges is a necessary but not sufficient step for addressing clinical disparities with American Indians and Alaska Natives.

TABLE 6.1	Methods for Providers to Aid in Reducing Health Disparities During Clinical Interactions With American Indian and Alaska Native Patients

- Become familiar with shared cultural elements of American Indian and Alaska Native populations.
- Develop knowledge about the culture, history, and customs of the specific the tribal groups you are working with.
- Gather a detailed cultural history during the initial assessment that includes tribal background, first language spoken (tribal vs. English), current languages spoken and identity of patient's primary language, traditional practices in the home and developmental environments, current engagement in traditional practices, spiritual history, and past and current use of traditional healing.
- Consider acculturation level of patient and how this affects patient's cultural identities and expression and communication of distress.
- Listen carefully to patients whose primary language is a tribal language when conversing in English for words that may represent differing concepts.
- Be respectful of a narrative style of communication and adapt clinical interviews for this style when warranted.
- Become attuned to patients' processes of communication with authority and be careful not to assume politeness is correlated with treatment compliance.
- Involve family when possible as appropriate in treatment.
- Assess patient's current use of traditional healing practices and desire to have traditional treatment incorporated into current treatment. For interested patients, consider collaborations with traditional healers in the community.

Solving these challenges requires not only gathering relevant data to develop new models but promoting these solutions through advocacy. Addressing the fundamental economic and systems disparities inherent in the mental health treatment of American Indians and Alaska Natives is a complex, intricate, and lengthy process. Solutions targeted initially at the patient-provider level, as opposed to the systems levels of clinical disparities, are easier to implement, can be funded on a small scale, require less political advocacy, and have the potential to diffuse upward to a system-wide level.

Among the more exciting recent developments is the use of live interactive videoconferencing, telepsychiatry, to provide mental healthcare to remote and rural populations. Telepsychiatry holds particular promise for American Indians and Alaska Natives because of the rural, remote, and dispersed nature of many of these communities. Over the past decade, the AIANP developed telepsychiatry clinics to provide services and to test the effectiveness of this technology. An accumulating body of evidence at the AIANP demonstrates the capacity of telepsychiatry to provide reliable psychiatric assessments and treatments with equivalent levels of satisfaction, comfort, and cultural sensitivity in direct care for American Indians and Alaska Natives (13). A growing series of AIANP telepsychiatry clinics in partnership with the Department of Veterans Affairs provides ongoing care for American Indian veterans struggling with posttraumatic stress disorder on rural reservations in the Northern Plains. As these clinics currently grow from 1 to 13 tribes in the region, they serve as a demonstration of how clinically implemented solutions can diffuse throughout treatment systems (14).

Another example of leveraging technology to address disparities is the AIANP's Native Telehealth Outreach and Technical Assistance Program (NTOTAP). The "digital divide" throughout much of rural America disproportionately affects American Indian and Alaska Native communities (Native Digital divide) (15). Even when sufficient technological infrastructure is present, community members often lack the technical skills or experience to use these resources. This often forces community members to use programs designed for and implemented by those who are not familiar with their communities. Furthermore, the dissemination of relevant healthcare information takes a "top-down" approach in which government agencies dictate the focus of these efforts. NTOTAP trains Native community members at the lay and professional levels (including providers) in the use of technology to address local healthcare needs. The program imparts technical knowledge and skills that enable participants to develop healthcare training for community-wide and regional dissemination. NTOTAP has completed eight multimedia-based projects (e.g., Web sites, interactive CD-ROMs, and video focusing on a variety of health concerns) that have been disseminated throughout rural communities (15). NTOTAP demonstrates how technology can be used to address provider training, enhance community involvement in healthcare, and involve communities in creating and distributing best practices discussed below.

Collaboration between traditional healers and behavioral health providers represent another important area for clinical disparities. Significant percentages of American Indian and Alaska Native use traditional healers. In the previously discussed AI-SUPERPFP study, the use of traditional healers by participants with DSM-IV behavioral disorders was high: 34% to 49% in the past year (6). Indeed, 16% to 32% of users of biomedical services for emotional problems had also seen a traditional healer (7). In a different study of American Indian veterans, service utilization rates for the two groups of veterans (Northern Plains vs. Southwestern) were compared across biomedical and traditional healing. The VA facilities were closer and more available in the Northern Plains than in the Southwest, causing significantly lower use of VA facilities for Southwest veterans. Southwest veterans had higher use of traditional services, erasing the overall health service difference with the Northern Plains, indicating that type of service use (biomedical vs. traditional) varied on the basis of availability (16).

These findings support the importance of making both behavioral health services and traditional services available to American Indian and Alaska Native patients. We strongly encourage providers to seek active collaboration with traditional healers when treating patients who use or are interested in such services. We recently created a set of guidelines that outlines recommendations for mental health providers seeking active collaboration with traditional healers (12). Several programs and systems around the country are already engaging in this work, which can be used to further enhance models and frameworks (12).

There is an increasing trend in the U.S. general population to adopt evidence-based medicine, best practices, and individualized medicine. Several important issues affect the implementation of evidence-based practices with American Indian and Alaska Native populations. The data underpinning evidence-based mental health practices rarely includes minority populations or considers cultural factors that affect treatment and outcomes. We simply do not know how applicable evidence-based practices are for American Indian and Alaska Native populations, what adaptations may be needed to render these practices acceptable and relevant for this population, and the impact these adaptations could have on treatments, processes, and outcomes (17). Furthermore, the generally accepted ranking of evidence, with the highest level being the randomized controlled trial, does not adequately account for cultural variation, the rich narrative and experiential traditions of Native culture, and the contribution of qualitative data. Although evidence-based medicine could prove to be a powerful tool for reducing clinical disparities among American Indians and Alaska Natives, its application in this population begs for further investigation. We need realistic models and methods of community collaboration, together with cultural adaptation and assessment of evidence-based practices.

The U.S. Government has a special obligation, based on both the historical record and negotiated treaties, to address mental health disparities specific to American Indians and Alaska Natives. This work should proceed with both a "top-down" and a "bottom-up" approach. The resource deficit must be addressed. Provider training and increased availability, the integration of cultural practices, and improving treatment practices can help to reduce clinical disparities. Tailoring technologies, traditional healing, and evidence-based medicine to Native communities builds on current advances in medicine and the growing belief that these practices can improve outcomes for this unique population.

References

1. Bureau of Indian Affairs. Indian entities recognized and eligible to receive services from the United States Bureau of Indian Affairs. *Fed Reg* 2008;73(66):18553–18557.
2. U.S. Department of Health and Human Services, Department of the Surgeon General, SAMHSA. Native American Indians: Fact Sheet: SAMHSA; 1999.
3. Shore J, Bloom J, Manson S, et al. Telepsychiatry with rural American Indians: Issues in civil commitments. *Behav Sci Law* 2008;26:1–14.
4. U.S. Commission on Civil Rights. *A Quiet Crisis: Federal Funding and Unmet Needs in Indian Country.* Washington, DC, 2003.
5. U.S. Department of Health and Human Services. *Mental Health: Culture, Race and Ethnicity: A Supplement to Mental Health: A Report to the Surgeon General.* Rockville, MD: U.S. Department of Health and Human Services, 2001.
6. Beals J, Manson SM, Whitesell NR, et al. Prevalence of DSM-IV disorders and attendant help-seeking in two American Indian reservation populations. *Arch Gen Psychiatry* 2005;62(1):99–108.
7. Beals J, Novins DK, Whitesell NR, et al. Prevalence of mental disorders and utilization of mental health services in two American Indian reservation populations: Mental health disparities in a national context. *Am J Psychiatry* 2005;162(9):1723–1732.
8. American Psychiatric Association. *Diagnostic and Statistical Manual of Mental Disorders, Fourth Edition (DSM-IV, text revision).* Washington, DC: American Psychiatric Association, 2000.
9. Garroutte EM, Kunovich RM, Jacobsen C, et al. Patient satisfaction and ethnic identity among American Indian older adults. *Soc Sci Med* 2004;59(11):2233–2244.
10. National Center for Post-Traumatic Stress Disorder. *Wound Spirits Ailing Hearts: Manual Two.* Vol 3 & 4. Salt Lake City, UT: Employee Education System Department of Veterans Affairs, 2000.
11. Dixon M, Roubideaux Y, eds. *Promises to Keep: Public Health Policy for American Indians and Alaska Natives in the 21st Century.* Washington, DC: American Public Health Association, 2001.
12. Shore JH, Shore JH, Manson SM. American Indian healers and psychiatrists: Building alliances. In Incayawar M, Wintrob R, Bouchard L, eds. *Psychiatrist and Traditional Healers; Unwitting Partners in Global Mental Health.* Hoboken, New Jersey: John Wiley & Sons; 2009.
13. Shore J, Brooks E, Savin D, et al. Acceptability of telepsychiatry in American Indians. *Telemedicine and e-Health* 2008;14(5):339–344.
14. Shore JH, Manson SM. A developmental model for rural telepsychiatry. *Psychiatr Serv* 2005;56(8):976–980.

15. Dick RW, Manson SM, Hansen AL, et al. The Native Telehealth Outreach and Technical Assistance Program: A community-based approach to the development of multimedia-focused health care information. *Am Indian Alsk Native Ment Health Res* 2007;14(2): 49–66.
16. Gurley D, Novins DK, Jones MC, et al. Comparative use of biomedical services and traditional healing options by American Indian veterans. *Psychiatr Serv* 2001;52(1):68–74.
17. Sheehan AK, Walrath-Greene C, Fisher S, et al. Evidence-based practice knowledge, use, and factors that influence decisions: Results from an evidence-based practice survey of providers in American Indian/Alaska Native communities. *Am Indian Alsk Native Ment Health Res* 2007;14(2):29–48.

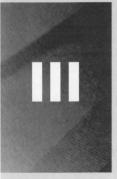

III Disparities Among Gender and Sexual Minorities

7 Women

Caroline E. Fisher and Roslyn Seligman

 INTRODUCTION

The concept of gender difference has historically been fertile ground for controversy and remains so. From the Divine Feminine of the Tantrists to the helpless waif of the Victorian era, social definitions of womanhood have always abounded. Early 20th century medical writings discuss the "weaker" sex in the face of clear evidence of women's hardiness and resiliency. The need for able-bodied workers during World War II forced women to reconsider their self-concept, their social role, and their physical abilities. The feminist movement of the 1970s created the illusion that women were "just like" men. Many otherwise rational people missed the critical difference between women being just like men in needs and rights and women being biologically the same as men. Gender must necessarily be understood as the intersection of two realities: one biological and one sociological. Women are women based on their biological makeup and women are women based on the social roles and expectations they have. A woman's psychological presentation is necessarily a response to both, to nature and nurture, to environment and experience.

As more precise research is undertaken, the biological differences between men and women become more evident and concrete as well as complex and intricate. Women present with different biological risks for mental illness, different presentations of symptoms, different responses to medications—including side effects—and different natural histories (1–4). The complexity of a woman's biological makeup and how it changes over time, cyclically and longitudinally, is

63

becoming better understood. We are coming to recognize that old studies obtaining data only from men (and by men) do not generalize to patients of both genders. Clinical presentation is the summation of myriad variables, and women are truly physiologically different than men.

On the other hand, social beliefs about women may subtly change the clinical interpretation of the patient's presentation as well as the research data. For example, women are more likely to be diagnosed with depression and less likely to be diagnosed with alcoholism. They are more likely to be prescribed pharmaceuticals and more likely to experience side effects from them, but less likely to have the side effects addressed by their doctor (4).

The lens of social expectations colors not only our interpretation of data but also more pragmatic realities. Availability of resources, social connectedness, and income all have an association with overall health, and all vary significantly by gender (2,5,6–8). Three out of four women in the United States make less than $40,000 per year and women still earn, on average, 77 cents for each dollar a man earns, from doctors to janitors (9). Women are more likely to be single heads of households with children and are more likely to suffer financially from divorce. This inequality necessarily affects women's mental health, mental health risks, and mental health treatment.

Because the data are many but the conclusions are few, this chapter attempts to address some of the issues that must be considered in treating women and ways in which the astute psychiatrist can provide better care to the female patient.

◤ DIAGNOSIS

Mental illness affects men and women differently. Prevalence of diagnoses differs by gender, as does presentation and course of specific illnesses. Women are more likely to experience comorbidities. In addition to innate biological differences between the sexes, social and environmental differences between men and women are compelling as explanations for the variation in prevalence. The research and data are colored, however, by social assumptions and prejudices. The data have been gathered historically by men in answer to questions posed by men, questions that may be in and of themselves based on faulty data or assumptions about women.

To say that a woman is not a man would seem a statement of the obvious. No society in history has ever denied this self-evident fact; indeed, a child of 3 years of age can identify gender and give evidence to defend her conclusion. No community has questioned this, either; no community but one: the scientific. For decades, science treated women as men. They were assumed to suffer disease at the same rate and with the same symptoms as men, to follow the same course of disease, and to respond as men do to medications and treatment. The exception was the reproductive system, and women were acknowledged to have a uterus and therefore uterine concerns. Historically, the uterus was thought to be the seat of all differences between the sexes, an organ of mystery and danger. The prevailing idea for several generations was to remove it as soon as possible.

Long after, it became clear that there were gender differences in the collected medical data; many researchers did not include women in studies or stratify their data by gender. The common reason cited for pharmaceutical studies was that they could not put the potential fetus at risk if a woman in a study became pregnant. The National Institutes of Health began to require collection of data on women in NIH-funded studies only within the last two decades, in response to several FDA-approved drugs, such as thalidomide, which had catastrophic and unanticipated effects on fetal development. Yet, a surveyor of the medical literature today might still have difficulty determining effectiveness and safety of medications for women. Similarly, diagnosis has been equally clouded. It is only the future DSM-V, to be released in 2011, that will assess the research on gender differences in mental illness and that only after much lobbying by the women of the APA. Previous editions have made scant references to gender, but perhaps only because of scant data.

The woman-as-man theory gave way to the concept that a woman is a man-who-gets-pregnant. This resulted in a relative bounty of information about mental health issues surrounding pregnancy and childbirth, at least for women. (The effect on men of pregnancy and childbirth is only starting to be realized, and just as 10% to 15% of new mothers are likely to become depressed, new fathers are similarly at risk for depression after the birth of a child [10]). Careful study of the course of mental illness surrounding pregnancy and childbirth has brought about a better understanding of the natural history of mental illness in women at other ages as well. Women may also be more at risk for the rapid cycling type of bipolar disorder (4). This line of exploration has led to interesting excursions into research on hormonal precipitants of bipolar disorder. That said, there is some research to suggest that the effect of biology and reproductive state on mental illness in women is less important, and may even disappear, when research controls for differences in psychosocial status.

Like bipolar disorder, schizophrenia may follow an entirely different course in women than in men. Women appear to demonstrate better premorbid functioning, present with initial onset somewhat later in life, and have better self-care skills such as shopping, cooking, and cleaning. (One could argue this is innate or merely over-learned.) Women may experience more positive symptoms of schizophrenia as well. If women with schizophrenia become homeless, they are more at risk for victimization, both sexual and physical, than similar men (4). As prevalence rates for schizophrenia are the same for men and women, whether the differences in presentation are caused by biochemistry, experience, or both remains to be determined.

There is a dearth of information on women outside of the context of childbearing. Only recently has research been designed to look at women without assuming they are like men, and slowly a picture of women begins to emerge. Historically, one of the major complaints against studying gender separately has been that it confuses social agendas with scientific ones and that gender differences are attributable not to scientific realities but to social roles: it is all about who does the dishes, and there is no place for that in the medical research. The counterargument is that women are physiologically different, as is obvious by the fact of menstruation, and that those physiological differences are worthy of research. Ironically, the emerging research suggests that there are clear physiological differences between genders that affect mental illness and that there are consequences of social roles and prejudices on the development, treatment, and course of mental illness.

Several large epidemiological studies have been or can be stratified by gender, and differences in prevalence rates are becoming more evident. Women are approximately twice as likely to suffer depression or anxiety as men, according to the European Study of the Epidemiology of Mental Disorders, the National Comorbidity Study, and the National Comorbidity Study Replication (11–13). They are more likely to experience comorbid conditions, usually also depression or anxiety of some kind, which in turn increases the burden of disease. They are about an eighth as likely to abuse alcohol or have antisocial personality disorders. They are more likely to develop an eating disorder. There does not appear to be much of a difference, in most studies, in prevalence of the psychotic disorders or bipolar disorder in women compared with men.

Depression is thought to be the fourth leading cause of disease burden worldwide, despite inexpensive, low-risk, and effective treatments (4). The NCS-R data indicate that one in five women will experience depression during their lives, a rate higher than breast cancer (10). The course of depression in women also diverges from that of men. Women are likely to have a more severe, chronic course. They are more likely to experience decreased libido as well as atypical symptoms such as oversleeping and overeating. Although alcoholism is more prevalent in men overall, women who are depressed are more likely to develop alcoholism than are their male counterparts. Physical pain is more frequently present in depressed women than in depressed men. Female gender itself is a risk for relapse of depression (4).

Female depression has public health consequences for more people than just the patient. Overall, depression in females is most likely to occur during the ages of 25 to 44 years, ages when women are likely to be building careers and raising children (5,9,13,14). This presents a double public health burden: depressed mothers are less able to care for their children and connect with them emotionally, so the children may also be at risk for later psychopathology. Women tend to be the primary caretakers of children and the elderly and carry the majority of responsibility for the household (8). It seems likely, therefore, that medical complications and morbidity of elderly dependents would increase in households of depressed women. Similarly, depression is likely to impede a woman's career, causing further disparity between the incomes of men and women and adding additional risk factors for further depression, such as financial stresses and lack of decision-making capacity. Single motherhood is one of the strongest predictors of mental health morbidity, followed by poverty. Comorbid substance abuse is also detrimental to parenting, caretaking, and employment. As the adage goes, "if Mama ain't happy, ain't nobody happy."

When considering the prevalence of anxiety disorders in women, it is helpful but dismaying to separate out posttraumatic stress disorder (PTSD) from other anxiety disorders. Women are more likely to experience all types of anxiety disorders than men, but they are more likely to experience PTSD in part because they are more likely to experience trauma (4,7,15). Trauma caused by combat exposure is no longer the sole purview of males but even during our current troubled times, combat exposure is still fairly uncommon. Much more common is interpersonal violence and childhood sexual abuse. Women are more likely to be the victims of both childhood sexual abuse and interpersonal violence, both clear risk factors for later psychopathology. Increased trauma experience is not the entire explanation for the increased rate of PTSD, however. Women are twice as likely to develop PTSD after exposure to trauma than men are, indicating an array of causes and interactions (5,7).

Other anxiety disorders are more common in females as well. One possible reason for this is the higher comorbidity in females with mental illness. Women with depression often develop a comorbid anxiety disorder, and women with an anxiety disorder frequently develop depression. Panic disorder seems to be the most common comorbid anxiety disorder, with onset of panic predictive of subsequent depression and vice versa. Women are more likely than men to have three or more lifetime disorders (1,14).

Suicide is a risk of both depression and anxiety. Suicide is the second leading cause of death (after motor vehicle accident) for persons ages 25 to 34 years and the third leading cause of death in adolescents ages 10 to 24 years. Although women are known to attempt suicide more often than men, they are less successful in completing suicide, and the death by suicide rate is about one-fourth of that of men. For women, the most common method is poisoning, followed by gunshot. Interestingly, about two-thirds of women who complete suicide had been diagnosed with a mental illness, a somewhat higher rate than men (15).

Eating disorders are overwhelmingly more prevalent in females versus males. This may be due, in large part, to the pressures modern society puts on women to be beautiful, to be thin, and to be successful. Around middle school, children become intensely intolerant and critical of themselves and one another as they strive to "fit in" by adopting the values of their peers. Social strata become more important, and exclusion is the dominant form of determining social strata. Many women with eating disorders describe a sense of superiority over their peers who are unable to control their weight. This system depends on the social value of thinness, however, and more exposure to media depicting the value of thinness seems to increase the risk of developing an eating disorder. Kids who are taught to value beauty and thinness less may be able to find healthier outlets for their competitive needs.

Discrepancies in diagnosis between men and women may differ between large, population-based surveys and the doctor's office. Survey data are collected by trained workers with standardized questionnaires, whereas doctors vary in their sophistication, approach to diagnosis, and available time. Most mental illness of all kinds, including schizophrenia, is not treated by psychiatrists but by primary care doctors, social workers, other types of professionals, or not at all. In turn, most primary care doctors have had minimal training in psychiatry, possibly no more than a few short weeks in medical school. Because women present with mental illness differently than the "textbook" case and suffer a different course, their symptoms may not be recognized by primary care doctors. The stereotypes of women interfere with correct evaluation and diagnosis.

Therefore, the careful practitioner who wants to be accurate with diagnosis will need to recognize the risks of too few data and too many social constructs of women, and plan accordingly. First, it is necessary to recognize that it is not fully understood how the average woman presents and therefore one must consider unusual presentations of disorders. As this is an emerging field, the savvy psychiatrist will devote some regular study to keep up with new data as they develop. Second, psychiatrists need to ask about comorbidities without preconception. Comorbidities in women such as panic and substance abuse should be assumed to be widely present. Third, careful attention must be paid to risk factors as they develop. Patients who experience interpersonal violence should be screened for later presentation of mental illness, as well as patients with stressful lives, women with little control over their circumstances, poor job satisfaction, multiple family responsibilities, and little time for themselves. Finally, screening for common disorders such as anxiety and depression should be done with the same regularity as screening for other medical disorders such as breast cancer (monthly), diabetes (annually), and heart disease. After all, depression may be more disabling than any of those.

TREATMENT

In considering treatment of women, it is necessary to understand their biological and social susceptibilities. Women are more vulnerable to the physical effects of medication, and they are more vulnerable to the social effects of treatment or lack thereof. Women are more likely to access care if they have it, but they are less likely to have access to care. Women are more sensitive to environmental changes such as loss of social networks and are more willing to take part in support groups and activities (2,4,5,7).

In the United States, mental health treatment is tied to private health insurance. Women work in lower-paying jobs with fewer benefits, on average, than their male counterparts (9). This results in fewer women having access to mental health coverage as a part of their employer-sponsored health insurance. With lower wages and more dependents at home, women's discretionary income is also less, so out-of-pocket payment for mental healthcare is more difficult for women as well. Although the poorest women may well be more likely to qualify for public health insurance (Medicaid) by virtue of having dependents, many more women fall into the gap of the working poor who neither qualify for public assistance nor receive health insurance benefits at work. This disparity in health insurance is likely to follow a woman throughout her life: by working lower-paying jobs, salary increases, retirement savings, and employer contributions to retirement are lower, resulting in a lower standard of living and less access to healthcare in old age as well as youth. A woman's longer life expectancy makes this situation doubly detrimental.

If mental healthcare is accessible, however, women are more likely than men to use it (5). This may have more to do with the stereotypes internalized by men than women. It appears that women are more willing to seek care and more willing to continue care if care is available. Further, women are more likely to make the mental healthcare decisions for their families than men are. Women do seem accepting of help from various arenas: friends and family, but also psychiatrists and other professionals.

What treatment is offered does differ somewhat between the genders. Women are more likely than men to be prescribed psychotropic medications and are also more likely to use them. Women are less likely to be hospitalized (4). It is hard to know what happens in the doctor's office. It may be that men are more likely to refuse medication when offered and hence are less likely to be prescribed medication rather than a perception of the doctor that women need medication more than men, or perhaps women are more comfortable with the idea of taking medication and therefore more likely to ask for a prescription.

One thing that is becoming evident is that women are affected by exogenous substances differently than are men. Alcohol is probably the best-studied substance with a clear pharmacokinetic difference between genders and yet it is still not well understood (3). Females demonstrate differences in absorption, distribution, and elimination of alcohol, and the net result is a higher blood alcohol content than males after equivalent ingestion. This may be caused by the differences in body composition, women having proportionately less body water than men. However, other hypotheses have been explored, including differences in first pass metabolism, effects of sex hormones on metabolism, and relative liver size.

Women also appear to have differences in the pharmacokinetics of other substances, including psychotropic medication (2). This may be the explanation for the observation that women are more susceptible to side effects in general, and particularly to side effects of antipsychotic medication. In turn, side effects make it hard for a person of either gender to sustain treatment. Women are noted to have more positive symptoms of schizophrenia (4), although whether this is caused by an inherent difference in the presentation of the disease in women or caused by side effect–induced noncompliance—or some other cause—remains to be determined. One can even question the data cited above that women are more likely to take psychotropic medication. Perhaps they are less willing to admit that they do not take it as prescribed. Pharmacokinetic differences are an area of cutting-edge understanding of the clinical consequences of gender on pathophysiology, yet it also is an area that can be affected by social expectations.

Finally, when considering treatment, the effect of treatment on a woman's larger life must also be carefully thought out. Sometimes social stereotypes cause psychiatrists to be short-sighted. Pregnant women are encouraged by well-meaning people to discontinue or delay psychiatric medications without thought for the consequences of the worsening mental illness on either mother or child. A pregnant woman taking lithium is at risk of delivering a child with birth defects, but a pregnant woman who is in the throws of depression and takes an overdose is at risk for death, her fetus is at risk for death, and both are at risk for permanent morbidity. Breast-feeding is healthier than bottle feeding, but deferring antidepressant treatment to allow for breast-feeding may be counterproductive: a depressed woman, even if she is breast-feeding, may not bond or care for her child well. Maternal depression during a person's childhood is a risk factor for later psychopathology in adulthood. Yet, women are told to wait to start medication "until after the baby," even in cases of significant risk of severe mental illness, leading to needless suffering of mother and child.

Little attention has been paid to the consequences of treatment on the rest of the woman's social context. For instance, many antidepressants cause decreased libido, especially in women. For some partners, lack of sexual intimacy may be an acceptable situation or necessary evil in exchange for a woman's recovery. For others, this may signify rejection of the partner, which in turn may undermine the relationship. If the relationship is troubled to begin with, or worse yet violent, this seemingly innocuous side effect may set in motion a cascade of worsening circumstances from withdrawal of emotional intimacy to divorce to assault. Similarly, the sense of responsibility that many women internalize for home and family may discourage a woman from seeking treatment if she feels it is going to be detrimental to her family, from lost time, job risk, stigma, etc. Inroads are being made, however, in programs that recognize the realities of womanhood and support women in all of their roles.

Therefore, the sensitive psychiatrist will need to consider all the complexities of being a woman when planning treatment. Barriers to treatment, whether financial or emotional or time-related, need to be considered and addressed with the patient. Risk-benefit analyses need to consider more than just physical consequences of pharmaceutical agents and take into account the sequelae of pharmaceutical and nonpharmaceutical treatments. Side effects need to be carefully inquired about, as well as the consequences of those side effects. The individual, patient-centered, biopsychosocial formulation–driven treatment plan remains the best means to eliminate treatment disparities in all underrepresented groups, not just women. Understanding the patient precisely combats bias and is more likely to result in appropriate treatment.

PREVENTION

Prevention of mental illness in women can be divided into primary prevention, or what measures can we take to ensure that women do not develop mental illness, secondary prevention, or what we can do to identify and treat the early manifestation of mental illness, and tertiary prevention, meaning how to mitigate the detrimental effect of established mental illness.

Primary prevention of mental illness is only emerging as an approach in the medical field, although the concept of *wellness* has taken hold of popular attention and spawned an entire industry. Many people in and out of psychiatry are unaware of the possibility of primary prevention of mental illness, and many react dismissively at the concept. The concept of primary prevention is challenging to the profession for good reason: for decades, psychiatry has struggled to convince the public that mental illnesses are real biological illnesses and not merely character flaws. To prevent people from developing mental illness, however, psychiatry cannot yet offer a clear biological target or pathophysiology. Instead, our best understanding of what prevents or mitigates the experience of mental illness is a series of behaviors, many of which used to be considered moral virtues! However, although the fundamental pathophysiology of mental illness must be biological—we exist no other way—behavioral treatments are effective and so are behavior-based prevention measures. In fact, most successful public health campaigns targeting illness of all kinds are behavior-based and often occur before pathophysiology is understood. HIV is one example if this.

Primary prevention of mental illness in women involves not merely reducing the disparities in treatment of women's mental illness but in treatment in women in society (16). It is estimated that if social disparities between genders were eliminated, the burden of disease of depression alone would have enormous economic benefit to society: businesses would have better productivity and less absenteeism, physical and mental healthcare costs would be reduced, entitlement programs such as Aid to Dependent Children and Families would be less costly, and one can even argue that public schools would need to spend less on behavior and emotional support programs for their students.

First, financial equality is truly a public health concern (9). By placing a gratuitous financial burden on women, society also endangers itself. There are several aspects, however, to address: the first and perhaps most hopeful, is the reality of equal pay for equal work. Each generation moves closer to equivalent salary rather than gender-based discrimination. That is, women who came of age in the 50s and 60s make about 60 cents for every dollar a man makes in a particular field, women who came of age in the 80s make about 80 cents on the dollar, and women who are coming of age now are making 95 cents on the dollar. However, occupational segregation remains: some jobs are considered more appropriate for women, and these jobs tend to pay less. Teaching and nursing are still very female dominated, but even within more "masculine" jobs like medicine, there is occupational segregation. Women now dominate obstetrics/gynecology and pediatrics, and they are beginning to dominate psychiatry and family medicine. All are relatively lower-paying medical specialties. Men still dominate surgery, especially orthopedics, and most higher-paying subspecialties. People have argued this is because women do not want to work as hard or put in as many hours or because they want to raise children. The obvious counterargument is that men should also not be expected to sacrifice their personal lives, and especially their children, to their career. Although a somewhat strange idea to the older generations, the younger generations, both men and women, are beginning to demand more "lifestyle" considerations from their employers, including time and resources for caring for children.

Interpersonal violence is a thornier problem. Public health initiatives targeting interpersonal violence have had excellent penetration into society and have changed social perception of what is acceptable. Primary care doctors are taught to ask about domestic violence, women's shelters are widely available, and popular media depicts abusive spouses as villains. Similarly, educating young people about what constitutes rape, how to say no assertively, and even rudimentary self-defense has empowered women in how they can negotiate sexual intimacy. If the sexual abuse scandal in the Roman Catholic Church has any silver lining, it is that it allowed America to openly discuss and reflect on the devastation that childhood sexual abuse creates. Yet domestic violence, rape, date rape, and sexual molestation persist. It may be because underlying social causes have not been addressed: the conditions of poverty, social disenfranchisement, and substance abuse have not only failed to get better but have gotten worse. Social disenfranchisement and substance abuse, and possibly poverty, are problems that have their roots in childhood.

One way to address primary prevention of interpersonal violence, therefore, is to prioritize children. The way children are currently treated in the United States is shameful and necessarily contributes significantly to social disenfranchisement, substance abuse, interpersonal violence and a host of other social ills. Schools are overcrowded and underfunded, even as politicians parrot a commitment to education. Public day care in the United States is virtually nonexistent, resulting in parents struggling to find affordable day care and often resorting to unlicensed, inadequate, and sometimes unsafe situations. Lack of social commitment to children has resulted in a network of poorly funded child protection agencies that are not able to protect children. Foster care situations are often as bad, or worse, than the homes the children were taken from, and children are moved repeatedly from place to place: a certain recipe for attachment problems, disenfranchisement, bad behavior, and even less stable situations. Parenting itself is given little support. State educational curricula often require students to receive education in personal finance, drivers training, nutrition, and sexuality, but never even the most rudimentary behavior plan. Sex education may be controversial, but parenting education is taboo.

Prioritizing children would benefit their mothers and would go far toward both primary and secondary prevention of mental illness. Regular "health visitors" (state-sponsored parenting coaches) to new mothers have been shown to reduce child abuse and increase parents' sense of competency and satisfaction (17). Free or low-cost child care can provide a woman the ability to work or go to school, which in turn can strengthen her self-esteem, improve her financial prospects, and perhaps allow her the freedom to leave an abusive spouse. A well-funded school can be a refuge for children, a means of education and screening for mental illness, and a place to teach coping skills, resiliency, negotiation with peers, and even sound parenting.

Early childhood screening for mental retardation and autism are well established. School-based mental health screening initiatives are mounting in several states, and evidence suggests that violent tendencies in early childhood persist into adulthood if not addressed, but are also amenable to early interventions. Bullying in school is becoming recognized as a significant source of emotional strife, and children who bully are now being recognized as being as at-risk for mental illness as are bullying victims. By addressing bullying in childhood, the incidence of bullying in adulthood, including domestic violence, is likely to be reduced. Schools are appropriate places to teach the coping and interpersonal skills that self-injurious young women lack, as well as ways to cope with feelings of sadness and disappointment and ways to recognize depression and anxiety. Stronger, happier, more empowered girls and boys are less likely to use drugs and alcohol, less likely to become depressed, less likely to have children before they are ready, and more likely to pursue higher education.

OTHER ISSUES: ETHNICITY, RELIGION, AND GENDER

Although many congregations are able to adapt the traditional view of women to accommodate women's changing roles in society, many other congregations instead emphasize the defined roles for woman as they are portrayed in the Bible: subservient and domestic. The rise of evangelical Christian sects, for example, has included an institutionalized sexism that can have tragic consequences to a woman's health, safety, and mental health. More pervasive and insidious, however, is the very mainstream definition of a "good" woman as a subservient wife, mother, helper, and caregiver. This view, common to most religions, reflects the social demands made on women to be exactly that. Similarly, religions can at times promote the concept of mental illness as sin or divine retribution for sin, so that women may feel that their symptoms are caused by their failure to live up to the religious ideal of womanhood.

That said, belief in a higher order is often cited as promoting a sense of well-being, and involvement in a religious group can be a means of social support and satisfaction. Many congregations of various kinds have become resources for women experiencing domestic violence, safety nets for emotional support, and even sources of job training and childcare. Religion is not a straightforward issue, and thus a sensitive psychiatrist will evaluate with the patient the meaning of mental illness within the context of the patient's religion, the meaning of the patient's religion in her larger social context, and whether the patient's faith can be an aid to recovery.

When considering the effect of ethnicity in women, one must consider the additive effect of membership in multiple minorities. Further complications occur when a female member of an ethnic minority is also a member of a minority religion. Women who are members of other underrepresented groups may well get the worst of each.

A desire to defend her religion or ethnicity may hinder a female patient's willingness to disclose her symptoms or psychosocial situation. Alternatively, she may be discouraged from seeking treatment from a nonminority psychiatrist lest she present her minority in a bad light. This is more likely true in insular groups or groups about which there is strong distrust in the majority community. These women are at significant risk of going without treatment, and therefore outreach to the community as a whole may be beneficial, as well as a scrupulously nonjudgmental and open approach by the psychiatrist. The treating psychiatrist should bear in mind the multiple and sometimes conflicting ideals of cultures within cultures.

SPECIAL POPULATIONS

Several populations of women have been touched on above, and many more can be identified; however, this section will focus on incarcerated women. This group is large, underserved, and face specific disparities in mental health treatment that are microcosms of the larger disparities between genders and the causes of these disparities.

Historically, there have been gender differences in rates of incarceration, but women are catching up: the rate of incarceration of females is growing faster than that of males. Women tend to be arrested on drug charges and nonviolent charges more than men are, and men are more likely to have more serious criminal histories (18). Most any prison psychiatrist will tell you, however, that female prisoners are much more impaired than male prisoners. They are more likely to have psychiatric illnesses, have suffered trauma, and to use "hard" drugs. Studies bear this out, and some interesting findings about the profile of the female offender emerge (18). They are more likely than not to be mothers. They are more likely to have been introduced to drugs by their partners and more likely to use drugs as a means to escape abusive relationships. They are more likely than the nonincarcerated population to have been abused physically or sexually in childhood. In short, the social disparities—domestic violence, sexual abuse, lack of treatment for substance abuse and mental illness, etc.—that could be targets for the prevention of mental illness could also be public health targets for the prevention of crime and recidivism. Not surprisingly, recidivism in these women responds to intensive psychiatric and psychosocial intervention better than to mere incarceration.

CONCLUSION

Beliefs about women are so ingrained that scientific understanding of women has been severely distorted, and therefore so has diagnosis and treatment of mental illness in women. Generations of male investigators framing questions about women based on faulty assumptions has created confusion about what is fact and what is artifact. Biased research questions generate biased information, which then creates biased interpretation of symptoms, which in turn biases the understanding of diagnosis and treatment and thus the information gathered. The one thing that can be concluded with any certainty is that the time has come to gather data about women without assumptions and with frank acknowledgment of our biases. Science needs to design studies to minimize our presumptions about what a woman is and instead allow us to find out. The clinical psychiatrist must take into account the nascent scientific information about gender and mental illness, while at the same time manage the pitfalls of stereotype by asking more thoroughly about comorbid symptoms and their meanings for the patient. The biopsychosocial formulation can be used to help understand the effects of treatment on the female patient, such as impact on family life, social stigma, religious meaning, and available supports. The psychodynamic formulation can be used to help understand the meaning of the symptoms, illness, treatment, and course for the individual woman. Side effects of pharmaceuticals should be strongly suspected until proven otherwise, and frank discussions are key to medication compliance. Prevention strategies can and must focus on decreasing social disparities between men and women, including equalizing salary, occupational distribution, and access to healthcare. As well, primary prevention must prioritize the health, safety, and education of children: elimination of domestic violence and childhood sexual abuse will go a very long way toward decreasing mental illness and criminality in both genders. Home visitors to new parents, availability of quality child care, and strengthened school systems are ways to both prevent and monitor for mental illness while reducing the strain on women. Women of different religions and ethnicities should be welcomed with open minds and a willingness to understand the meaning of mental illness within their own context without judgment. In so many ways, women have gained in society, and in so many ways, they have not.

References

1. Afifi M. Gender differences in mental health. *Singapore Med J* 2007;48:385–391.
2. Clayton AH. Gender differences in clinical psychopharmacology. *J Clin Psychiatry* 2005; 66:1191.
3. Ramchandani VA. Research advances in ethanol metabolism. *Pathol Biol (Paris)* 2001; 49:676–682.
4. World Health Organization, Department of Mental Health and Substance Dependence. *Gender disparities in mental health.* Available online at: http://www.who.int/media/en/242.pdf. Accessed January 8, 2009.

5. Kendler KS, Myers J, Prescott CA. Sex differences in the relationship between social support and risk for major depression: A longitudinal study of opposite-sex twin pairs. *Am J Psychiatry* 2005;162:250–256.

6. Phillips SP. Defining and measuring gender: A social determinant of health whose time has come. *Int J Equity Health* 2005;4:11.

7. Stewart DE. The international consensus statement on women's mental health and the WPA consensus statement on interpersonal violence against women. *World Psychiatry* 2006;5:61–64.

8. Stewart DE. Social determinants of women's mental health. *J Psychosom Res* 2007;63: 223–224.

9. DeNavas-Walt C, Proctor BD, Smith IC, U.S. Census Bureau. Income, poverty, and health insurance coverage in the United States, 2006, Washington, DC: Bureau of Census; 2007.

10. Matthey S, Barnett B, Howie P, et al. Diagnosing depression in mothers and fathers: Whatever happened to anxiety? *J Affect Disord* 2003;74:139–147.

11. Alonso J, Angemeyer MC, Bemert S, et al. Prevalence of mental disorders in Europe: Results from the European study of the epidemiology of mental disorders (ESEMeD) project. *Acta Psychiatr Scand Suppl* 2004:420:21–27.

12. Kessler RC, Demler O, Frank RG, et al. Prevalence and treatment of mental disorders, 1990 to 2003. *N Engl J Med* 2005;352:2515–2523.

13. Kessler RC, Berglund P, Demler O, et al. Lifetime prevalence and age-of-onset distributions of DSM-IV disorders in the national comorbidity survey replication. *Arch Gen Psychiatry* 2005;62:593–602.

14. Narrow WE, Rae DS, Robins LN, et al. Revised prevalence estimates of mental disorders in the United States: Using a clinical significance criterion to reconcile 2 surveys' estimates. *Arch Gen Psychiatry* 2002;59:115–123.

15. Karch DL, Lubell KM, Friday J, et al. Surveillance for violent deaths: National violent death reporting system, 16 states, 2005. *PMID* 2008;57:1–45.

16. Radke AQ, Burke M, Chahan S, eds. *The Integration of Public Health Promotion and Prevention Strategies in Public Mental Health Report*. National Association of State Mental Health Program Directors Position Statement Reports; 2004.

17. Adams C. Health visitors' role in family mental health. *J Fam Health Care* 2007;17; 37–38.

18. Messina N, Burdon W, Hagopian G, et al. Predictors of prison-based treatment outcomes: A comparison of men and women participants. *Am J Drug Alcohol Abuse* 2006;32;7–28.

8 Gay Men

Jack Drescher

INTRODUCTION

It has been almost four decades since the American Psychiatric Association (APA) removed homosexuality from the Diagnostic and Statistical Manual in 1973 (1). Soon afterward, the American Psychological Association and the National Association of Social Workers endorsed a similar, nonpathologizing view of homosexuality. In 1992, the World Health Organization removed homosexuality from the International Classification of Diseases (ICD) as well.

These diagnostic changes were a watershed in a gradual if not astonishing cultural shift in scientific and popular thinking. The 19th century's medical case history model viewed homosexuality (among other forms of nonheterosexual, nonreproductive sexual activities) as psychopathological. The 21st century view, in part based on empirical data and in part on social justice issues, sometimes implicitly and at other times explicitly deems same-sex attractions and relationships as being within the normal range of human sexual expression. However, it was only after 1973, when science and medicine added their imprimatur to this paradigm shift that the pace of changing social attitudes quickened. Since the 1973 APA decision, there has been so much of an increase in the social acceptance of gay people that many countries and U.S. states that once criminalized same-sex behavior now have laws allowing gay marriage or other new forms of legal arrangements to protect gay people and their families.

In the aftermath of these diagnostic and social changes, there has been a gradual shift in efforts by mainstream mental health professionals away from either trying to "cure" or "prevent" homosexuality to an increased focus on the mental health needs of gay patients. It is difficult, at this time, to state with precise scientific accuracy what exactly those needs may be. Although there has been a growing literature and an increased interest in addressing the mental health needs and concerns of gay, lesbian, bisexual, and transgender (GLBT) patient populations, research efforts to better understand, determine, and prioritize those needs have been and continue to be hampered by a dearth of centralized public health approaches.

This chapter first outlines some of the factors that make it difficult to research and assess mental health disparities for gay, lesbian, and bisexual (GLB) patients as a group. After discussing the limitations, this chapter highlights what is presently known and hypothesized about some of the mental health disparities affecting gay male populations. The chapter concludes with suggestions about what can be done to overcome existing obstacles to further research to increase our scientific and clinical knowledge in ways that can reduce mental health disparities.

FACTORS HINDERING RESEARCH ABOUT GLB POPULATIONS

Among the factors that currently affect scientific research about GLB populations are sample bias, social invisibility, subgroup differences within GLB populations, the problem of distinguishing behaviors from identities, the stigma associated with homosexuality, and political opposition to sex research. Although these obstacles are parsed separately, they are interrelated to each other and reflect the broader social issues affecting GLB populations that have nothing to do with research about mental health disparities per se. As some researchers have persuasively argued, factors that make this research difficult, such as stigma and political opposition to gay rights, may also be a contributing factor to the mental health disparities themselves (2,3).

SAMPLE BIAS

Much of the early mental health literature studying gay populations relied on convenience samples. Study subjects were reachable because they either attended venues such as GLBT political organizations, were readers of particular magazines, or went to gay Internet sites or bars (4). Although these studies did not rely on random selection or large population-based samples, they showed higher rates (when compared with the general heterosexual population) of depressive disorders, suicidal ideation, anxiety disorders, substance use disorders, and eating disorders in some homosexual populations (2). However, the absence of credible, random-sample, large population studies that would permit and include identification of openly GLB subjects made it difficult to verify the findings first obtained from biased sample studies.

SOCIAL INVISIBILITY

The colloquial term for describing GLB people who hide their sexual identities is "being in the closet." However, being in the closet is not just about a gay person's unwillingness to reveal his or her sexual minority status. The "closet" is constructed of diverse factors; some hiding relates to an individual's psychology and other kinds of hiding are embedded in the cultural context in which the individual lives (5). What sometimes appears from the outside as a gay person hiding can alternatively be interpreted as either the heterosexual environment's active avoidance of direct looking or discouragement of disclosure. The most explicit enactment of this social phenomenon is codified in the U.S. military's "don't ask, don't tell" policy: gay people in military service hide their sexual identities ("don't tell") and their heterosexual superiors are not allowed to deliberately seek out information about their sexual identities ("don't ask"). In a social matrix where the subject of homosexuality is deliberately avoided, commendable service by gay people in the military is rendered invisible and stereotypes about the "harmful" effects of allowing gays to be open in the military are perpetuated.

A "don't ask, don't tell" approach also infuses large population surveys as they also usually treat gay people as invisible. For example, the U.S. 2000 census included a category of "unmarried partner" and reported that there were more than 600,000 same-sex couples who identified themselves as heads of households. However, it is not clear whether these numbers actually reflect who is and who is not a gay couple.

Census 2000 not only omitted asking respondents any direct questions about their sexual orientation or sexual identity; in those instances in which same-sex couples did respond on the census form to the "married" category, the U.S. Census Bureau flagged their responses "as invalid" to comply with the 1996 Federal Defense of Marriage Act (DOMA) that instructs all federal agencies only to recognize opposite-sex marriages (6). Although at the time of this writing gay marriages are now legal in Connecticut and Massachusetts, and 18,000 gay couples were married in California in late 2008, the implementation of DOMA precludes the counting of any of these marriages in the upcoming 2010 census (7). Other legal alternatives to marriage for gay people in other parts of the United Stateers, such as civil unions (New Hampshire, New Jersey, Vermont) and domestic partnerships (California, Maine, Oregon, Washington), are unlikely to appear in the 2010 census as well.

One of the most significant examples of diminished gay visibility in the public health arena was in a 2001 report dealing with mental health issues among minority groups: *Mental Health: Culture, Race, and Ethnicity: A Supplement to Mental Health: A Report of the Surgeon General.* This 219-page report includes only two references to sexual orientation. In reference to "a mix of barriers deterring minorities from seeking treatment or operating to reduce its quality once they reach treatment" (p. 4), acknowledges, "The cumulative weight and interplay of all of these barriers, not any single one alone, is likely responsible for mental health disparities. Furthermore, these barriers operate to discernibly different degrees for different individuals and groups, depending on life circumstances, age, gender, sexual orientation, or spiritual beliefs." The second reference is made in an effort to define "culture," acknowledging that there may be some individuals who "may identify with other social groups to which they feel a stronger cultural tie such as being Catholic, Texan, teenaged, or gay" (p. 9). With its focus on racial and ethnic minorities, the rest of the report appears to omit even the possibility that a GLBT identity might constitute membership in a cultural minority.

In an effort to break through the invisibility barrier and determine the prevalence of GLB people in the general population, Black et al. (4) looked at cumulative data from three large data sets. Among the studies they looked at was the National Health and Social Life Survey (NHSLS), a 1994 large-scale study of sexuality in the United States (8) believed to offer the most reliable and recent estimates of the prevalence of homosexuality in the United States. That study found that 2.7% of the 3159 men and 1.3% of the 1749 women surveyed had participated in same-sex sexual behavior during the preceding year, and 4.9% of men and 4.1% of women had done so since age 18; 7.7% of men and 7.5% of women reported having experienced sexual desire for someone of the same sex; and 2.8% of the men and 1.4% of the men reported a homosexual or bisexual identity. These figures varied considerably across groups based on age, marital status, education, religion, race, and place of residence. Further analysis by Black et al. (4) of the 1990 U.S. census data suggests that the NHSLS prevalence rates cited above may be two to three times higher among gay people in the 20 largest U.S. cities.

Invisibility exists in the clinical setting as well. The most mundane example can be found in the routine forms patients are asked to fill out in either a clinic or a psychiatrist's office. Such forms usually list the option of describing oneself as "single, married, widowed, or divorced." There are few medical forms today that mention any of the several types of already legalized gay relationships like "domestic partnerships" or "civil unions." As a result of this social invisibility, assessing the health and mental health needs of gay patients is an ongoing problem as both a public policy issue and at the individual, clinical level.

SUBGROUP DIFFERENCES

A significant barrier to sampling sexual minorities stems from the fact that they are not all members of a homogenous group (3). For example, there are GLB people who feel more closely identified with some other aspect of their social identity, such as race or ethnicity; alternatively, others may accept a "double minority status" (i.e., Asian and lesbian) or even a multiple minority status (i.e., African American, Muslim, bisexual). Further complicating matters, it is likely that the mental health needs of GLB individuals will vary across differences in age (i.e., teenagers as opposed to the elderly), gender (differences between gay men and lesbians, between bisexual men and bisexual women), race, ethnicity, socioeconomic status (i.e., ability to access and afford care), and the social milieu (i.e. urban versus rural) in which members of sexual minorities live.

PROBLEMS OF DEFINITION: DISTINGUISHING BEHAVIOR FROM IDENTITY

Another confounding factor in determining the mental health needs of gay patients centers on how one defines the populations at risk. Black et al. (4) noted that different large-scale surveys try to determine the sexual orientation of their subjects by asking questions like "Have you ever had a same-sex partner?" or "Have you had as many same-sex partners as opposite-sex partners since age 18?" Other efforts to define survey subjects as "gay" or "homosexual" assumed they were so if they had exclusively same-sex sex either over the previous year or over the last 5 years. Some surveys ask subjects directly whether they think of themselves as "heterosexual, homosexual, bisexual, or something else." The drawbacks of these approaches include:

1. The conflation of sexual behavior with a sexual identity and using behavioral patterns to define who is and who is not gay;
2. The use of arbitrary time frames. For example, is a male subject "gay" if he has been having sex with men for 6 months? A year? Five years?
3. These approaches assume that subjects either understand the questions being asked or are willing to accept or admit to socially stigmatized identities regardless of their actual sexual behaviors.

In the realm of HIV assessment, treatment, and prevention, questions about how one defines sexual behaviors and identities are paramount and, unfortunately, are in need of greater refinement. For example, it is difficult to create public health messages intended to educate about, present the spread of, and encourage treatment of HIV if the messages do not reach their target audience(s). For example, not all men who engage in sexual activity with other men identify as "gay," so the HIV treatment community has adopted a descriptive term for this population: "men who have sex with men" or MSM. MSM are a heterogeneous group, and a recent study of this patient population illustrates the difficult and complex relationships between behavior and identity. Pathela et al. (9) published a population-based sample of 4193 men in New York City. Their study focused on self-reported sexual identity and sexual behavior and found "behavior-identity discordance" among 9.4% of the 2717 "straight-identified" men they surveyed. What was the nature of the discordance? The latter group reported having sexual intercourse with at least one man (and no women) in the year before they were surveyed. The study also found that among the 206 MSM, 72.8% of them identified themselves as "straight."

In their discussion of the results, the authors noted "Foreign-born men who have sex with men . . . were less likely than U.S.-born men to identify as gay, suggesting that rather than misunderstanding the question regarding identity, foreign-born men in New York City who have sex with men were reluctant to associate their behavior with a gay identity" (pp. 422–423). Further complicating matters of definition, 70% of the straight-identified MSM reported that they were heterosexually married. Members of this group were likely to have fewer sexual partners than gay-identified MSM but they were also less likely to use condoms or to be tested for HIV. Findings like these demonstrate the difficult challenges public health officials and epidemiologists face in trying to identify the subjects they wish to identify and study.

STIGMA ASSOCIATED WITH HOMOSEXUALITY

The above-noted discordances between sexual behavior and sexual identity are often attributed to the social stigma attached to homosexuality. Despite the social gains of the last four decades, there are many places where open expressions of a gay identity meet with disapproval. This complicates efforts to ascertain the full extent of the mental health needs of this population because existing social opprobrium or an anticipated expectation of disapproval may prevent respondents from openly identifying as members of a sexual minority (8). In addition, there are institutional settings such as the U.S. armed forces, prisons, or socially conservative religious universities where public knowledge of a gay person's sexual orientation could have such adverse consequences as loss of employment, loss of status, expulsion from one's community, loss of limb, or loss of life. Under "don't ask, don't tell," a lesbian soldier seeking treatment for an anxiety disorder who reveals her sexual identity to a military psychiatrist may face possible discharge.

Non-American cultural prejudices against homosexuality may also play a role in determining who identifies as gay. As Pathela et al. (9) note, "foreign-born men who have sex with men may be subject to the social and cultural contexts of the countries in which they were born and thus may be reluctant to acknowledge homosexuality or use a more narrow definition of what homosexuality constitutes" (p. 423). Significantly, they note the growth in the foreign-born population of New York City, where 36% of the population was born in countries other than the United States, with a third of them estimated to have emigrated from Latin America and another third from Asia. Another recent, troubling finding (10), undoubtedly resulting from stigma about homosexuality, is that among 452 MSM respondents, 175 (39%) had not disclosed to their healthcare providers that they were attracted to or had sex with other men.

OPPOSITION TO SEX RESEARCH

There is significant political opposition, in the United States and other countries, to government funding for sex research in general and for research about sexual minorities in particular. In one telling example, a broad population study (8) was originally to be federally funded as a survey of 20,000 people. Because of political opposition, federal funding was withdrawn, alternative financial support was sought, and, because of a lowered amount of replacement funding, only about 5000 people were surveyed (11).

Hunt (11) sees opposition to sex research needed for formulating both mental health and public health policies as stemming from the influence of "religious and political conservatives" (p. 206) who view epidemiological sex research—or any sex research—as:

1. Unnecessary because such individuals feel current sexual knowledge is adequate
2. Damaging to families because they believe that asking questions about sexual practices will encourage people to engage in those practices
3. Immoral as such research tends to normalize sexual practices that their religious beliefs label as sinful
4. Inconsistent with shrinking the role of government and a waste of tax dollars.

Hunt quotes one U.S. Senator who saw sex research as a subterfuge for other political agendas having nothing to do with public health policy: "These sex surveys have not—have not—been concerned with scientific inquiry as much as they have been concerned with a blatant attempt to sway public attitudes to liberalize opinions and laws regarding homosexuality, pedophilia, anal and oral sex, sex education, teenage pregnancy, and all down the line" (Congressional Record, September 12, 1991, S12861, S12862; Cited in Hunt, 1999, p. 189). This opposition can also be found in the executive branch of government as well. In his 2007 testimony to Congress, former Surgeon General Richard Carmona said executive office officials "repeatedly tried to weaken or suppress important public health reports because of political considerations" and that during his 2002 to 2006 tenure he was not allowed "to speak or issue reports about stem cells, emergency contraception, sex education, or prison, mental, and global health issues" (12).

MENTAL HEALTH DISPARITIES AFFECTING GAY MEN

Despite the obstacles mentioned above, and given the available research, it is possible to highlight some of the most salient mental health disparities currently believed to affect gay men. A more comprehensive review can be found in Wolitski et al. (3).

Cochran et al. (13) found that GLB populations were more likely to see a mental health provider in the previous year (19% of gay or bisexual men vs. 8% of heterosexual men and 33% of lesbian or bisexual women vs. 11% of heterosexual women). More recently, Cochran and Mays (14) maintain that these groups "represent a vulnerable population for prevalent mental health morbidity, especially major depression, substance use disorders, anxiety disorders, and suicide attempts. As well, studies document a higher perceived need for mental health services among gay and bisexual men than their heterosexual counterparts" (p. 98).

MOOD DISORDERS

A large, Dutch population survey (15) found higher rates of mood disorders in homosexual men (defined as such on the basis of self-reports of having had sex with other men in the previous year): 17% vs. 5% in heterosexual men. A U.S. study (13) examining psychiatric morbidity and self-identified sexual orientation found gay and bisexual men had higher rates of major depression in the previous year (31% compared with 10% in heterosexual men).

ANXIETY DISORDERS

Sandfort et al. (15), in their Dutch population survey, also found higher rates of anxiety disorders among gay men when compared with heterosexuals (20% vs. 8%). Cochran et al. (13) found an increased rate of panic disorder (18% vs. 4%). Gilman et al. (16), using same-sex sexual behavior as a marker for sexual orientation, also found increased rates of anxiety disorders in gay men.

SUBSTANCE ABUSE DISORDERS

One controversy in this area of epidemiological research is the prevalence of substance abuse in the gay community. Gilman et al. (16) found higher rates of drug abuse and dependence in homosexual men. Ostrow and Stall (17), in a recent review of the this literature, argue that even without larger population studies, there are sufficient data to raise concerns about an increased use of "sex-specific" drugs (intended to enhance sexual pleasure) among gay men, including "poppers" (alkyl nitrites), crystal methamphetamine, ecstasy (MDMA), cocaine, ketamine, and GHB (gamma-hydroxybutyric acid). These authors find that gay men are significantly more likely to smoke than are heterosexual men and that despite stereotypes about gay bar culture and alcoholism, the prevalence of alcohol-related problems or heavy drinking does not vary much between gay men and their heterosexual peers.

SUICIDE

Since the 1990s, there is a growing literature on suicide risk among gay adolescents. Remafedi (18), in a survey of 255 15- to 25-year-old men who had sex with another man in the previous year, found a third of respondents reported at least one suicide attempt, and 4.7% attempted suicide in the previous year. He found suicide attempts more prevalent among African Americans and urban residents. Silenzio et al (19), analyzing the National Longitudinal Study of Adolescent Health (2001–2002), labeled subjects describing themselves as bisexual, mostly homosexual, or exclusively homosexual as "LGB." They found LGB respondents reported higher rates of suicidal ideation and suicide attempts than non-LGB respondents controlled for race, gender, and age. Their analysis showed problem drinking, problem drug use, and depression associated with elevated risk for suicidal ideation and suicide attempts among non-LGB respondents and that whereas problem drinking and depression increased risk for suicidal ideation among LGB respondents, drug use did not. Ryan et al. (20) compared young LGBT adults reporting higher levels of family rejection during adolescence to be 8.4 times more likely to report attempting suicide and 5.9 times more likely to report high levels of depression when compared with peers from families reporting either no or low levels of rejection. There are also data (14) suggesting rates of thinking about suicide and rates of attempted suicide may be higher among gay men when compared with heterosexual men.

SOURCES OF DISTRESS

Sources of distress among GLB populations that may affect the presentation of mental problems in this population can include awareness of sexual orientation difference, acceptance of sexual orientation difference, decision-making regarding "coming out," creating supports, integration of GLB identity and other aspects of a personal identity, and confronting social bias. Other sources of distress may lead to mental health disparities, including (i) coping with antihomosexual attitudes such as heterosexism, internalized homophobia, and moral condemnations of homosexuality; (ii) legal sanctions and the absence of civil equality such as the right to marry and protection from antidiscrimination laws (21); and (iii) antigay violence.

THE DIAGNOSTIC AND STATISTICAL MANUAL

Since the 1987 removal of ego-dystonic homosexuality from the DSM-III-R, the diagnostic manual remains mostly silent about homosexuality The current DSM text sections do not address associated risk factors as they relate to GLB patients among its many diagnostic categories. It should be noted that although a homosexual orientation has not been shown to "cause" psychiatric illness, it may nevertheless be a risk indicator of illness just as age, race, gender, and socioeconomic status may be risk factors associated with psychiatric disorders.

ADDRESSING MENTAL HEALTH DISPARITIES

Although the obstacles toward increasing greater understanding of mental health disparities for gay men and other sexual minorities are not insignificant, having been identified, they can be directly addressed and in some cases overcome.

POPULATION STUDIES

Given that sexual minority populations in the United States may number in the millions, more broad-based population surveys of their mental health needs are required. Such studies need to remove the bureaucratic invisibility cloak that has been placed over gay people and to ask questions, both about sexual identity ("Does the subject identify as gay?") and behavior ("What is the gender of people with whom the subject is having sex?"). The 2010 U.S. Census would be a likely place to begin asking questions about sexual identity, allowing respondents to self-identify as "heterosexual, homosexual, bisexual, or other." In addition, asking GLB census respondents if they are in legal same-sex marriages, civil unions, or domestic partnerships would be useful to epidemiologists and other researchers wishing to identify and analyze data related to mental health and marital status (21).

INCREASED AWARENESS OF MULTIPLE MINORITY STATUS

Patients who are members of ethnic, racial, and religious minorities may also openly identify or be in the closet as gay, lesbian, or bisexual. Consequently, they may have to contend not only with antihomosexual attitudes but with racial and ethnic prejudices as well. The invisibility of GLB people in the general population is often greater among some racial, ethnic, or religious groups. Data on multiple minority status could be of vital importance to clinicians, researchers, and demographers, and raising awareness of these often-overlooked individuals can be done through education, such as presentations about sexual and other minority diversity at professional meetings across all interested disciplines.

 ## INCLUSIVE CLINICAL SETTINGS

The clinical setting, either in public and private offices, should provide an atmosphere of inclusiveness for gay patients. The use of self-reporting forms for patients that neutrally inquire about sexual identities and family arrangements (i.e., relationship of emergency contact to patient) and acknowledge legal relationships that are not officially a marriage can help reassure a GLB patient of greater acceptance in the clinical setting.

 ## COMBATING STIGMA ASSOCIATED WITH HOMOSEXUALITY

APA policies repeatedly emphasize the harmful effects of stigma, and the organization has worked incessantly, with various degrees of success, to remove the social stigma associated with mental illness. Since the 1973 removal of homosexuality from the DSM, APA has also worked to combat the stigmatization of homosexuality and opposes discrimination against gay people (1). In 2005, the APA took a position in support of civil marriage equality for gay people. APA and other mainstream mental health professions continue to issue position statements whose intent is to reduce the stigma associated with same-sex relationships. Increasing outreach between mainstream mental health organizations and the leaders of racial, ethnic, and religious communities that condemn homosexuality may also help to reduce stigma experienced by the GLB members of these groups.

 ## RECOMMENDATIONS FOR THE DIAGNOSTIC AND STATISTICAL MANUAL

Notations about sexual orientation, sexual identity, and adjustment to should be considered for inclusion in Axis IV, both generally and related to specific domains such as primary support group, education, housing, access to health care, and occupational, economic, and legal issues. It is also recommend that descriptive text be added in the forthcoming DSM-V to include pertinent aspects of psychiatric disorders in GLB populations. This includes variations in the presentation of disorders in GLB populations including differential prevalence rates, typical patterns of evolution of disorders in GLB populations, and illustrative examples in GLB populations to clarify diagnostic criteria.

References

1. Drescher J, Merlino JP, eds. *American Psychiatry and Homosexuality: An Oral History.* New York: Harrington Park Press, 2007.
2. Sandfort T, Bakker F, Schellevis F, et al. Sexual orientation and mental and physical health status: Findings from a Dutch population survey. *Am J Public Health* 2006;96:1119–1125.
3. Wolitski RJ. Stall R, Valdiserri, RO, eds. *Unequal Opportunity: Health Disparities Affecting Gay and Bisexual Men in the United States.* Oxford: Oxford University Press, 2008.
4. Black D, Gates G, Sanders S, et al. Demographics of the gay and lesbian populations in the United States: Evidence from available systematic data sources. *Demography* 2000;37(2): 139–154.
5. Drescher J. *Psychoanalytic Therapy and the Gay Man.* Hillsdale, NJ: The Analytic Press, 1998.
6. U.S. Census Bureau. *Technical Note on Same-Sex Unmarried Partner Data from the 1990 and 2000 Censuses,* nd (retrieved August 10, 2008, available at http://www.census.gov/population/www/cen2000/samesex/index.html).
7. Lee C. Census won't count gay marriages. *Washington Post,* July 18, 2008 (July 26, 2008, available at http://www.washingtonpost.com/wp-dyn/content/article/2008/07/16/AR2008071602566.html).
8. Laumann EO, Gagnon JH, Michael RT, et al. *The Social Organization of Sexuality: Sexual Practices in the United States.* Chicago: University of Chicago Press, 1994.
9. Pathela P, Hajat A, Schillinger J, et al. Discordance between sexual behavior and self-reported sexual identity: A population-based survey of New York City men. *Ann Intern Med* 2006;145(6):416–425.
10. Bernstein K, Liu K-L, Begier E, et al. Same-sex attraction disclosure to health care providers among New York City men who have sex with men. *Arch Intern Med* 2008;168 (13):1458–1464
11. Hunt M. *The New Know-Nothings: The Political Foes of the Scientific Study of Human Nature.* New Brunswick, NJ: Transaction Publishers, 1999.
12. Harris G. Surgeon General sees 4-year term as compromised. *The New York Times,* July 11, 2007 (retrieved July 27, 2008, available at http://www.nytimes.com/2007/07/11/washington/11surgeon.html).
13. Cochran S, Sullivan J, Mays V. Prevalence of mental disorders, psychological distress, and mental health services use among lesbian, gay, and bisexual adults in the United States. *J Consult Clin Psych* 2003;71:53–61.
14. Cochran SD, Mays VM. Prevalence of primary mental health morbidity and suicide symptoms among gay and bisexual men. In: Wolitski RJ, Stall R, Valdiserri RO, eds. *Unequal Opportunity: Health Disparities Affecting Gay and Bisexual Men in the United States.* Oxford: Oxford University Press, 2008; 97–120.
15. Sandfort T, de Graaf R, Bijl R, et al. Same-sex sexual behavior and psychiatric disorders: Findings from the Netherlands Mental Health Survey and Incidence Study (NEMESIS). *Arch Gen Psychiatry* 2001;58:85–91.
16. Gilman S, Cochran S, Mays V, et al. Risk of psychiatric disorders among individuals reporting same-sex sexual partners in the National Comorbidity Survey. *Am J Public Health* 2001;91:933–939.
17. Ostrow DG, Stall R. Alcohol, tobacco, and drug use among gay and bisexual men. In: Wolitski RJ, Stall R, Valdiserri RO, eds. *Unequal Opportunity: Health Disparities Affecting Gay and Bisexual Men in the United States.* Oxford: Oxford University Press, 2008; 121–158.
18. Remafedi G. Suicidality in a venue-based sample of young men who have sex with men. *J Adolesc Health* 2002;31(4):305–310.

19. Silenzio VM, Pena JB, Duberstein PR, et al. Sexual orientation and risk factors for suicidal ideation and suicide attempts among adolescents and young adults. *Am J Public Health* 2007;97(11):2017–2019.

20. Ryan C, Huebner D, Diaz RM, et al. Family rejection as a predictor of negative health outcomes in white and latino lesbian, gay, and bisexual young adults. *Ped* 2009;123: 346–352.

21. Herdt G, Kertzner R. I do, but I can't: The impact of marriage denial on the mental health and sexual citizenship of lesbians and gay men in the United States. *Sex Res Soc Policy* 2006;3(1):33–49.

9 Lesbians

Nimisha Gokaldas and Khakasa Wapenyi

DEFINITIONS

The most common definition of a lesbian is a woman who is romantically, erotically, and sexually attracted exclusively to other women. In psychiatry, when speaking of the "lesbian population" it is important to distinguish descriptive versus operational definitions: the literature shows that the majority of self-identified lesbians have had sexual contact with a male partner during their lifetime (1). For research purposes, lesbians are often defined as women who have sex with women (WSW); however, this definition is reductive and potentially overinclusive (i.e., bisexual women would be included). When thinking about lesbian patients, it is important to distinguish sexual identification from behavior or orientation (and gender). A lesbian's self-identification might not correspond with her behavior and vice versa. In terms of gender, most people are aware that lesbians do not identify cross-gender (i.e., lesbians may be masculinized or "butch," but they do not identify as male or take the role of "the man in the relationship"). In addition, different cultures, as well as ethnic/racial minorities, may have different terms or concepts for women who are defined in the predominant Western culture as "lesbians."

Sappho, a 6th century Greek poet who lived on the island of Lesbos, is generally credited with originating the idea of the "lesbian." Sappho wrote homoerotic, sensual poems addressed to women (an alternative term to lesbian is "sapphist"). The term "lesbian" in its modern usage was coined in 1890; however, the adjective "lesbian" was recognized in the 1590s as a group of "homosexual females" from the island of Lesbos (2). Historians stress that same-sex relationships between women were not always sexualized, as in the concept of the "Boston marriage" that blossomed during the first wave of Westernized feminism during the 1920s. During the second wave of Westernized feminism of the 1970s, activists argued that lesbian relationships ranged from sexual to platonic and were more broadly defined as same-sex relationships between women that did not fall within the traditional heterosexual marital paradigm (3). Recently, the term "woman identified woman" has been created to refer to a woman or girl who had experienced a "girl crush" or a fervent, romantic infatuation for another woman or girl. These infatuations are nonsexual and do not lead to the development of longer-term same-sex attractions or relationships (4).

Lesbian self-definition and behavior, including sexual practices, can be quite diverse. Early psychiatric theory conceptualizes lesbian orientation and psychosexual development as gender confusion or inversion and formal pathologizing of same-sex orientation until 1973 (when homosexuality was removed as a disorder from DSM III).

This history, taken with ongoing practice by a subset of psychiatrists to change same-sex orientation via "reparative therapy," reveals why some lesbians may be wary of psychiatry as a profession. It behooves us as psychiatrists, clinicians, scientists, and therapists to be respectfully curious about our lesbian patients' internal world as well as how they live their lives on a day-to-day basis. This is especially important because so little research has specifically focused on lesbian mental health.

COMING OUT

When looking at mental health needs in the lesbian population, the first thing to consider is the "outness" of the patient. Being "out" means becoming aware and acknowledging one's own gay identity as well as disclosing that identity to others. A widely accepted model of coming out described by Cass involves six discrete stages that an individual goes through in the coming out process. These six stages include identity confusion, identity comparison, identity tolerance, identity acceptance, identity pride, and identity synthesis (5). These stages allow for women to eventually accept their sexuality as an aspect of their self and acknowledge this to those around them. These stages are not necessarily linear, and not all must be experienced to come out. What must be recognized when looking at coming out models such as the one above are that they are Westernized concepts that might not apply to non-Westernized individuals.

There are differences among the genders in regard to sexual identity milestones, with women generally labeling themselves as gay before actually having a same-sex experience, unlike their male counterparts, who generally pursue sex prior to coming out (6). Both sexes took approximately 10 years from first same-sex attraction to first disclosure, with women being more emotionally oriented and coming out occurring at an average age of 18.

There are only a handful of studies that specifically look at mental health in relation to the outness of the subject. A recent study suggests that lesbians who were not out are twice as likely to experience suicidal ideation and an increased risk of suicidal attempts and that lesbians experienced more stress as teenagers than their heterosexual counterparts (7). The stress experienced as teenagers may have to do with the coming out process, which can be confusing and stigmatizing. We know that discriminatory behavior is associated with psychological distress and mental illness, and hostility and abuse toward those coming out may lead to depression and anxiety (8). This discrimination can cause lesbians to stay "in the closet" rather than disclose their sexual preferences to themselves and others. This continued suppression of one's sexual desires and identity may lead to self-loathing and hatred that can manifest in poor coping mechanisms and mental illness. An older study found that suicide attempts decreased considerably after adolescence and coming out (9). This decrease in suicide associated with adolescence and coming out underlies the importance of the process for self-awareness and self-acceptance.

During the coming out process, it is not uncommon for the individual to experience an adjustment disorder, be it predominantly depressed or anxious type. The process of coming out may take months to years, and attention should be paid to where in the process the individual identifies as being in. Lesbians may be out only to themselves or only other lesbians and friends and may take years to come out to family, or vice versa. These types of scenarios are very real and contribute to lesbians having adjustment disorders that affect their lives and relationships. It appears that lesbians are more likely to use psychotherapy for depression than their heterosexual or bisexual counterparts (7), and this may be the best avenue to discuss the coming out process and its impact on mental health.

This author argues that more studies need to pay attention to the outness of the individual to fully assess their mental health risks. In addition, we as practitioners must be willing to ask these questions of our patients rather than assume outness, which is done routinely on the basis of first impressions and outness of the patient to the provider.

LESBIAN YOUTH AND SUICIDE

Adolescents in general are a high-risk group for suicide, but same-gender sexual orientation is an independent risk factor on suicidal ideation and attempts. In fact, the literature supports that the lesbian, gay, bisexual, and transsexual (LGBT) demographic is at an increased risk of suicidal behaviors and an increased risk of drug and alcohol use and mental illness. There are no studies specific to lesbians; rather, the literature focuses on LGBT youth in general.

Before a discussion about suicide can begin, we must recognize that LGBT youth also have higher rates of substance abuse and mental illness as compared with their peers/heterosexual counterparts. However, in a recent study, drug use and depression were associated with adverse outcomes among heterosexual youth but not among LGBT youth (10). At first glance, this appears to be counterintuitive because there is an increase in depression and substance abuse among LGBT adolescents. Yet, this study suggests that the struggle lesbian adolescents face that may lead to suicidal behaviors are independent of their drug use and depression. This does not imply that drug use and depression are not risk factors for suicide, rather, that these factors are not the sole issues that drive LGBT youth to suicidal behaviors.

What is the cause for an increase in suicidal behavior among lesbian youth? Some have argued that there may be higher rates of victimization and abuse, especially during adolescence among lesbians. Hostility is recognized, whether self-inflicted or perpetrated by others, as a risk factor for suicide, and self-destructive behaviors appear to be a maladaptive coping strategy to deal with stress. In addition, various psychological factors such as a sense of isolation, low levels of social support, and frequent stressful life events may lead to an increase in suicide rates (8). It is unclear, however, if the lack of social support is a direct result of sexual orientation.

In a Minnesota study, more than half of LGBT students had thought of suicide, and 37% had reported an attempt (11). Homosexual youth are 2 to 3 times more likely to commit suicide than their heterosexual peers. This study went on to look at protective factors associated with a reduced risk of suicide and found that LGBT youth had significantly lower levels of protective factors than their peers. Some of these protective factors such as teacher caring, other adult caring, and school safety are amendable to change and should be considered for targeting interventions in this high-risk population. Other protective factors such as family connectedness are more intricate and may be more difficult to target in these populations.

In addition, the social pressures and lack of role models must be considered when looking at adolescents struggling with their sexuality. Adolescence is a time of such social pressure, and with heterosexuality continuing to be the norm and the high probability for some aspect of internalized homophobia, coming out can be extremely daunting and isolating. Continued education and safe LGBT environments within schools could minimize the suicide risks these youth face.

Overall, adolescence is a time of increased substance abuse, depression, and suicidal ideation and attempts, but with the addition of same-sex gender orientation, the risk for suicide increases substantially.

ANXIETY DISORDERS

In reviewing the literature, lesbians report high levels of anxiety, up to 79% in certain samples, yet it is unclear whether they as a group experience anxiety disorders at higher rates (12). Looking at the sparse available data, researchers have found the most common psychiatric disorders among lesbians to be anxiety and depressive disorders. Of the anxiety disorders, generalized anxiety disorder, social anxiety, and posttraumatic stress disorder (PTSD) appear to be most common (13). Some risk factors for anxiety include (i) job-related discrimination and/or harassment, (ii) intimate relationship conflicts, (iii) discord with the family of origin, (iv) financial stressors, (v) child care and custody issues, and (vi) perceived lack of social support. As would be expected, PTSD is significantly associated with being the victim of antilesbian hate/bias crime (14).

Because of experiences of stigma, discrimination, harassment, ostracism, and abuse, lesbians may present with complaints of stress, worry, and fear. These complaints and negative experiences may overlap with the signs and symptoms of idiopathic anxiety disorders. The culturally competent psychiatrist would endeavor to elicit from the history whether the anxiety experienced by her lesbian patient were stress related to external factors (or internalized homophobia) as compared with an anxiety disorder per se. Granted, at times, this is not an easy task. However, if the anxiety symptoms do not meet criteria for a specific anxiety disorder, psychiatrists would do well to focus the therapeutic work on potentially adverse factors particular to lesbians. In addition to the above, these factors may include narcissistic deficits, low self-esteem, internalized homophobia, lack of familial and/or social support, and inadequate, unsatisfactory, or absent attachments (15).

DEPRESSIVE DISORDERS

Lesbians have been called "invisible" in terms of research examining clinical depression (14). Lesbians have at least similar prevalence rates of depressive disorders compared with the general American female population (lifetime prevalence rates range from 33% to 66%) (15).

Certain depression risk factors specific to lesbians have been identified: (i) lack of romantic relationship, (ii) satisfaction with relationship status, (iii) hate or bias-crime victimization, (iv) history of sexual or physical abuse, (v) self-esteem level, (vi) social support level (particularly partner support), (vii) rejection of negative stereotypes (of lesbians), (viii) acceptance of positive sexual minority identity and (ix) identification with her lesbian community (15).

In the differential diagnosis of depressive disorders in lesbian patients, psychiatrists must be aware that higher rates of alcohol use disorders (as compared with heterosexual women) may directly affect rates of affective disorders seen in the lesbian community. A careful substance use history correlated with presenting signs and symptoms will help discern whether the diagnosis points more toward a secondary substance-induced depressive disorder. If alcohol appears to be the culprit, dual diagnosis treatment is crucial. In treatment planning, psychiatrists should be cognizant that lesbians might have better outcomes and decreased relapse rates if treated by LGBT-affirmative treatment providers or settings.

Although we do know that lesbian teens have higher rates of suicidality than their heterosexual peers, we do not know whether this applies to adult lesbians.

Homophobia (externalized and internalized) may negatively affect a lesbian's self-esteem and directly cause increased stress, distress, and impairment. We may hypothesize that with America's decreasing levels of homophobia, rates of depression in the lesbian community may decrease. With greater lesbian visibility (in society and the media) and more widespread acceptance of same-sex relationships (marriage equality, professional advancement, improved civil/human rights, religious/spiritual sanction), lesbians may have less reason to direct negative effects toward the self, engage in self-destructive/risky behaviors, and/or isolate, all factors associated with clinical depression. As previously noted, self-acceptance and coming out may have positive effects in terms of mental health, including reducing the risk for depression.

SUBSTANCE ABUSE AND DEPENDENCE

The trend of an increase in drug use in LGBT adolescents' population continues into adulthood; specifically, tobacco dependence and alcohol abuse/dependence. Most studies on other drugs target focus on and investigate the gay male population; however, a small study from New York suggests lesbian and bisexual women have an increase use of methamphetamine, cocaine, MDMA, ketamine, GHB, and LSD during their lifetime (16). This study is biased in that it specifically looked at dance club attendees, who may skew the data because this population may not represent lesbians in the general population.

In regard to nicotine dependence, studies show that both adolescent and adult lesbians have higher smoking rates than their heterosexual peers. In adolescents, it appears that girls with a history of abuse, violence within the family, depressive symptoms, and stressful life events are more at risk for regularly smoking (17). In fact, there are numerous studies that confirm that younger lesbians (>50 years old) are 3 times more likely to smoke than their heterosexual counterparts. Lesbians in adulthood report an increased level in stress and depression as contributing factors for their nicotine dependence. It would not be much of an extrapolation to say that nicotine dependence that starts in youth continues into adulthood despite other factors such as higher education and successful careers among lesbians.

Nicotine dependence has a large impact on healthcare costs and should be carefully monitored and cessation encouraged among lesbians who continue to smoke. However, care should be taken in regard to new nicotine partial agonists used to help patients quit smoking because this may precipitate depression and suicidal ideation among this high-risk group.

In regard to alcohol abuse and dependence, there appear to be differences among bisexual women and lesbians regarding consumption (18). Heterosexual females had the lowest rates of drinking alcohol; however, they also had less childhood sexual abuse, early alcohol use, and depression. Bisexual women appeared to have higher rates of alcohol consumption than lesbians; however, sample sizes were very small, and more studies among these subgroups would be useful.

There is evidence that lesbians have increased rates of excessive alcohol use compared with heterosexual females. Other risk factors such as family history of alcoholism and drug abuse, rape and childhood sexual abuse, and report of having made a suicide attempt were higher in lesbians (19).

There is no clear understanding of continued nicotine and alcohol abuse/dependence among lesbians, but the literature supports multiple factors that may contribute to these issues. What is clear is that high risk of substance abuse and dependence begins at an early age and continues despite higher education and successful careers among lesbians. Interventions would best be started during adolescence with regard to drug education and surveillance to minimize continued substance abuse into adulthood.

TAILORED PSYCHIATRIC CARE

Lesbians access healthcare services less often than do heterosexual women, and the barriers to care are multifactorial. Barriers to care may be structural, financial, personal, or cultural and often result in lesbians being underserved when it comes to mental healthcare. Half of LGBT adults have withheld their sexual orientation from their healthcare provider. One-quarter of LGBT individuals have withheld sexual behavior information from their healthcare provider (20). Lesbians report experiences of stigma, harassment, discrimination, ostracism, abuse or, at worst, assault with disclosure (either voluntary or involuntary) of their sexual orientation. Lesbians have described experiences of perceived stigma, institutionalized homophobia, and discrimination in access to certain healthcare services (e.g., fertility treatments).

Institutionalized, professional, or personal homophobia within the psychiatric community may be seen in (i) lack of specific training for psychiatric trainees in providing culturally competent care for lesbians, (ii) lack of medical training in mental health problems pertinent to lesbians (higher rates of alcohol and tobacco abuse, internalized homophobia, same-sex intimate partner violence, "lesbian bed death," diversity in sexuality and sexual dysfunction), (iii) negative countertransference or discomfort in discussing topics related to lesbians, or (iv) outright disapproval or moral condemnation of lesbians. More ubiquitously, lesbians may not disclose their sexual orientation if their psychiatrist assumes a heterosexual background in taking the clinical history, which may reinforce a "closeted" individual to remain so.

These factors emphasize the importance of approaching psychiatric sexual history taking in a manner that promotes healthy disclosure. When taking a sexual history, the use of gender-neutral or "inclusive" language, as well as open-ended questions about identity, behavior, and orientation, encourages a broader range of disclosure. An affirmative, nonjudgmental tone is essential, with positive feedback with welcoming disclosure. Normalizing disclosure of minority sexual orientation with encouragement and follow-up questions elaborating on our patient's unique life experience can be therapeutically ameliorative in establishing and maintaining rapport.

Some openly lesbian and gay psychiatrists suggest that selective disclosure of the psychiatrist's sexual orientation to their certain lesbian patients may be therapeutically beneficial (21). Regardless of the sexual orientation of the individual psychiatrist, all psychiatrists must strive to create a setting and develop a therapeutic alliance that provides lesbian patients with culturally competent care addressing their specific mental health needs. We can cultivate the concept of a "safe space," where external realities of homophobia, stigma, ignorance, and intolerance are temporarily lifted so that lesbian patients may feel free to explore whatever troubles them without fear of negative repercussions (22).

The dearth of research on lesbian mental health is exacerbated by the fact these studies have historically focused on Caucasian, urban/suburban, adolescent or adult, middle class lesbians with at least a high school education. For lesbian patients who are apart of other minority communities, care should be taken to tailor psychiatric services for their unique needs. Individuals from ethnic/racial minority, socioeconomically disadvantaged, rural, disabled, or immigrant populations who identify as lesbians may have poorer mental health outcomes (23) and therefore warrant multifaceted assessment (i.e., narrative cultural formulation) (24) to examine how diverse cultural factors may affect their mental health. These women may struggle with the triple burden of discrimination based on gender, sexual orientation combined with another minority status. However, some authors argue that lesbians who have a strong bond within their minority community might better adapt emotionally over the long term; that is, if they have previously successfully negotiated coping with adversity caused by their (other) minority status. Of equal importance is access to translation services or culture brokers for lesbians whose primary language is not English. This is essential for at least two reasons: (i) being able to effectively communicate and (ii) being equipped to assess cultural nuances/differences in language when describing female same-sex relationships. Integrating cultural formulation into the standardized clinical diagnostic evaluation will go a long way in developing a more in-depth and comprehensive psychiatric assessment and treatment plan.

Mental health clinicians cannot generalize about the optimal disclosure or "out" status for an individual lesbian. Some can achieve a level of emotional well-being with different levels of disclosure: full or partial (i.e., choosing to selectively disclose to friends, family, workplace colleagues, religious/spiritual group members or sexual partners, or any combination of the above). One can adopt the use of selective-disclosure as an adaptive response to a homophobic society or environment (25).

In conclusion, with improved psychiatric and medical education about lesbian health, a commitment by the psychiatric research community to examine lesbian mental health, and the individual psychiatrist's dedication to ensure culturally competent care for our lesbian patients, we can begin to address the clinical disparities in psychiatric care for lesbians.

References

1. Laumann EO, Gagnon JH, Michael RT, et al. *The Social Organization of Sexuality: Sexual Practices in the United States.* Chicago: University of Chicago Press, 1994.
2. Downing C. *Myths and Mysteries of Same-sex Love.* New York: Continuum Publishing Co., 1989.
3. Rich A. *Dream of a Common Language 1974–1977.* New York: Norton, W. W. & Company, Inc., 1993.
4. Rosenbloom S. *She's So Cool, So Smart, So Beautiful: Must Be a Girl Crush.* Available at http://www.nytimes.com/2005/08/11/fasion/thursdaystyles/11CRUSH.
5. Cass VC. Homosexual identity formation: A theoretical model. *J Homosex* 1979;4(3): 219–235.
6. Savin-Williams RC, Diamond LM. Sexual identity trajectories among sexual-minority youths: Gender comparisons. *Arch Sex Behav* 2000;29(6):607–627.
7. Koh AS, Ross LK. Mental health issues: A comparison of lesbian, bisexual and heterosexual women. *J Homosex* 2006;51(1):33–57.
8. Gilman SE, Cochran SD, Mays VM, et al. Risk of psychiatric disorders among individuals reporting same-sex sexual partners in the national comorbidity survey. *Am J Public Health* 2001;91(6):933–939.

9. Sorenson L, Roberts SJ. Lesbian uses of and satisfaction with mental health services: Results from Boston Lesbian Health Project. *J Homosex* 1997;33(1):35–49.5

10. Silenzio VM, Pena JB, Duberstein PR, et al. Sexual orientation and risk factors for suicidal ideation and suicide attempts among adolescents and young adults. *Am J Public Health* 2007;97(11):2017–2019.

11. Eisenberg ME, Resnick MD. Suicidality among gay, lesbian and bisexual youth: The role of protective factors. *J Adolesc Health* 2006;39(5):662–668.

12. Rogers TL, Emanuel K., Bradford J. Sexual minorities seeking services: A retrospective study of the mental health concerns of lesbian and bisexual women. *J Lesbian Studies* 2003;7: 127–146.

13. Cochran SD, Mays VM, Sullivan JG. Prevalence of mental disorders, psychological distress and mental health services use among lesbian, gay, and bisexual adults in the United States. *J Counsel Clin Psychol* 2003;71:53–61.

14. Kerr SK, Emerison AM. *A review of lesbian depression and anxiety.* In Mathy RM, Kerr SK, eds. *Lesbian and Bisexual Women's Mental Health.* Binghamton, NY: The Hawthorn Press Inc; 2003:143–162.

15. Grossman AH, Kerner MS. Self-esteem and supportiveness as predictors of emotional distress in gay male and lesbian youth. *J Homosex* 1998;35(2):25–39.

16. Parsons JT, Kelly BC, Wells BE. Differences in club drug use between heterosexual and lesbian/bisexual females. *Addict Behav* 2006;31(12):2344–2349.

17. Simantov E, Schoen C, Klein JD. Health-compromising behaviors: Why do adolescents smoke or drink? Identifying underlying risk and protective factors. *Arch Pediatr Adolesc Med* 2000;154(10):1025–1033.

18. Wilsnack SC, Hughes, TL, Johnson TP, et al. Drinking and drinking-related problems among heterosexual and sexual minority women. *J Stud Alcohol Drugs* 2008;69(1): 129–139.

19. Roberts SJ, Grindel CG, Patsdaughter CA, et al. Lesbian use and abuse of alcohol: Results of The Boston Lesbian Health Project II. *Subst Abuse* 2004;25(4):1–9.

20. Diamant AL, Wold C. Sexual orientation and variation in physical and mental health status among women. *J Women's Health* 2003;12:41–49.

21. Langdridge D. Gay affirmative therapy: A theoretical framework and defense. *J Gay Lesbian Psychother* 2007;11(1/2):27–44.

22. Crowley C, Harré R, Lunt I. Safe spaces and sense of identity: Views and experiences of lesbian, gay and bisexual young people. *J Gay Lesbian Psychother* 2007;11(1/2):127–144.

23. Solarz A. Institute of Medicine, National Academy of Sciences. Lesbian health: Current assessment. Washington, DC: National Academy Press, 1999.

24. Gaw A. *Cross-Cultural Psychiatry.* Washington, DC: American Psychiatric Publishing, 2001.

25. Igartua KJ. Therapy with lesbian couples. *Can J Psychiatry* 1998;43(4):391–396.

10 Bisexuals

Serena Yuan Volpp

INTRODUCTION

The notion that people could be defined by their sexual desires and behaviors, that is, that there was such a person as "a homosexual" or "a heterosexual" began to appear in medical discourse in the mid to late 19th century (1). As Harvard professor Marjorie Garber points out in her comprehensive book *Bisexuality and the Eroticism of Everyday Life*, the meaning of the word bisexuality has changed over time. In current times, bisexual generally refers to a person who is sexually attracted to both men and women. In the 19th and early 20th centuries, however, bisexual referred to being of two sexes. Through his career, Freud, for example, used the term bisexuality in various ways: as having two sets of sexual organs, as having both a male and a female psyche, as having a fluid, divided sexuality, and, as desiring both men and women as sexual partners (2).

In the late 19th century, the sexologist Havelock Ellis used this earlier notion of bisexuality to help explain homosexuality, or what was called "inversion" at the time. Using the heterosexual paradigm, he hypothesized that a male invert's "feminine" side desired men, whereas the female invert's "masculine" side desired women. The person who was attracted to both sexes was described as a "psychosexual hermaphrodite" by the sexologist Richard von Krafft-Ebing. By the end of the first decades of the 20th century, the term "bisexual" had become to mean both the prior notion of two sexes in one individual as well the person who was attracted to two sexes (2).

Freud conceptualized bisexuality as an intrinsic, original state at birth. He hypothesized that as a child matured, he or she would repress the homosexual attraction as per societal expectations (2). (Garber points out that this idea was originally that of Freud's friend Wilhelm Fliess [2].) Early in his career, in keeping with the 19th-century scientific belief that humans were constitutionally bisexual (of two sexes), Freud felt that bisexuality was anatomically or biologically determined. He later shifted to a belief that bisexuality was psychologically and culturally determined.

The mid-20th century brought us the famed Kinsey reports (*Sexual Behavior in the Human Male* and *Sexual Behavior in the Human Female*) (3,4) with their seven-point scale of sexual attraction (from 0, or exclusively heterosexual, to 6, or exclusively homosexual). Interestingly, although those in the category of 1 through 5 were presumably bisexual to various degrees, the word "bisexual" was not used in the scale—the 3 rating, for example, was described as "equally heterosexual and homosexual." Although the reports scandalized the American public by exposing the degree to which Americans had engaged in same-sex fantasy and activity, the researchers in fact found a high rate of bisexuality (2). The rate of "overt experience" with and "psychologic response" to both sexes was 46% in the men (3) and 28% in the women (4).

As seen even in the Kinsey reportage, in current usage, bisexuality encompasses different meanings. Just as with homosexuality or heterosexuality, there are different components of sexuality, including sexual desire, sexual behavior, and sexual identity. The Kinsey study was reporting on desire/fantasy and behavior together. Studies that include bisexuality as an epidemiologic variable more often than not conflate these different facets, as will be discussed below.

Unlike homosexuality, bisexuality was never classified as a mental illness. In both scientific and political discourse, bisexuality is often either subsumed under homosexuality or left out altogether (5). In one of the biggest "sex studies" in the United States since the Kinsey report, Laumann et al.'s *The Social Organization of Sexuality: Sexual Practices in the United States*, bisexuality is not even listed in the index (6). This chapter attempts to redress this historical elision and omission.

EPIDEMIOLOGY

The data on the incidence of bisexuality are difficult to compare, given the variation of definitions of bisexuality. The data from the Kinsey report are listed above. Two more recent large studies have been that of Laumann et al. (6), mentioned above, which surveyed residents of the United States through the National Health and Social Life Survey, and that of Sandfort (7), which surveyed people in 10 European nations. Laumann et al. (6) found the prevalence of bisexual behavior among men to be between 0.7% and 5.8% (in the previous year and since puberty, respectively), whereas Sandfort found a rate between 0.6% and 8.6% (in the previous year and over lifetime, respectively) (7). For women, the prevalence of bisexual behavior was found to be between 0.3% and 3.7% by Laumann (6), and between 0.1% and 3.9% by Sandfort (7).

Estimates of those who claim bisexual identity are generally lower than estimates of those who report bisexual behavior. Laumann et al. reported that less than 1% of those surveyed identified as bisexual (0.8% of men, 0.5% of women) (6). In a smaller community-based study of 4824 adults in Australia, Jorm et al. found that the percentage of adults self-defining as bisexual varied with age—for the age 20- to 24-year-old group, the prevalence of bisexual identity was 1.8% in men and 2.7% in women, for the 40- to 44-year-old group, the prevalence of bisexual identity was 0.8% in both men and women (8).

Reports of bisexual behavior and identity have been found to be higher in African American and Latino men than in white men in the United States (5). In a study done by the CDC, demographics of men with AIDS were analyzed. Of the 65,389 men who had reported sex with men since 1977, 26% were bisexually active, and bisexual behavior was more common in black (41%) and Hispanic (31%) than in white (21%) men (9). Note that these subjects are all men who reported sex with men. A more detailed discussion of ethnic minorities is found toward the end of this chapter.

METHODOLOGICAL PROBLEMS WHEN DISCUSSING DISPARITIES IN MENTAL HEALTH IN THE BISEXUAL POPULATION

As one can infer from the above discussion about definitions and epidemiology, one of the primary challenges in any discussion of sexual orientation and disparities in mental health is definitional. This challenge is even more pronounced when conducting research on or discussing the research on the bisexual population. Dimensions measured include, but are not limited to, sexual attraction, sexual behavior, and sexual identity. Different subpopulations are sampled, depending on the dimension used. Whether one dimension of sexual orientation is more highly correlated to disparities in mental health than the others is currently unknown. As Cochran and Mays (10) point out, studies that only measure behavior may not use individuals without recent sexual activity, which may bias results around mental health correlates in various ways, depending on the outcome of interest. They also note that studies that only use the behavioral dimension may include generally heterosexual individuals with some same-sex activity related to sexual impulsivity; this could then inflate prevalence of disorders associated with impulsivity, for example.

The biggest challenge in terms of discussing mental health disparities in the bisexual population is the lack of studies that separate out the bisexual population. Bisexuals are commonly grouped together with gay men or women (i.e., lesbians) based on behavior—many studies pool together all men who have sex with men, for example, even if some of these individuals have engaged in sexual activity with women as well. Studies have at times collapsed homosexuals and bisexuals together in their results and discussion even if they have identified bisexuals separately in their sample (11,12).

Another problem in studying bisexuals and mental health is that of sampling. Many studies, especially through the mid-1990s, used convenience sampling, that is, finding people who identify themselves as gay, lesbian, or bisexual through places such as gay and lesbian community centers, gay bars, or gay and lesbian events. Depending on the source, these subpopulations could be biased; for example, those at a gay pride event may be overall less distressed than those who are not comfortable enough to go to such an event, or data from those found at a gay bar or club may be biased toward overuse of substances. Only more recently, researchers have taken advantage of population-based surveys that include a measure of sexual orientation. Although these surveys reduce selection bias and often include a heterosexual group as a comparison, the sample sizes of nonheterosexuals are usually very small, which means that in practice, bisexuals are usually grouped with gay men or lesbians.

Response bias may also be a factor, whereby those who identify as sexual minorities may be more likely to report potentially stigmatizing information, such as a history of suicide attempts, for a few reasons. There is some evidence that sexual minorities are more likely to have received counseling than heterosexuals (13), which may make them less defensive about disclosing mental health problems to researchers. As well, many sexual minorities go through a self-reflective period of recognizing and coming to terms with their sexual orientation, which again may allow them to be more open about sharing psychological or mental health issues. As Ilan Meyer points out, the so-called "coming out" process may also serve as a focal point for recall "that could lead to recall bias that exaggerates past difficulties" (14). Publication bias is also an issue, whereby studies with positive findings, showing increased rates of mental disorders in sexual minorities, whether homosexual or bisexual, may be more likely to be published than those with negative findings.

MENTAL HEALTH ISSUES

As Dodge and Sandfort note in their 2007 review article, the few studies that have examined bisexuals as a separate group often have found elevated rates of mental health problems as compared with homosexuals and heterosexuals (5). I will describe these studies.

MOOD AND ANXIETY DISORDERS

In a community-based study in Australia with 4824 adults (71 bisexual, 78 homosexual) conducted by Jorm et al. (8), participants self-defined their sexual orientation through a single question. The study found that bisexuals scored higher on measures of anxiety, depression, and negative affect than homosexuals or heterosexuals, with the homosexual group scores in between the bisexual and heterosexual groups. Bisexuals reported more childhood adversity, more current adverse life events, less positive support from family, more negative support from friends, and more financial difficulties than the heterosexual group. Compared with the homosexual group, the bisexual group reported more current adverse life events and more financial difficulties. Note that HIV status and variables related to stigma and/or discrimination were not addressed.

Warner et al. (12) reported on a cross-sectional survey of 1258 self-identified gay, lesbian, and bisexual individuals (including 85 bisexual men and 114 bisexual women) in England and Wales. Bisexual men scored significantly higher than gay men on the Clinical Interview Schedule (CIS-R), which assesses presence of symptoms associated with depressed mood and anxiety. However, when the scores were dichotomized to clinical case (12 and above)/no case (11 and below), there was no statistically significant difference between gay men and bisexual men. There were also no significant differences found between bisexual and lesbian women. Rates of cases overall were high in the sample as a whole: case rates were 42% for gay men, 52% for bisexual men, 43% for lesbians, and 46% for bisexual women, compared with previously reported community rates of 12% in men and 20% in women. Note that this survey sample was recruited through a snowball sampling method that can bias recruitment toward those who are willing to participate in the research topic (in this case, sexuality and well-being); it is possible that the subjects were more psychologically distressed than the general gay/lesbian/bisexual population.

What about bisexual adolescents? In a rare study of adolescents that separated out individuals with both-sex partners from individuals with same-sex-only and opposite-sex-only partners, Udry and Chantala (15) reported on data from the National Longitudinal Study of Adolescent Health, using a school-based sample of 20,745 adolescents enrolled in grades 7 through 12. Bisexuality was defined behaviorally. Although boys with same-sex only partners were more likely to report being depressed than boys with opposite-sex only partners, boys with partners of both sexes were not more likely to report being depressed than boys with opposite-sex only partners. However, the girls with partners of both sexes were more likely than girls in the same-sex only and opposite-sex only groups to report being depressed.

SUICIDE

The gay, lesbian, bisexual population has been found in many studies to have a higher rate of suicidal ideation and suicide attempts than the general population. Only a few studies have separated out the bisexual population. Paul et al. (16) studied 2881 men who have sex with men (MSM) in the United States. Sexual orientation was determined by behavior and/or self-identification. All men either reported having had sex with a man since age 14 or self-identified as gay or bisexual. Of the sample, 9% reported themselves to be bisexual (84% reported themselves as homosexual or gay, 4% as other, and 3% as heterosexual). Suicidal plans and attempts were highest among those identified as bisexual or "other." Thirty percent of bisexuals reported having had a suicide plan, versus 25% of "other" MSM, 20% of homosexual/gay MSM, and 17% of heterosexual MSM. In terms of suicide attempts, 21% of "other" MSM and 16% of bisexual MSM reported a previous suicide attempt, versus 12% of heterosexual MSM and 11% of homosexual/gay MSM.

Jorm et al. (8), in the above-mentioned Australian study, also found that bisexuals scored higher on suicidality measures than homosexuals or heterosexuals. Here the difference between the bisexual and homosexual groups was not statistically significant, but the suicidality ratings were significantly higher in both the bisexual group and the homosexual group than in the heterosexual group.

In Warner's study in England and Wales (12), more than half of the bisexual group (55% of the men and 57% of the women) had considered suicide, and a quarter to a third (27% of the men and 33% of the women) had attempted suicide. Although high, these rates were not significantly different than those of the gay men and lesbian groups.

Turning again to adolescents, in a compilation of four population-based high school studies (the Youth Risk Behavior Surveys) in Vermont and Massachusetts, sexual orientation was defined behaviorally. Robin et al. (17) found that the prevalence of suicide attempts requiring medical attention in the previous year was highest among students with both-sex partners. In Vermont, the prevalences were 4.5% for students with opposite-sex partners, 5.6% for students with same-sex partners, and 26.8% for students with both-sex partners. In Massachusetts, they were 4.5%, 7.8%, and 31.6%, respectively. Since they found that students with both-sex partners reported a much higher rate of being forced to have sexual intercourse in their lifetime, the authors controlled for this variable, as well as age and gender in logistic regressions. The students with both-sex partners still had significantly higher odds of having made a suicide attempt requiring medical attention over the students with opposite-sex partners (OR = 4.84; 95% CI, 2.95–7.96 for Vermont, OR = 5.06, 95% CI, 2.74–9.34 for Massachusetts), whereas the odds ratio for the students with same-sex partners were not statistically different than the students with opposite-sex partners.

Udry and Chantala (15) also found that female adolescents with both-sex partners reported higher rates of suicidality than females with same-sex-partners, females with opposite sex-partners, and females without any sex experiences. However, the males with both-sex partners did not have a significantly higher probability of reporting suicidal thoughts than the males with opposite-sex partners.

In a unique study, Mathy et al. (18) compared bisexual men and women with transgender individuals on several mental health variables. This was a secondary analysis of data that had been collected on the Web site of a major news organization. The sample used for this analysis consisted of 1457 bisexual males, 792 bisexual females, and 73 transgender individuals (current gender unspecified). They reported higher rates of prior suicidal ideation and past suicide attempts among bisexual women and transgender individuals than among bisexual men. Note that the results of this study cannot be said to be representative of the bisexual or transgender population at large, or even of bisexual and transgender Internet users. However, it does point to the need for further studies comparing bisexual men with bisexual women as well as with transgender individuals to better understand the effect of gender and gender identity.

VIOLENCE

In Robin et al.'s study of adolescents in Vermont and Massachusetts (17), a higher percentage of students with both-sex partners reported having carried a weapon in the prior 30 days (48% in Vermont and 49% in Massachusetts) than students with opposite-sex partners (25%, 26%) and students with same-sex partners (23%, 34%). Students with both-sex partners had greater odds than their peers with opposite-sex partners of being in a physical fight during the prior 12 months and of being threatened or injured with a weapon at school. Note that students with same-sex partners in Vermont were significantly less likely than their peers with opposite sex partners either to carry a weapon (OR = 0.54; 95% CI, 0.33–0.90) or to have been in a physical fight (OR = 0.62; 95% CI, 0.42–0.90). The implication here is that adolescents with same-sex partners only versus adolescents with both-sex partners may be distinct subpopulations.

ALCOHOL AND DRUG USE

In Robin et al.'s study (17), students with both-sex partners were more likely than students with opposite-sex partners to report ever using cocaine (Vermont OR = 4.43; 95% CI, 3.34–5.88, Massachusetts OR = 3.86; 95% CI, 2.56–5.83). The odds of using marijuana were also more than twice as high for students with both-sex partners over students with opposite-sex partners. Students with same-sex partners were comparable to students with opposite-sex partners in their cocaine use in Vermont, and slightly more likely to use cocaine than their peers with opposite-sex peers in Massachusetts. In Udry and Chantala's study of 20,745 7th through 12th graders, in which sexual orientation was defined through sexual behavior, boys with both-sex partners were more likely than boys with same-sex only or opposite-sex only partners to report cigarette smoking, alcohol use, and any illegal drug use (15). Bisexual female adolescents were found to be at higher risk for cigarette smoking, alcohol use, and any illegal drug use than any of the other female groups as well. Note that both bisexual males and females were found to be at higher risk for selling sex for drugs or money than any of the other groups; that is, either the individuals with same-sex-only partners or the individuals with opposite-sex-only partners.

What about adults? Meyer et al. (19) published a study recently which examined variability within a gay, lesbian, and bisexual population. Eighteen percent of the 388 respondents identified as bisexual. DSM-IV diagnoses were made with a computer-assisted interview. Fifty-one percent of those with a self-reported bisexual identity reported a substance use disorder, leading to an adjusted odds ratio of 1.8 (95% CI, 1.0, 3.0) for a substance use disorder in bisexuals as compared with lesbian or gay individuals. However, in Warner et al.'s study (12), lifetime use of drugs and hazardous drinking was similar between bisexual men and women and gay men and lesbians, and gay men were more likely than bisexual men to have used drugs in the prior month.

EATING DISORDERED BEHAVIOR

In Robin et al.'s study of adolescents in Vermont and Massachusetts (17), students with both-sex partners were significantly more likely than opposite-sex peers to engage in vomiting and using laxatives for weight control (Vermont OR = 3.46; 95% CI, 2.35–5.08, Massachusetts OR = 5.87; 95% CI, 3.37–10.20). Students with same-sex partners were more likely to engage in these practices than students with opposite-sex partners in Vermont, but not in Massachusetts.

In French and colleagues' study of eating disordered behavior in adolescents (11), the authors collapsed the self-identified homosexual and bisexual groups together for their statistical analysis although they reported raw numbers separately. They did this despite having more bisexual individuals (131 male, 144 female) than homosexual participants (81 male, 38 female). Their findings that "homosexual males" were more likely to report poor body image, frequent dieting, and binge/purge behaviors than heterosexual males includes bisexual males. They stated that frequent dieting (five or more times per year) was the only measure that differed significantly between homosexual and bisexual males, with 8.9% of the homosexual males endorsing this measure compared with 4.6% of the bisexual males. In terms of raw data, the bisexual male group was between the heterosexual and homosexual male group terms of poor body image and binge eating. Results for the females were not significant except for body image of the "homosexual" group being less likely to perceive themselves to be overweight and more likely to report a positive body image than the heterosexual group. In terms of the raw data, the bisexual group ratings were in between the heterosexual and homosexual group on these measures.

MENTAL HEALTH SERVICE UTILIZATION

I was unable to find any studies addressing healthcare access and service utilization of the bisexual population in specific. I will thus describe some data available about sexual minorities in general. Cochran and colleagues (13) analyzed data from the McArthur Foundation National Survey of Midlife Development in the United States (MIDUS), which was a population-based study of over 3000 adults between the ages of 25 and 74 years. They found that gay-bisexual men were more likely than the heterosexual men to have seen a mental health provider in the prior 12 months (adjusted OR = 3.38; 95% CI, 1.05–5.41), as were lesbian-bisexual women compared with heterosexual women (adjusted OR = 3.37; 95% CI, 1.41–8.08). Both sexual minority groups were also more likely than their heterosexual counterparts to have seen a general physician for a mental/emotional complaint, and to have attended a self-help group in the prior 12 months. Note that despite the sample size of over 3000 adults, there were only 37 individuals in each of the gay-bisexual groups (male and female), which illustrates why it is difficult to separate out the bisexual group for analysis in these types of population-based studies.

The study of Heck et al. (20), which described healthcare access as found in a probability sample (the 1997–2003 National Health Interview Survey), reported that women in same-sex relationships are at higher risk of poor access to healthcare. In the survey, sexual orientation was not ascertained per se; participants were described as either being in a same-sex relationship (SSR) or opposite-sex relationship (OSR), depending on the gender of and relationship with other household members. Thus, bisexual women could either be in the SSR group or the OSR group, depending on whom they were in a relationship with at the time of the survey. SSR women were less likely than OSR women to have health insurance coverage, were more likely to have unmet medical needs because of the cost, were less likely to have seen a medical provider in the prior year, and were less likely to have a usual source of healthcare, this despite overall being more highly educated and more likely to be employed than the OSR women. SSR men, on the other hand, were more likely than OSR men to have seen a healthcare provider in the past year, even after controlling for self-reported health status. This study represented the partnered population, which is more likely to have access to healthcare than single individuals (12% of male and 17% of female SSR had health insurance through a domestic partner or someone else). Note that coverage by health insurance is influenced by marital status. In the 2003 National Health Interview Survey, only 12.6% of married people were uninsured, compared with 26.9% of people who had never been married and 31.7% of those living with a partner (21).

Note that none of these studies are qualitative, that is, none of them describe the experience of the participants. Certainly, there are multiple first-person narratives about difficulties finding providers who are knowledgeable about bisexuality (e.g., do not make assumptions such as that all bisexual people have sex with men and women simultaneously). I will speak more specifically to the issue of "biphobia" below.

MENTAL HEALTH AND BISEXUAL ETHNIC MINORITIES

There are few studies on mental health issues in ethnic minorities within the sexual minority population; of those that exist, the quality is variable. For bisexuals, unfortunately, this is even more the case. Many have written about the complexity of holding multiple minority statuses and the potentially negative consequences thereof on mental health, especially vis-à-vis the experience of discrimination. This includes racial discrimination from the general population, and also more specifically from within the gay, lesbian, bisexual community, and discrimination based on sexual orientation or homophobia both from the heterosexual community at large and from within one's own racial or ethnic group.

There are some data to suggest that sexual minorities from nonwhite communities may be more reluctant to identify as gay, lesbian, or bisexual and/or to disclose this identification. In the Laumann study (6) of sexual practices in the United States, for example, there was a striking difference by race/ethnicity in the proportion of people who claimed a homosexual or bisexual identity in relation to those who admitted to having had same-sex desire. For white men, this percentage was 40.5%, that is, 40.5% of men who reported same-sex desire identified as homosexual or bisexual. For black men, this was 22.2%; for Hispanic men, 26.6%. For Asian men, 0% identified as homosexual or bisexual despite 17.1% admitting to same-sex desire. For women, the trend was similar. Over the last 10 years or so, the phrase "down low" has come to refer to black men who are behaviorally bisexual (have sex with other men as well as women), but who identify as heterosexual. Note that this occurs in all communities, but because of the proliferation of discussion in the media about this phenomenon in regard to rates of HIV infection in the black community, the term has come to be used almost exclusively in relation to the black community (22). Theories relating to the lower rates of identification and disclosure of sexual minority status within racial/ethnic minority communities include cultural expectations around family role obligations, fear of ostracization from families, and conflicts over religion and same-sex desire. Given the complexity of issues in these varied ethnic communities, a much longer discussion is deserved.

Studies, however, have been inconclusive about whether gay, lesbian, bisexual ethnic minorities do have worse mental health outcomes than either the white sexual minority population or the heterosexual ethnic minority population. Again, in terms of national or regional probability surveys, these data are not available for the bisexual community specifically. One such study, the National Latino and Asian American Survey (NLAAS), used self-reported markers of sexual orientation status, including identity and recent reports of sexual experiences, in a sample of 4407 Latinos and Asian Americans in the United States (23). Unfortunately, the results for bisexuals were grouped together with the lesbian and gay samples. Lesbian and bisexual women were more likely to have a recent (OR = 1.94; CI, 1.17, 3.21) and lifetime (OR = 1.63; CI, 1.04, 2.55) history of depressive disorders and recent history of drug abuse or dependency (OR = 12.05; CI, 1.10, 132.08). Gay and bisexual men were more likely than heterosexual men to report a suicide attempt within the last year (OR = 6.43; CI, 1.63, 25.36), but no significant differences were found in lifetime or recent prevalence of psychiatric disorders. The numbers were too small to separate the Latino and Asian American groups for analysis. Although problematic to make a direct comparison to other studies, the authors did some comparisons to the National Comorbidity Survey (NCS) of Gilman et al. (24), which was also a population-based survey examining rates of psychiatric disorders that included a measure of sexual orientation. In comparison with sexual minorities in the NCS, lower rates of psychiatric disorders were found in the Latino and Asian American sexual minority group. Thus, although Latino and Asian American sexual minorities may be at higher risk for psychiatric disorders than their non-sexual minority counterparts, their ethnicity may be protective to some degree.

EXPLANATIONS FOR DISPARITIES

The research described above cannot be summarized easily. The findings are not consistent. However, there does seem to be a trend that overall bisexuals are found to have higher rates of mental health issues than their homosexual or heterosexual counterparts. If we accept this trend, how might we explain it?

First, a there exists a caveat about research on sexual orientation and mental health in general. As Herek and Garnets point out, mental health issues in the heterosexual population are not attributed to a person's heterosexuality per se, even if the issues are manifested in sexual feelings or behaviors (1). The mental health issues in a nonheterosexual population, likewise, should not a priori implicate the person's sexual orientation as the cause of the issue or problem.

Theories that have been generated about disparities in mental health in minorities include the psychological effects of "minority stress," social stigma, isolation, discrimination, alienation, and violence. The experience of stigma and victimization by the gay, lesbian, bisexual population has been well documented. Since many of the published population-based studies that include data on sexual minorities were not designed to answer the question of why disparities exist, studies with questions about mental health generally have not included questions that relate to discrimination or stigma. One study that did include several of these variables in addition to some mental health indicators was the National Survey of Midlife Development in the United States. As reported by Mays and Cochran (25), sexual orientation was self-identified (heterosexual, homosexual, or bisexual); however, the homosexual and bisexual populations were pooled together in the analysis. The homosexual/bisexual group reported lifetime and day-to-day experiences of discrimination at higher rates than the heterosexual group, and about 42% attributed the discrimination in whole or in part to their sexual orientation. When discrimination was controlled for in the analysis, associations between sexual orientation and the presence of any psychiatric disorder was attenuated. Thus, elevated rates of mental health issues could be caused by the experience of discrimination, as opposed to any factors intrinsic to sexual orientation.

Warner's cross-sectional survey in England and Wales (12) was able to speak to the bisexual experience more specifically. Eighty-three percent of respondents (gay/lesbian/bisexual) reported having experienced at least one act of hostility or discrimination, including damage to property, personal attacks, or verbal insults in the past 5 years, or insults or bullying at school. Having been attacked in the past 5 years and having been bullied at school were associated with attempted suicide. Having been attacked or insulted in the past 5 years, and having been insulted at school were factors associated with higher scores on the Clinical Interview Schedule. Although the bisexual group experienced similar levels of hostility, they were less likely to attribute the discrimination to their sexuality.

A unique issue for the bisexual population is the fear of bisexuals themselves, or so-called "biphobia," from both the heterosexual and the gay/lesbian community. In 2002, Herek published the first empirical study based on a national probability sample that examined heterosexuals' attitudes toward bisexuals (26). In this telephone survey, 1335 respondents were asked to use a thermometer rating from 0 to 100 to describe their feelings toward various social and demographic groups. Overall, feelings toward bisexuals were lower, or less favorable, than toward any other group, including religious, racial, ethnic, and political groups, except for injection drug users. Previous qualitative studies have suggested numerous explanations for negative attitudes toward bisexuals, including assuming that bisexuals are as a group sexually nonmonogamous or promiscuous, fearing bisexuals as vectors of HIV and other sexually transmitted diseases, and feeling anxious about the challenge to the heterosexual/homosexual dichotomy. Hostility toward bisexuals from gays and lesbians has also been described and written about. Many members of the gay and lesbian community resent bisexuals for maintaining "heterosexual privilege" by dating people of the opposite sex. Some gays and lesbians feel that bisexual people are actually gay but afraid to fully "come out" as gay. Thus, feelings of stigmatization or discrimination from both "sides"—straight and gay—may contribute to feelings of psychological distress.

The predominant paradigm of a dichotomized sexuality—heterosexual versus homosexual—has political and social implications in terms of bisexuals finding a community. Psychologically, not having a clear "either/or" orientation may serve as an internal stressor. Note that in Warner et al.'s study (12), gay men were more likely than bisexual men to have recognized their sexual orientation early in life: 26% of the gay men stated they were aware of their sexual orientation by age 10, compared with 8% of the bisexual men. The women, in keeping with other reports, reported being aware of their sexual orientation on average somewhat later, but there was still a difference at the younger end: 15% of the lesbians were aware of their orientation by age 10, compared with 9% of the bisexual women.

Accepting and claiming one's sexual identity may have an impact on levels of psychological distress. In the California Quality of Life Survey conducted in 2004 to 2005 (27), sexual orientation was self-identified and was divided into four categories: lesbian or gay, bisexual, history of same-sex partners with current heterosexual identity (homosexually experienced heterosexual), and heterosexual. The "homosexually experienced heterosexual" would, in most other studies, be classified as bisexual. Among women, bisexual women reported the highest level of psychological distress (as measured by the Kessler Psychological Distress Scale), followed by homosexually experienced heterosexual women, lesbians, and, last, heterosexual women. After controlling for demographic variables, lesbian and bisexual women still had higher psychological distress levels than heterosexual women. Among men, a similar pattern was seen. Homosexually experienced heterosexual men had the highest level of psychological distress, followed by bisexual men, gay men, and then exclusively heterosexual men. After adjusting for confounding, both homosexually experienced heterosexual men and gay men continued to have higher levels of psychological distress than heterosexual men. Thus, in both men and women, those with bisexual identity or behavior reported higher levels of psychological distress than gay men or lesbians prior to adjusting for demographic differences. Yet, these findings suggest that those who label themselves as bisexual and those who label themselves as heterosexual but who have same-sex sexual experience may be two different subgroups in terms of their levels of psychological functioning or levels of distress.

Nondisclosure of sexual minority identity to others has been shown to be a risk factor for depression (28). Warner et al. (12) found in their study that the bisexual group was less likely to be open with their friends and family about their sexuality than were the gay men and lesbians; for example, 77% of the gay men and 74% of the lesbians said their mothers were aware of their sexuality versus 38% of the bisexual men and 39% of the bisexual women. Whereas 84% of the gay men and 86% of the lesbians stated they were "open with all or most friends," only 44% of the bisexual men and 53% of the bisexual women endorsed that item. Without further details, we do not know how the bisexual group represented their identity to friends and family. It is possible, for example, that some people present to heterosexual family members as "straight," while presenting as "gay" to their gay and lesbian friends. Regardless, the inability to be "known" to friends and family for who they feel themselves to be likely takes a psychological toll.

Before ending this section, the studies on adolescents deserve a special caveat. Adolescents are still in an active process of identity formation. Although adolescents with bisexual behavior may be particularly stressed psychologically if they feel they do not have a dichotomized group identity (gay or straight), without more longitudinal studies of sexual identity development, we do not know whether adolescents with bisexual behavior represent either future adults who have bisexual behavior or future adults who identify as bisexual. In Robin et al.'s study of adolescents (17), the Massachusetts survey measured both sexual behavior and sexual identity. They noted that the two did not match; 73% of the students with both-sex partners labeled themselves as gay, lesbian, bisexual, or unsure, and 80% of the students with same-sex partners labeled themselves as heterosexual. They question whether the students in the same-sex partners group had lower rates of at-risk behaviors than the students in the both-sex partners group because they were less likely to identify themselves in the sexual minority. They also raise the question of whether having both-sex partners in adolescence may be part of a cluster of interrelated risk behaviors.

CONCLUSION

When not left out altogether, the bisexual population has been subsumed under the gay and lesbian population not only politically, but also scientifically. As this chapter demonstrates, mixing in bisexuals with gays and lesbians obscures potentially important differences among the sexual minority population. If, as many of the studies described here show, bisexuals are actually more vulnerable than gays and lesbians to different forms of psychological and psychiatric distress, grouping them together not only artificially raises described rates of mental disorders for gays and lesbians, but also hides a population in need of more study and more clinical attention.

To elucidate further the mental health needs of bisexuals, future research must distinguish bisexuals from homosexuals and heterosexuals. Even within the bisexual population, as the discussion of the Robin et al. study and the California Quality of Life Study (17, 27) shows, multiple measures of sexual orientation should be used to gain a better sense of the disparities between sexual behaviors and sexual identities and how each construct is associated with markers of mental health. More careful attention to the intersections of sexual and gender identities will also be helpful in answering questions about what factors make bisexuals vulnerable to mental health issues. Only when we understand these vulnerabilities will we truly be able to provide culturally competent care for this population.

References

1. Herek GM, Garnets LD. Sexual orientation and mental health. *Ann Rev Clin Psychol* 2007;3:353–375.
2. Garber M. *Bisexuality and the Eroticism of Everyday Life*. New York: Routledge, 2000.
3. Kinsey AC, Pomeroy WB, Martin CE, et al. *Sexual Behavior in the Human Male*. Philadelphia: W.B. Saunders, 1948.
4. Kinsey AC, Pomeroy WB, Martin CE, et al. *Sexual Behavior in the Human Female*. Philadelphia: W.B. Saunders, 1953.
5. Dodge B, Sandfort TGM. A review of mental health research on bisexual individuals when compared to homosexual and heterosexual individuals. In: Firestein BA, ed. *Becoming Visible: Counseling Bisexuals Across the Lifespan*. New York: Columbia University Press, 2007:28–51.
6. Laumann EO, Gagnon JH, Michael RT, et al. *The Social Organization of Sexuality: Sexual Practices in the United States*. Chicago: University of Chicago Press, 1994.
7. Sandfort TGM. Homosexual and bisexual behavior in European countries. In: Hubert MC, Bajos N, Sandfort TGM, eds. *Sexual Behaviour and HIV/AIDS in Europe*. London: UCL, 1998:68–105.
8. Jorm AF, Korten AE, Rodgers B, et al. Sexual orientation and mental health: Results from a community survey of young and middle-aged adults. *Br J Psychiatry* 2002;180:423–427.
9. Chu SY, Peterman TA, Doll LS, et al. AIDS in bisexual men in the United States: Epidemiology and transmission to women. *Am J Public Health* 1992;82:220–224.
10. Cochran SD, Mays VM. Prevalence of primary mental health morbidity and suicide symptoms among gay and bisexual men. In: Wolitski RJ, Stall R, Valdiserri RO, eds. *Unequal Opportunity: Health Disparities Affecting Gay and Bisexual Men in the United States*. New York: Oxford University Press, 2008, 97–120.
11. French SA, Story M, Remafedi G, et al. Sexual orientation and prevalence of body dissatisfaction and eating disordered behaviors: A population-based study of adolescents. *Int J Eating Disord* 1996;19(2):119–126.

12. Warner J, McKeown E, Griffin M, et al. Rates and predictors of mental illness in gay men, lesbians, and bisexual men and women: Results from a survey based in England and Wales. *Br J Psychiatry* 2004;185:479–485.
13. Cochran SD, Sullivan JG, Mays VM. Prevalence of mental disorders, psychological distress, and mental health services use among lesbian, gay, and bisexual adults in the United States. *J Consult Clin Psychol* 2003;71:53–61.
14. Meyer IH. Prejudice, social stress, and mental health in lesbian, gay, and bisexual populations: Conceptual issues and research evidence. *Psychol Bull* 2003;129:674–697.
15. Udry JR, Chantala K. Risk assessment of adolescents with same-sex relationships. *J Adolesc Health* 2002;31:84–92.
16. Paul JP, Catania J, Pollack L, et al. Suicide attempts among gay and bisexual men: Lifetime prevalence and antecedents. *Am J Public Health* 2002;92(8):1338–1345.
17. Robin L, Brener ND, Donahue SF, et al. Associations between health risk behaviors and opposite-, same-, and both-sex sexual partners in representative samples of Vermont and Massachusetts high school students. *Arch Pediatr Adolesc Med* 2002;156:349–355.
18. Mathy RM, Lehmann BA, and Kerr DL. Bisexual and transgender identities in a nonclinical sample of North Americans: Suicidal intent, behavioral difficulties, and mental health treatment. *J Bisexual* 2004;3(3/4):93–109.
19. Meyer IH, Dietrich J, Schwartz S. Lifetime prevalence of mental disorders and suicide attempts in diverse lesbian, gay, and bisexual populations. *Am J Public Health* 2008;98(6): 1004–1006.
20. Heck JE, Sell Randall L, Sheinfeld Gorin Ṣ. Health care access among individuals involved in same-sex relationships. *Am J Public Health* 2006; 98(6):1111–1118.
21. Cohen RA, Coriaty-Nelson Z. Health insurance coverage: Estimates from the National Health Interview Survey, 2003. Hyattsville, MD: National Center for Health Statistics, 2004.
22. Malabranche DJ. Bisexually active black men in the United States and HIV: Acknowledging more than the "Down Low." *Arch Sex Behav* 2008;810–816.
23. Cochran SD, Mays VM, Alegria M, et al. Mental health and substance use disorders among Latino and Asian American lesbian, gay, and bisexual adults. *J Consult Clin Psychol* 2007,75:785–794.
24. Gilman SE, Cochran SD, Mays VM, et al. Risk of psychiatric disorders among individuals reporting same-sex sexual partners in the National Comorbidity Survey. *Am J Public Health* 2001;91:933–939.
25. Mays VM, Cochran SD. Mental health correlates of perceived discrimination among lesbian, gay, and bisexual adults in the United States. *Am J Public Health* 2001;91:1869–1876.
26. Herek G. Heterosexuals' attitudes towards bisexual men and women in the United States. *J Sex Res* 2002;39(4):264–274.
27. Cochran SD, Mays VM. Physical health complaints among lesbians, gay men, and bisexual and homosexually experienced heterosexuals: results from the California Quality of Life Survey. *Am J Public Health* 2007;97:2048–2055.
28. Ullrich PM, Lutgendorf SK, Stapleton JT. Concealment of homosexual identity, social support and CD4 count among HIV-seropositive gay men. *J Psychosom Res* 2003;54: 205–212.

11 Transgender Persons

Richard R. Pleak

INTRODUCTION

From the last decade of the 20th century and ongoing into the early 21st century, an increasing number of clinicians are being sought out by people for issues related to their gender identity. Most clinicians have had little, if any, training or experience in these issues when first approached for their help. This puts both the clinician and the patient at a disadvantage, a situation that can be rectified by an open, nonjudgmental approach and willingness to gain knowledge and experience as part of practice-based improvement and life-long learning. People who identity as having gender identity issues often face obstacles in terms of equal protection by nondiscrimination laws, access to general and gender-related healthcare; and societal discrimination and rejection. This chapter seeks to address these disparities of care and offer information and remedies for the clinician by separately exploring these issues in children, adolescents, and adults.

Although people with intersex conditions (disorders of sexual differentiation) may, not uncommonly, have confusion or dilemmas regarding their gender identity, their particular issues are beyond the scope of this chapter. For information about gender identity in intersex individuals, the clinician should consult resources such as the Intersex Society of North America (http://www.isna.org), books such as those by Money (1) and Cohen-Kettenis and Pfäfflin (2), and websites for individual intersex conditions.

TERMS

Many of the terms used in this chapter require brief definitions for how they are being used. Terms relating to gender issues seem to undergo transformation more readily than many other terms; meanings shift over short periods of time, and these terms are often used differently by many people. When any such terms are used by patients, colleagues, and researchers, a clinician should inquire how that person is using these terms, rather than wrongly assuming the meaning is the same as the clinician's.

Sex generally refers to biological determinants of maleness or femaleness, such as chromosomes, anatomy, gonads, hormones, and reproductive ability.

Gender generally indicates the cultural or societal characteristics of maleness or femaleness, such as clothing, hairstyle, jewelry, occupation, interests, and comportment. These characteristics change through time and between cultures; what is considered typical of a female today in one culture may be very different from the same culture several decades ago and may be very different for a divergent culture.

Gender identity is the internal sense of one's gender and is thought to be largely biologically determined.

Gender role is the outward manifestation of one's gender—what clothes or hairstyle or mannerisms a person expresses, which leads others to define that person's gender. Gender role is subject to control and modification by the individual and may be congruent or incongruent with one's gender identity. For example, a patient may present to the clinician dressed in pants, shirt, and tie, with a short haircut and beard, low voice, and masculine mannerisms, appearing typically male; however, this person may feel female inside.

Gender variant or *gender atypical* refers to behaviors and identity that predominately and persistently are different from what a society considers usual and customarily for one gender, transgressing the boundaries established for that gender. "Gender disordered," "gender dysphoric," and "gender-referred" were equivalent terms used in much of the literature from the 1960s through 1980, as no official diagnoses were applicable. From 1980 to 1994, the diagnostic terms gender identity disorder of childhood and transsexualism for adults were used, and from 1994 on, the diagnostic term gender identity disorder (GID) for both children and adults has been the official one in DSM-IV, the *Diagnostic and Statistical Manual of Mental Disorders, Fourth Edition* (3). Since there are no established criteria for when to use the terms *gender variant* or *gender atypical,* these terms may or may not describe the same person who would be diagnosed with GID or who meets subthreshold criteria for GID.

Transsexual is a term dating back to the early 20th century, which connotes a person who wishes to or has started or completed transitioning from one sex and gender to another, often through use of hormones and surgical procedures. A *transman* is a former female who is transitioning or has transitioned to being male, and a *transwoman* is a former male who is transitioning or has transitioned to being female.

Transgender is an umbrella term that gained use in the mid-1990s and, in this chapter, refers to people with cross-gender identity and/or behavior, including transsexual people as well as those who are not transitioning from one to another gender but somewhere in-between. Transgender individuals may never seek any medical interventions or may choose limited or substantial procedures to achieve a sense of what seems right for their gender identity.

Transvestite often is used psychiatrically to refer to those with an obligatory sexual fetish to cross-dress, gaining erotic arousal from the transgressive act of cross-dressing (i.e., transvestic fetishism). This is exclusively found in males. In lay terminology, the term may be applied to anyone (but more often men) who cross-dresses on more than just uncommon occasions, whether for occupational or other reasons, but generally excludes those who are transgender or transsexual. This may include drag queens and drag kings.

DEVELOPMENTAL ISSUES IN CHILDHOOD

Gender identity is usually consolidated around the age of 3 years, and most children will grow through life with a firm sense of themselves as boys or girls, as being masculine or feminine, which matches with their biological sex. A very small minority of children will feel different; their sense of gender will be incongruous with their biological sex, and as they develop their ability to identity the gender of others, they become increasingly aware that they themselves are different. These children may feel that they are the opposite gender from how they are being raised; they may feel that their anatomy is incorrect and wish that their genitalia would change or disappear; they may be much more attracted to toys and activities of the other gender; and they may be more comfortable having playmates of the other sex. For example, a child born and raised as a boy may show gender atypical or cross-gender play as early as age 18 months or 2 years, putting on his mother's shoes and jewelry; he may, by age 3 or 4, refer to himself as a girl, insist he is or will become a girl, have mostly girl friends, play with stereotypically feminine toys such baby or Barbie dolls, dress up as a girl, pretend to be female characters, draw girls more than boys, use feminine gestures and vocal inflections, and desire to wear feminine clothes and attire. Such a girl-identified boy may be said to be gender variant or gender atypical, or for diagnostic purposes to meet the criteria for gender identity disorder in DSM-IV (3). Most professionals with expertise in the area of childhood gender variance tend not use the terms transgender and transsexual to describe prepubertal youth because of the frequent fading of cross-gender identification with age. Likewise, some professionals avoid use of the DSM diagnosis of GID in children and adolescents because this lumps children and adults into the same category and because this diagnosis may result in discrimination against the individual should it appear in school or other records (4). This diagnosis is then reserved for use when needed for legal issues such as contesting child custody or to document need for certain types of treatment. The determinants of how and why gender variance or GID develop are not known but are thought to be primarily biologically based.

In most Western societies, there is more social difficulty for the boy or man who is feminine than for the girl or woman who is masculine. The girl who wears pants and has short hair and plays roughly with toy trucks and guns may be called a tomboy, and as such is more accepted in society than the "sissy" boy, who may wear a skirt and lipstick and carries a baby doll. This is one reason why fewer gender-variant girls than boys are seen professionally: it does not cause as much concern in the parents or in the school. Girls who are more likely brought to a clinician are those who have a greater degree of gender variance, who may insist that they are boys or wish to have a penis or refuse to wear girl's clothes, whereas boys may be brought in for lesser variance. This greater concern over the more rigid societal stereotypes for masculine norms may falsely give an impression that gender variance is more common in boys. Later in life, it appears that the number of women who identity as gender variant or transgender is about the same as the number of men who do so.

It is crucial for the clinician to understand that the majority of gender-variant children, whether boys or girls, do not grow up to be gender-variant adolescents or adults. Gender variance tends to fade, or "desist," between ages 8 to 12 years, for unknown reasons. If it does not fade by then, this gender variance is likely to be lifelong. For such individuals whose cross-gender identification persists past 13 years of age and who commonly become troubled by the onset of pubertal development of secondary sexual characteristics, the term transgender becomes apt. For those who wish to or who start transitioning from one gender to another, the term transsexual is apt.

Families with gender-variant children who seek professional advice or care do so particularly in the year or so before kindergarten. By age 4 years, many parents will become concerned that the "phase" of cross-gender identification and behavior is no longer a phase but more long-lasting, and they fear that their child may become a victim of discrimination when they go off to school. Parents seek ways to keep their child safe from bullying and harassment by schoolmates and by the adults in school. By this time, there commonly is dysfunction within the family caused by differences in opinion and approaches to the child's cross-gender behavior, and constant attention to gender issues may define many of the family interactions. Occasionally, parents will have concerns more focused on their child's ultimate development into adulthood; they may be apprehensive regarding possible adult outcomes such as homosexuality or transsexuality. Families who do seek out a psychiatrist or therapist with substantial experience working with gender-variant children will find very few anywhere (aside from a few major cities such as Toronto, Amsterdam, London, New York, and Washington, DC), and this paucity of experienced clinicians can interfere with the family accessing care. Most families who do come in will be seen by a clinician with no or limited initial experience in this area.

Children who display cross-gender behaviors are frequently the target of disdain and bullying, especially by peers 8 to 12 years of age, who are concrete and rigid in thinking and liable to be more openly judgmental. This bullying may be subtle or overtly physical and dangerous. Not infrequently, school personal do not intercede with the same diligence when peer harassment is directed at gender variance as they do when it is directed at racial or religious characteristics. A teacher or school authority may let a derogatory comment about being "gay" or a "sissy" slide by but quickly intervene when there is a racial slur; sometimes the adults in a child's environment will join in the harassment. Gender-variant children and their bullying peers pick up from these adult models that cross-gender behavior and identity are not acceptable. Children who are not as able to adapt to such negative surroundings by moderating their cross-gender behaviors are more likely to be bullied and suffer more. Thus, gender-variant children who are less able to conform, less able to consider consequences, and less able to control their impulses are at greater risk. This includes children with attention-deficit/hyperactivity disorder, impulse control disorder, and mood disorders. These are the children more likely to be brought to clinicians for evaluation and treatment. Clinicians can provide a valuable service by working with the schools to decrease ostracism of the child, sometimes by holding in-school training and education sessions, and involving school-focused organizations such as the Gay, Lesbian, and Straight Education Network (GLSEN). Having the teacher's ratings for control, impulsivity, attention problems, and self-esteem is very helpful in assessing difficulties in these arenas. The clinician can help families with a gender-variant child by assessing the functioning of the family and assist with restoring or establishing healthy family activities with less focus on gender-related issues, while enhancing control and promoting adaptive functioning.

The desistence of gender variance from childhood through adolescence that occurs in most gender-variant youth is speculated to be caused by a confluence of factors, such as the beginning surges of pubertal hormones, more flexible thinking with consideration of alternatives as abstract reasoning develops, consolidation of moral development, and the negative reactions by peers and society. Therapy has not been shown to have much if any effect on ultimate gender identity but may be extremely beneficial in how the child and family function. It is not possible to predict which gender-variant children will become transgender adults or nontransgender adults, nor which gender-typical children will become nontransgender adults or transgender adults. Much benefit can be gained over time with supportive education regarding the various adult outcomes for children, whether gender variant or gender typical, as ultimately becoming gay men, heterosexual men, heterosexual women, lesbian women, transsexual men, or transsexual women. Approaches to therapy that focus on denying or punishing cross-gender behavior and identity are generally counterproductive and may be harmful, as are approaches that totally embrace cross-gender behavior and identity because they disregard the eventual outcome of most gender-variant children.

DEVELOPMENTAL ISSUES IN ADOLESCENCE

When cross-gender behavior and identity persist past the age of 13 years, it then is considered to be life-long in almost all people. This is a minority outcome for children with gender variance: about 10% to 20% of children will have continued gender variance into adolescence (5,6). Approximately two-thirds of gender-variant children will grow up to be nontransgender homosexual or bisexual adults, and about a quarter will grow up to be nontransgender heterosexual adults (the reverse is not the case: most homosexual and most heterosexual adults do not have a history of childhood gender variance, and thus the popular equation of gender variance in childhood with adult homosexuality is erroneous) (7). There are some male teenagers who may develop cross-gender identification during pubertal years without having had recognizable gender variance as a child. For these few adolescents, the origins of gender confusion may be part of a developing transvestic fetishism: the initial cross-gender behaviors in these individuals is more centered on erotic arousal when wearing female undergarments and/or fantasizing about being female, and this has been called auto-gynephila (8). Over time, this eroticism may fade and the person finds that he feels more true to self when dressed in female clothing other than just underwear, as his gender identity shifts from being male to female. This shift may occur during adolescence or even much later in life, as autogynephilia or transvestism evolves into transgenderism.

The degree of unease and discomfort with identity and body image that a gender-variant youth has as secondary sexual characteristics develop is considered to be a hallmark for predicting persistence of gender variance (9,10). This can be seen as early as Tanner stage 2 (breast budding in girls, testicular and penile enlargement in boys). Girls may try to hide breast development by wearing loose clothes or by binding the breasts; boys may try to tuck their penises in. As puberty continues, teenagers may try to mask other changes by modifying hair, voice, and clothing. As their unease grows, transgender teenagers may become more isolated, less likely to be social with peers, and sometimes avoiding situations that place them at risk for persecution, such as attending school. Without support and guidance, these teens can suffer from low self-esteem and depression and may become suicidal: the risk for attempted and completed suicide in transgender teenagers is estimated to be considerably more than average. The adolescent may seek out ways to escape these problems, including drug use, unprotected sex, self-injurious behaviors, and other jeopardous behaviors. Teenagers who show cross-gender behaviors are at greater risk for being rejected, thrown out of their homes and becoming homeless, and being the victims of violence and even murder (11). In contrast, transgender teenagers with supportive families, networks, and therapists, who attend accepting schools, and who are more flexible in adapting their behaviors to potentially dangerous situations can have very positive outcomes as their transgender identity solidifies.

Transgender teens, like their gay and lesbian counterparts, often have derailed psychosexual development caused by social ostracism of their engaging in normal sexual behaviors (7). They are less able to openly partake in crushes, dating, romance, holding hands in school hallways, and being in social cliques without encountering scrutiny and reprisal. The result can be further isolation, sexualization of relationships, and prolonged confusion about sexual and gender issues. Finding safe, accepting, nonsexual social situations and groups for the transgender teen is a challenge that the clinician can help with. Often, social solace can be found in arts and theater groups and in some progressive religious organizations. Adolescents will frequently seek social contacts and information on the Internet, which can be an excellent source for this but also can be risky and replete with false information. An adolescent, or a parent, who does an Internet search using terms such as transsexual or transgender will find a plethora of pornographic websites and danger for predation and exploitation. Astute clinicians can guide teens and their families to appropriate websites conducive to education and social support.

With the anatomical transformations of puberty, many sexual characteristics become permanent—hair distribution, voice lowering, breast enlargement, penile size, and so on. These features will require major modification by surgical and hormonal means for postpubertal people who decide to pursue sex reassignment. Since the 1990s, some groups, such as the one Cohen-Kettenis leads in the Netherlands, have offered earlier treatment to transgender adolescents before the ultimate development of Tanner stage 6 (9). This is done by administration of pubertal blocking hormones to halt sexual development in selected adolescents after reaching Tanner stage 2 and who have been carefully screened for consistency of transgender identity since early childhood, absence of major psychiatric illness, and positive familial support. As puberty is blocked, the teenager's gender identity is reassessed in therapy over time, and if the adolescent continues to be transgender and certain of the desire to transition physically, then hormones to promote opposite sex sexual development can be given at age 16 years. Generally, surgical procedures are deferred until age 18 years. In the United States, access to such sex reassignment procedures may be hampered by insurance denials, and the unreimbursed costs of transition may be beyond reach for many families (10,11). This is not a hindrance to care in countries such as the Netherlands and Canada. Because of these barriers, some transgender adolescents in the United States will turn to obtaining illicit (and often impure) hormones from the Internet or street and may attempt perilous procedures such as autocastration. Risks for exposure to infection, including human immunodeficiency virus and hepatitis, are high if needles are shared for injecting hormones.

There is not yet international consensus for the Netherlands approach to give hormones to halt puberty by Tanner stage 2. The generally accepted Standards of Care (SOC) developed by the Harry Benjamin International Gender Dysphoria Association (now known as the World Professional Association for Transgender Care, WPATH) undergo revision every few years to address the changing needs of transgender people, cultural shifts, and advances in healthcare (12). The SOC pertaining to adolescents provide valuable updated information and recommendations to guide clinicians in ethical and responsible care.

ISSUES IN ADULTHOOD

Transsexual and transgender adults have greater access to healthcare and mental healthcare than gender-variant children or adolescents, primarily because of the far larger number of available clinicians. Even so, access to experienced providers is seldom adequate in most areas. Experienced mental health clinicians can be located through organizations such as WPATH, but oftentimes, the less-experienced clinician will be the one to continue to provide care. The transgender adult often presents to mental health providers to gain access to sex reassignment procedures by endocrinologists and surgeons. In previous versions of SOC (12), the individual had to live full time as the opposite sex and be in therapy for a specified duration before the clinician could write a letter documenting agreement for the person to be prescribed hormones or scheduled for surgery; these criteria have been modified in the most recent revision of SOC. This can place the mental health provider into the role of a gatekeeper, and has come under strong criticism by the transgender community as an impediment to self-determination of care and different from decision-making capacity for other aspects of one's healthcare (13). It remains important for the mental health clinician to assess the transgender adult's preparation for receiving hormones and surgery and to provide counseling about the procedures, benefits, side effects, and risks of sex reassignment, which may take considerable time in therapy with the individual and the family or significant others in the person's life. It is also paramount for the therapist to be in contact with the endocrinologists and surgeons to optimize the process and outcome of transitioning. Although some treatment results and surgical procedures are easily reversible, many others are not (e.g., voice lowering with testosterone, removal of hair by electrolysis, mastectomy, and orchiectomy); thus, regret and later decisions that sex reassignment was not the right choice can impose significant difficulties for the individual in costs, risks, and functioning.

In the past, sex reassignment was popularly regarded as being a one-time procedure—a person went off to a sex reassignment center and days or weeks later returned as transformed into the opposite sex. This was never the case and belies the long period of preparation the transsexual person accomplishes on the road to transition—coming out as transsexual to others, living as the opposite gender at home and work, being in therapy, working on changing sex designations on legal documents such as driver's licenses, initiating hormones, fighting discrimination, and planning an altered life. Centers for sex reassignment thus primarily accomplished several surgical and bodily procedures at one time. These centers are fewer in number than two decades ago; and most localities have never had a nearby center, surprisingly including New York City. Since the 1990s, there has been a growing movement by transsexual adults to no longer travel to these centers but rather to have procedures done locally or in various places and over a more extended period of time. This has created a sea change in both access to care and provision of care. Transitioning may be done much more according to one's readiness for and ability to afford certain procedures, with greater time to adjust to life changes. Transitioning becomes less an "all or nothing" regimen, and thereby more open to variation: the transition for some becomes less from one sex to the other than a transition away from one sex to a less-defined in-between area of gender fluidity; hence the term transgender suites many who are not going entirely from male to female (MTF) or female to male (FTM). A transgender individual may elect to have low-dose hormones to promote certain sexual characteristics without any surgery; he may have a hysterectomy, mastectomy, and nipple repositioning but not phalloplasty; she may have breast augmentation but not vaginoplasty and may keep her penis. The opportunities that are now more readily available to transgender adults create greater flexibility but also more uncertainty for some; this also creates greater confusion for many clinicians in understanding transgender adults and knowing how to help them. It is essential for therapists to update themselves on the most current changes in the field and newest revisions of the SOC. This is easily done via the Internet or attending local and national meetings for transgender care.

Without assistance, families with transgender members can find it overwhelming to adapt to the transperson's transitioning. Some spouses may be supportive but may no longer find themselves sexually attracted to the transperson; some spouses may be hostile and initiate divorce proceedings and custody battles; some become depressed and withdraw from the family; and sometimes parental alienation syndrome occurs (14). Gender therapists find it vital to work with family members; sometimes, therapy is better accepted by the family when another therapist is engaged. Support organizations like PFLAG (Parents, Families, and Friends of Lesbians and Gays) can be extremely valuable for family members of transgender people, but it may take some time and effort for family members to accept this support. Children of transgender parents go through major periods of confusion and reappraisal as they try to view their father as becoming a woman or their mother becoming a man; it may be exceedingly formidable for them to see their father dressed as a woman. One simple thing becomes a vexing dilemma for the children: what to call a transitioned parent in public—using "mom" in public for a transman can be quite challenging; to start calling their mother "father" is burdensome and is distressing to the father; therefore some children may stop using terms like "mom" and "dad" in public, to the chagrin of the parent. Support and information for children through these difficult adjustments should be offered by the therapist and can be obtained from PFLAG and other organizations.

The young transgender adult may continue to be going through some of the major developmental tasks of adolescence because of the derailed development mentioned above and may still question and be confused about his or her gender identity and other life issues. The clinician must be aware of this prolonged adolescence as a possible confound in therapy, but this also may afford an enhanced ability to help the person achieve a positive gender identity.

Advancing transgender identity affirmation for ultimate emotional well-being should be the primary overall goal for the therapist and patient (15). Working together to achieve this goal is a journey that encompasses persevering over disparities and barriers to care, overcoming discrimination and fostering safety, expansion of knowledge and expectations, and joint learning and discovery. This journey for both clinician and patient can be inspiring and meaningful, and hence immensely rewarding (16–21).

References

1. Money J. *Gay, Straight, and In-Between: The Sexology of Erotic Orientation*. New York: Oxford University Press, 1988.
2. Cohen-Kettenis PT, Pfäfflin F: *Transgenderism and Intersexuality in Childhood and Adolescents*. Thousand Oaks, CA: Sage Publications, 2003.
3. *Diagnostic and Statistical Manual of Mental Disorders, Fourth Edition, Text Revision (DSM-IV-TR)*. Washington, DC: American Psychiatric Association Press, 2000:576–582.
4. Pleak RR. Ethical issues in diagnosing and treating gender-dysphoric children and adolescents. In: Rottnek M, ed. *Sissies & Tomboys: Gender Nonconformity & Homosexual Childhood*. New York : University Press, 1999:34–51.
5. Zucker KJ. Gender identity disorder in childhood and adolescence. *Ann Rev Clin Psychol* 2004;1:467–492.
6. Drummond KD, Bradley SJ, Peterson-Badali M, et al. A follow-up study of girls with gender identity disorder. *Dev Psychol* 2008; 44(1):34–45.
7. Pleak RR, Anderson DA. Observation, interview, and mental status assessment (OIM): Homosexual. In: Noshpitz JD, Harrison SI, Eth S, eds. *Handbook of Clinical Child and Adolescent Psychiatry, Volume 5: Clinical Assessment and Intervention Planning*. New York: John Wiley & Sons, 1998:563–575.

8. Blanchard R. Early history of the concept of autogynephilia. *Arch Sex Behav* 2005;34(4): 439–446.

9. Cohen-Kettenis PT, Delemarre-van de Waal HA, Gooren LJ. The treatment of adolescent transsexuals: Changing insights. *J Sex Med* 2008;5(8):1892–1897.

10. Spack N. *An Endocrine Perspective on the Care of Transgender Adolescents.* American Psychiatric Association 161st Annual Meeting. Washington, DC, May 2008.

11. Pleak RR. *Healthy Transteens 2007.* World Professional Association for Transgender Health Biennial Symposium. Chicago, September 2007.

12. The Harry Benjamin International Gender Dysphoria Association's Standards of Care for Gender Identity Disorders, Sixth Ed, Minneapolis, Minnesota; 2001.

13. Hale CJ. Ethical problems with the mental health evaluation standards of care for adult gender variant prospective patients. *Perspect Biol Med* 2007;50(4):491–505.

14. Green R. Parental alienation syndrome and the transsexual parent. *Int J Transgenderism* 2006;9(1):9–13.

15. Nuttbrock L, Rosenblum A, Blumenstein R. Transgender identity affirmation and mental health. *Int J Transgenderism* 2002;6(4):1–11.

16. Stryker S. *Transgender History.* Berkeley, CA: Seal Press, 2008.

17. Brown ML, Rounsley CA. *True Selves: Understanding Transsexualism, for Families, Friends, Coworkers, and Helping Professionals.* San Francisco: Jossey-Bass, 1996.

18. Winfield CL. *Gender Identity: The Ultimate Teen Guide.* Lanham, MD: Scarecrow Press, 2007.

19. Brill S, Pepper R. *The Transgender Child: A Handbook for Families and Professionals.* San Francisco: Cleis Press, 2008.

20. Ettner R, Monstrey S, Eyler AE, eds. *Principles of Transgender Medicine and Surgery.* New York: Haworth Press, 2007.

21. Roughgarden J. *Evolution's Rainbow: Diversity, Gender, and Sexuality in Nature and People.* Berkeley, CA: University of California Press, 2004.

Disparities Among Age Groups

12 Children and Adolescents

Andres J. Pumariega

INTRODUCTION

Do children have significant mental health needs? The question is somewhat rhetorical, but it is one that many in the United States, from parents to policy makers, continue to ask themselves. Many of the barriers to accessing children's mental health services are attitudinal. The adage "little people—little problems, big people—big problems" is one that still underlies many perceptions around the mental health needs of children and youth. Some of this is fueled by an idyllic image of problem-free childhoods that is still promoted in literature and popular media. Another source of barriers stem from the overall stigma of mental illness and emotional disturbance that is still closely held in our society, with many parents fear labeling of their children and the resulting stigma ascribed by peers, teachers, neighbors, and even extended family members.

Children and adolescents are also not accorded their due in terms of priority (and funding) for services. Above all, children do not vote, and parents are usually in their most demanding and least economically and politically potent stage of life. Additionally, adults with serious mental illness are far more visible (as a result of homelessness, whereas children are cared for by their families) and disruptive (because of their sheer size and knowledge) than children with mental or emotional disorders (and these are additionally contained within and by agencies and social institutions such as schools, child welfare/foster care, and juvenile justice agencies). It is then not surprising that funding for mental health services devoted to children and youth are estimated at around 11.68 billion dollars out of a total mental health expenditure of 85.4 billion, improved from past decades but far short of their proportion of the population (13.7% versus 25% of the population under the age of 18 (1). At the same time, shortages of child and adolescent psychiatrists as well as other child mental health professionals continue to grow annually as a result.

These imbalances and shortages are compounded by the reality that child and adolescent mental health services are more complex and challenging given the child's changing developmental needs (physical, psychological, and social), the critical importance of family engagement and involvement, the importance of the environmental context of treatment, and the simultaneous need for recovery from their illness/disorder and developmental progression/habilitation. These multiple developmental needs give rise to the child's and family's involvement with multiple agencies that often fight over "turf," including pre-eminence, ideological orientation of services, and financing for services, frequently involving the same child. Other phenomena that can arise from such fragmentation are parental confusion over agency requirements, or the child and family being caught between agencies as they engage in "cost-shifting" or "burden-shifting" with multiproblem children or population.

FINANCIAL BARRIERS

Financial considerations play important roles as barriers to access to care. The challenges around adequate access to health insurance are especially felt by young families with children, where the rates of being uninsured are high. The U.S. federal government increasingly used Medicaid funding to improve funding for children's mental health services, with a major boom in funding from the 1970s to 1990s. However, by the late 1900s to 2000s, as a result of the growth in mental health expenditures, Medicaid funding has been increasingly curtailed and the resources available to fund child mental health and human services are increasingly restricted. Spending on mental health treatment for children was estimated at $11.68 billion, or $172 per child, in 1998. Funding was provided by private insurance (47%), Medicaid (24%), state and local mental health agencies (21%), and other public insurance (3%) (1).

Approximately 18% of children and adolescents 18 years of age and under are enrolled in the Medicaid program (including up to 25% of those under 3 years of age). The great majority of these children and youth are poor, underserved children, often from ethnic minority backgrounds. Children from these populations experience higher levels of stressors (such as poverty, discrimination, and exposure to violence and trauma) and are likely to have higher levels of need for services. The cost of serving these populations of children and adolescents is in contrast to the high cost of the psychosocial morbidity they contend with, including lost productivity and the costs of welfare dependency and institutionalization (2).

These trends in reduced funding have also increased pressures on public child mental health and social service agencies to demonstrate improved clinical- and cost-effectiveness, increasingly turning to managed care approaches to finance and organize mental health and social services. For example, more than 60% of children who are Medicaid beneficiaries are under managed care plans, the largest beneficiary group in these programs. However, most managed care methods were developed with adult and private sector populations in mind and are usually accompanied by the privatization of services. Managed care methodology is being increasingly implemented within Medicaid-funded children's mental health services with the aim of reducing utilization and costs, including such newer approaches as restrictive formularies, level of care criteria, and restrictive case rates. When applied to public child mental health services, these approaches have often resulted in fragmentation of care and the shifting of the burden of services and cost to the other child-serving agencies and systems, with the potential for significantly increased morbidity. Such methodology is also being used to manage services funded by the child welfare system and juvenile justice systems, with significant potential impact on access to and quality of care (2). A result of these pressures for cost containment has been an exponential growth of class action lawsuits over the past 15 years against state Medicaid, educational, child welfare, and juvenile justice agencies for failing to meet Federal service mandates. However, rather than increase funding or make better use of resources, the response by the federal government has been to pursue legislation to undo many of the mandates associated with Medicaid, Title IX child welfare funding, and the Civil Rights for Institutionalized Persons Act (CRIPA), which are the bases of these lawsuits. A result of these pressures for cost containment has been an exponential growth of class action lawsuits over the past 15 years against state Medicaid, educational, child welfare, and juvenile justice agencies for failing to meet Federal service mandates. However, rather than increase funding or make better use of resources, the response by the federal government has been to pursue legislation to undo many of the mandates associated with Medicaid, Title IX child welfare funding, and the Civil Rights for Institutionalized Persons Act (3).

CULTURAL BARRIERS

Minority and immigrant children and youth face many barriers to effective mental healthcare. These include population barriers (socioeconomic disparities, stigma, poor health education, lack of documentation), provider factors (deficits in cross-cultural knowledge and skills and attitudinal sensitivity), and systemic factors (services location and organization, lack of culturally competent services, etc.). These barriers result in increased mental health disparities among these populations. Minority youth often reside in neighborhoods where services are often unavailable or they lack public or private insurance necessary to obtain mental health services. These issues are particularly acute among young children and among Latino youth (4). Hispanic families underutilize mental health services because of language and cultural barriers, whereas Asians-Americans experience shame around mental illness (5).

Stigma is a major barrier to seeking mental health services in general, and cultural beliefs play a large role in the perpetuation of stigma. Many cultures have major negative associations with any type of mental health assistance, often equating this with serious psychopathology and social undesirability. The fear of double-stigmatization (being culturally different as well as "crazy") also presents major barriers for diverse families and youth to accessing services. Some of these attitudes may originate historically in negative experiences with the mental health system by minority populations in the United States (including oppression) and by immigrants in their home nations (6). Diverse cultural groups' understanding of mental illness can vary significantly and influence their help-seeking behaviors, invoking spiritual, supernatural, sociological, and interpersonal explanatory models. Diverse families often view many behaviors as normative or volitional on the part of the child. They may have a more limited understanding of the mental health system than mainstream families, which can be compounded by limited English proficiency. All of these factors contribute to latter recognition of the severity of mental disorders in children and youth and to significant barriers to obtaining mental health services (7).

There is significant evidence that psychiatric disorders are frequently misdiagnosed among culturally diverse youth. Various studies have found an overdiagnosis of conduct disorder and underdiagnosis of internalizing disorders among minority youth (8). Misdiagnosis largely originates from difficulties that clinicians from majority and minority origins have in addressing cultural difference, including cognitive biases stemming from stereotyping, lack of systematic assessment, and lack of contextualization of information obtained in diagnostic assessments. The majority of care of mental healthcare is typically provided by primary care physicians who may have relatively little experience with psychiatric disorders in children and adolescents and have added disincentives such as decreased reimbursement for identifying a mental health versus a somatic health problem (9).

PREVALENCE OF MENTAL HEALTH SERVICES IN CHILDREN

The MECA Study (Methodology for Epidemiology of Mental Disorders in Children and Adolescents; Shaffer et al.) (10) estimated that almost 21% of children and youth experienced at least one mental, emotional, or addictive disorder associated with at least minimum impairment at any time. When significant functional impairment at home, school, or peers are taken into account, estimates drop to 11%, and when extreme functional impairment is the criterion, the estimates drop to 5%. Cumulative prevalence rates total up to 37% for all disorders by age 16 and vary across different disorders from 4% to 6% for attention deficit hyperactivity disorder, 10% to 12% for depressive disorders, 10% to 15% for anxiety disorders, and 12% to 15% for substance use disorders (11).

Mental health need is also higher among different at-risk groups of children and youth. Several studies have documented high rates of serious emotional disturbance among youth in the juvenile justice system, with estimates of approximately 50% to 70% (12). Many youth with mental disorders are typically referred to juvenile justice because of displays of aggressive or disruptive behaviors and after multiple disciplinary interventions in schools and out of home placements. There has also been increasing recognition that children in the child welfare system have extremely high mental health needs, with prevalence rates estimated at close to 50%, yet are significantly underserved with respect to mental health services. This is likely related to the high risk and level of exposure to trauma, poverty, and other adversities in this population. Other high-risk populations include students in special education (prevalence rates of approximately 70%) and in substance abuse services (60%) (13). Another high-risk population that is less recognized is that of children of women who have experienced maternal depression. The prevalence of postpartum depression is 8% to 15% overall within 1 year of birth. Longitudinal research has demonstrated the long-term impact on children from maternal depression, including estimated prevalence rates of emotional or behavioral disturbance of 50% to 80%, with increased risk for depression, separation anxiety, attention deficits, and conduct disturbances (14).

Among minority populations, some studies have suggested higher prevalence of psychiatric disorders such as depression, anxiety disorders, substance abuse, and even eating disorders (7). For example, the Youth Risk Behavior Survey of the Centers for Disease Control found a significant increase in the prevalence rates of sad mood and suicidality of Latino and African American youth as compared with non-Hispanic whites.

MENTAL HEALTH SERVICES UTILIZATION IN CHILDREN

Studies show that 75% to 85% of children with mental illnesses do not receive specialty mental health services, with most receiving no treatment at all. Based on three national surveys between 1996 and 1998, 5% and 7% of all children use any mental health specialty services in a given year. This average rate is similar to the rate among adults, but it obscures major differences across age groups. Only 1% to 2% of preschoolers use any services, but 6% to 8% of the 6- to 11-year age group and 8% to 9% of the 12- to 17-year age group do. There is substantial variation in mental health service utilization by type of insurance, ranging from 8.4% for Medicaid enrollees to 4.0% for the uninsured. Children on Medicaid are estimated to have more than 1300 specialty visits per 1000 children per year, compared with 462 specialty visits per 1000 children with private insurance, 391 visits per 1000 children with other types of insurance, and 366 visits per 1000 children with no insurance (1).

Mental heath utilization in children and youth can vary by type of disorder because of such factors as degree of recognition, expertise of clinicians, and availability of specialty services. For example, according to the 2006 National Survey on Drug Use and Health, 38.9% of youths aged 12 to 17 years with a major depressive episode in the past year received treatment (saw or talked to a medical doctor or other professional or used prescription medication). Among youths with major depressive disorder in the past year, 23.9% saw or talked to a medical doctor or other professional only, 2.1% used prescription medication only, and 12.7% received treatment from both sources for depression in the past year. On the other hand, approximately 20% of youth in the juvenile justice system utilize mental health services, significantly lower than their level of need (15).

Mental health utilization varies greatly across racial/ethnic groups. Latinos are the least likely of all groups to access specialty care (5.0%), even though Latinos and African American children have the highest rates of need (10.5%) (1). Cuffe et al. (16) found that African American youth receive significantly lower rates of treatment than whites and stay in treatment half the time as white children. Pumariega et al. (17) found that Latino children receive an average of half as many counseling sessions, whereas Hough et al. (18) found that Latino children receive significantly fewer specialty mental health services and at a later age than Caucasians and African Americans. These disparities have resulted in the overrepresentation of minority youth in other child service sectors such as special education, child welfare, and juvenile justice.

APPROACHES TO ADDRESS CHILD AND ADOLESCENT MENTAL HEALTH DISPARITIES

Over the past 20 years, there have been numerous approaches developed to improve access and effectiveness of children's mental health services. Several approaches are being used to improve the financing of children's mental health services at the Federal level. These have included the promotion of the State Children's Health Insurance Program (SCHIP) and Medicaid Expansion SCHIP (M-SCHIP) to expand children's health insurance coverage to uninsured children. Some states have used Home and Community-Based Services (HCBS) waivers or the Tax Equity and Financial Responsibility Act (TEFRA) option under Medicaid to expand Medicaid eligibility to children with mental disabilities who would not generally be covered by the program because of higher family income. These expansions help prevent the entry of children into state custody as a result of lack of coverage for mental illness and emotional disturbances by funding children to be treated in the community, so long as the cost of that care does not exceed the estimated cost of institutional care. The Early Periodic Screening Detection and Treatment mandate also provides for states to deliver medically necessary mental health services for children covered by Medicaid who have a mental disorder identified as part of periodic screening, with some states using behavioral health screening tools. Additionally, legislation sponsored by Congressman Patrick Kennedy is pending before Congress to address workforce shortages in child mental health disciplines through tuition support and payback for services options.

Community-based systems of care for children's mental health has been a service philosophy that has been increasingly promoted and adopted nationally to better address both access to care and effectiveness of services, including endorsement by the U.S. Surgeon General. The key principles of community systems of care include access to a comprehensive array of services, treatment individualized to the child's needs, treatment in the least restrictive environment possible, full utilization of family and community resources, full participation of families as partners in services planning and delivery, interagency coordination, the use of case management for services coordination, no ejection or rejection from services because of lack of "treatability" or "cooperation," early identification and intervention, smooth transition of youth into the adult service system, effective advocacy efforts, and nondiscriminating, culturally competent services. Community systems of care promote a flexible and individualized approach to service delivery for the child and family within the context of his/her home and community as an alternative to treatment in out-of-home settings while attending to family and systems issues that affect such care. These include access, utilization, child and family empowerment, financing, and clinical- and cost-effectiveness of mental health services provided to children and adolescents, as well as the functioning and effectiveness of systems of care for child mental health. Psychiatry, which was central in the traditional model, has only recently reengaged itself as a discipline in this new model. Psychiatrists face a major challenge in reaffirming their role in this model and integrating their developing clinical and scientific knowledge and skills base (19).

More recently, the Center for Mental Health Services (CMHS) Comprehensive Community Mental Health Services Program for Children and Their Families has funded more than 100 demonstration projects in diverse communities throughout the nation to implement systems of care. The goals of these programs have been to implement CASSP values, reduce out-of-home placements, reduce service fragmentation, and promote earlier mental health intervention to reduce functional morbidity. The current phase of the grant program emphasizes culturally diverse populations and early childhood grants. The multisite national evaluation of the Comprehensive Mental Health Services Program for Children and Their Families has shown improved child and family functioning, increased stability of living situation, and reduced cost of care when cost offsets in education, juvenile justice, child welfare, and general health are considered (20).

The system-of-care model appears to be beneficial in reducing use of residential and out-of-state placements and achieving improvements in functional behavior in youth with severe emotional and behavioral disorders who are served in multiple systems. However, questions remain about the effectiveness of such systems in relation to more traditional systems, which specific outcomes are most meaningful to measure in evaluating the model, and what the active ingredients are that produce desired outcomes. As a result, the focus has shifted from measuring system-level outcomes to measuring clinical and functional outcomes of individual children and the integration of evidence-based psychotherapy within community systems of care (19).

In addition to the community-based systems of care model, there have been several community-based evidence-based interventions that have demonstrated efficacy and effectiveness and are increasingly being implemented in child mental health programs. These include intensive case management, therapeutic foster care, partial hospitalization, and intensive in-home wraparound interventions. Other community-based interventions that show promise include school-based interventions, mentoring programs, family support and education programs, wilderness programs, crisis mobile outreach teams, time-limited hospitalization with coordinated community services, and family support services (19).

A recent salutary development in the area of interagency systems of care is the renewed interest in school-based services. These go beyond traditional school mental health consultation services and involve the colocation of health and mental health professionals within schools to provide a wide array of direct and indirect/preventive health and mental health services. School-based mental health services serve as an as ideal core service for a children's system of care, providing an excellent accessible portal of entry which is nonstigmatizing, and a naturalistic setting to observe behavior and integrate interventions into a child's environment. These services are often funded through blended Medicaid fee-for-service and managed care funding augmenting limited school funding. Several models have been implemented in communities such as Baltimore, Maryland, rural South Carolina, the state of Hawaii, and Charlotte, North Carolina, with documented success in reducing morbidity and increasing access to needed services (19).

Community-based treatment of adolescents with substance abuse disorders is both accessible and efficacious. There is considerable evidence for the use of day treatment, night programs, and school-based programs. Few such community-based programs and treatment modalities designed to treat the special needs of females, minority groups, and medically compromised individuals such as those with AIDS, but recent progress is being made in adopting the principles of cultural competence in the treatment of adolescent substance abuse disorders. Brief Strategic Family Therapy, an evidence-based family intervention, has been developed and tested with Latino and African-American youth (21). Ethnically specific programs for American Indian youth based on traditional values and rituals/ceremonies have also been developed and evaluated (22).

Comprehensive prevention programs for substance abuse among youth are being increasingly implemented with demonstrated effectiveness in community implementation. These typically include involvement at the school and community levels, outreach to families for participation, peer involvement, training for adult and peer leaders, and attention to multiple risk factors associated with substance abuse as well as supporting life skills training. Program components such as parental psychoeducation and monitoring programs and youth-adult partnerships that are usually part of integrated comprehensive multilevel approaches have demonstrated some limited effectiveness as stand-alone interventions. The Adolescent Alcohol Prevention Trial, a longitudinal multisite approach combining resistance skills and psychoeducation, has demonstrated reduction in mean levels and rates of growth for cigarette and alcohol use (21).

The early childhood population (generally ages 0 to 5, defined by their preschool-aged status) is a particularly vulnerable group of children for whom it has been shown that environmental risks can have significant long-term developmental impact, and that early intervention has the potential to be very beneficial over the long term. Until CMHS recently started funding of system-of-care projects for 0- to 6-year-olds, the early childhood age group had not benefited from system of care reform. Since many agencies are involved with young children, the system-of-care model that promotes integrated planning and service strategies is extremely suitable for this age group. System-of-care integrated service strategies may include such activities as providing mental health consultation to Head Start, Early Intervention, primary care practitioners, community health nurses, and child care workers; and providing mental health services to adults whose children are at risk of out-of-home placement (14).

Barriers to these efforts persist, however, some of which are related to funding and eligibility for services. Mental health agencies may be unable to provide services to children who do not yet meet the full criteria for a mental health diagnosis, and addressing the parents' mental health or substance abuse issues may not be possible if they are uninsured. To address this issue, the state and local funding agencies need to adopt alternative eligibility criteria for services, have contractual agreements with other child-serving agencies that obviate the need for formal diagnosis, or allow the parent to be the recipient of services. For young children who are already showing some early symptoms of disorder, use of a more age-appropriate Diagnostic System for Zero to Three, Revised (DC:0-3R) (23) is more likely to identify conditions making them eligible for services. A crosswalk to ICD-9 diagnoses is needed for billing under the Medicaid system, however. States such as Maine, Florida, Washington, and California have developed crosswalks from DC: 0-3 to ICD-9 diagnoses as part of their statewide early childhood plans. Another barrier is that there are few clinicians trained to diagnose and treat mental health conditions in very young children. States are beginning to invest resources in training to improve the skills of early childhood clinicians (14).

There are encouraging efforts toward enhancing and improving models of collaborative care between primary care and mental health providers, especially child and adolescent psychiatrists, to improve access. A few state Medicaid plans have adopted model or statewide programs to facilitate access to child mental health consultants by primary care practitioners. Some others have invested in training for primary care practitioners on EPSDT tools and referral procedures and support and consultative programs to enhance their function as mental health providers to high-risk populations. Other more formal models of collaborative care, using such technologies such systematic screening tools and telemedicine, are being evaluated and found to be effective in improving access to community-based care. More formal evaluation is needed on the use of nurse practitioners and physician's assistants as extenders in the delivery of child psychiatric services, though such are essential given the national shortage of child and adolescent psychiatrists (19).

An increasing consensus exists for delivering mental health services for ethnic/racial minority populations within the cultural competence framework. This framework indicates the need to identify and address the special mental health needs of diverse populations through both clinician-related factors (such as acquiring knowledge, skills, and attitudes that enable them to serve populations different from their own) and system factors (such as reviewing and changing policies and practices that present barriers to diverse populations, staff training around cultural competence, and the recruitment of diverse staff and clinicians for planning service pathways and delivering care). It also calls for the use of natural strengths and resources in concert with professional services that are protective and support children and families in diverse communities and cultures dealing with emotional disturbance. Cultural competence also includes the adoption of culturally specific therapeutic modalities (such as use of native healers or cultural mediators), mainstream modalities evaluated with diverse populations, and the appropriate use of language interpreters (7).

The cultural competence framework has been operationalized in consensus health and mental health cultural competence standards, such as the Center for Mental

Health Services standards. These standards address cultural adaptations and modifications in clinical processes (such as assessment, treatment planning, case management, and linguistic support) and system processes (such as staff training and development, access protocols, governance of service systems, quality assurance and improvement, and information management). There is beginning evidence that adopting such practices results in improved access to services and retention in treatment. The CMHS Comprehensive Community Mental Health Services Program for Children and Their Families has promoted the cultural competence model, with improved outcomes for children and youth of minority backgrounds correlating to the application of cultural competence principles. The CMHS system of care initiative has also developed a series of programs, Circles of Care, which are specially focused on the needs of American Indian children and youth. Several other community-based programs have adopted the cultural competence framework, such as Cognitive-Behavioral Intervention for Trauma in Schools (CBITS) (4,7).

CONCLUSION

Despite numerous approaches to address mental health disparities among children and youth, the United States faces an increasing gap between the mental health needs of its most vulnerable citizens and its capacity to deliver services. The challenge for this nation will be to address these increasing needs before they adversely affect its future integrity, productivity, and overall well-being. So far, approaches to reforming the children's mental health system in the United States have been piecemeal and fragmented, largely because of this nation's decentralized political structure and ambivalence toward mental health needs and services. Nationwide reform of a comprehensive nature, based on the lessons from the many promising practices that have been developed recently, is the best approach toward addressing what remains a national crisis.

References
1. Ringel JS, Sturm R. National estimates of mental health utilization and expenditures for children in 1998. *J Behav Health Serv Res* 2001;28(3):319–332.
2. Pumariega A, Nace D, England M, et al. Community-based systems approach to children's managed mental health services. *J Child Fam Stud* 1997;6:149.
3. Vaughan T, Pumariega AJ, Klaehn R. Systems of care under legal mandates. In: Pumariega AJ, Winters NC, eds. *Handbook of Child and Adolescent Systems of Care: The New Community Psychiatry.* San Francisco: Jossey Bass, 2003:414–431.
4. Kataoka SH, Zhang L, Wells KB. Unmet need for mental health care among U.S. children: Variation by ethnicity and insurance status. *Am J Psychiatry* 2002;159:1548–1555.
5. Ruiz P, Langrod J. Hispanic Americans. In: Lowisohn J, Ruiz P, Millman R, et al, eds. *Substance Abuse: A Comprehensive Textbook, third edition.* Baltimore: Williams & Wilkins, 1997.
6. Suite D, LaBril R, Primm A, et al. Beyond misdiagnosis, misunderstanding, and mistrust: Relevance of the historical perspective in the medical and mental health treatment of people of color. *J Natl Med Assoc* 2007;99: 879–885.
7. Pumariega AJ, Rogers K, Rothe E. Culturally competent systems of care for children's mental health: Advances and challenges. *Commun Ment Health J* 2005;41(5):539–556.
8. Nguyen L, Arganza G, Huang L, et al. The influence of race and ethnicity on psychiatric diagnoses and clinical characteristics of children and adolescent in children's services. *Cultur Divers Ethn Minority Psychology* 2007;13:18–25.

9. Rost K, Smith R, Matthews D, et al. The deliberate misdiagnosis of major depression in primary care. *Arch Fam Med* 1994;3(4):333–337.

10. Shaffer D, Fisher P, Dulcan MK, et al. The NIMH Diagnostic Interview Schedule for Children Version 2.3 (DISC- 2.3): Description, acceptability, prevalence rates, and performance in the MECA Study: Methods for the Epidemiology of Child and Adolescent Mental Disorders Study. *J Am Acad Child Adolesc Psychiatry* 1996;35:865–877.

11. Costello E, Mustillo S, Erkanli A, et al. Prevalence and development of psychiatric disorders in childhood and adolescence. *Arch Gen Psychiatry* 2003;60:837–844.

12. Rogers K, Pumariega AJ, Atkins DL, et al. Factors associated with identification of mentally ill youth in the juvenile justice system. *Commun Ment Health J* 2006;42(1):25–40.

13. Garland A, Hough R, Mccabe K, et al. Prevalence of -psychiatric disorders in youths across five sectors of care. *J Am Acad Child Adolesc Psychiatry* 2001;40:409–418.

14. Onunaku N. *Improving Maternal and Infant Mental Health: Focus on Maternal Depression*. Los Angeles: National Center for Infant and Early Childhood Health Policy at UCLA, 2005.

15. Pumariega AJ, Atkins DL, Rogers K, et al. Mental health and incarcerated youth, II: Service utilization in incarcerated youth. *J Child Family Stud* 1999; 8:205.

16. Cuffe S, Waller J, Cuccaro M, et al. Race and gender differences in the treatment of psychiatric disorders in young adolescents. *J Am Acad Child Adolesc Psychiatry* 1995;34(11): 1536–1543.

17. Pumariega A, Glover S, Holzer C, et al. Utilization of mental health services in a tri-ethnic sample of adolescents. *Commun Ment Health J* 1999;34:145–156.

18. Hough R, Hazen A, Soriano F, et al. Mental health care for Latinos: Mental health services for Latino adolescents with psychiatric disorders. *Psych Svcs* 2007;53:1556–1562.

19. Pumariega AJ, Winters NC, Huffine C. The evolution of systems of care for children's mental health: Forty years of community child and adolescent psychiatry. *Commun Ment Health J* 2003;39(5):399–425.

20. Foster EM, Connor T. Public cost of better mental health services for children and adolescents. *Psychiatr Serv* 2005;56:50–55.

21. Szapocznik J, Williams RA. Brief Strategic Family Therapy: Twenty-five years of interplay among theory, research and practice in adolescent behavior problems and drug abuse *Clin Child Fam Psychol Rev* 2000;3:117–134.

22. Pumariega AJ, Rodriguez L, Kilgus M. Substance abuse among adolescents: Current perspectives. *Addict Disord Treat* 2004;3:145–155.

23. Zero to Three. *DC:0-3R: Diagnostic Classification of Mental Health and Developmental Disorders of Infancy and Early Childhood*, Revised edition. Washington, DC: Zero to Three Press; 2005.

13 Adulthood

Ann Marie Sullivan and Charles T. Barron

INTRODUCTION

Adulthood is usually defined as the period of life from ages 18 to 65 years and encompasses the many complex roles individuals play in their families and community over this wide range of time. Two major characteristics of this phase of life are work, and its expected productivity to society, and caregiving as parents, partners, adult children, and friends. Mental illness occurring during this long and demanding phase of life can have a powerful impact on how an individual lives his or her adulthood. Similarly, the demands of adulthood have an impact on an individual's mental illness and may demand help and treatment specific to this phase of life.

Disparities in psychiatric care during this period of life have major implications for the individual, families, and society. Disparities in adulthood are present in all the expected areas: access to care; prevention; diagnosis and treatment; and outcomes of care. As discussed throughout this text, age, racial, ethnic, socioeconomic, cultural, gender, and sexual issues all have an impact during adulthood and affect disparities in care during this phase of life. The challenge for this chapter on adulthood is to integrate these issues with the key roles of work and caregiver and to emphasize the special challenges that disparities bring in adulthood.

We will begin the chapter with a general discussion of the disparities in mental healthcare as they affect adults and the key roles of adulthood. We will then look in more detail at three major mental illnesses that affect adults: major depression, schizophrenia, and substance abuse. We will discuss selected examples of the impact of disparities of care for each of these illnesses, who is affected, how it affects their roles as adults, and how it affects the care clinicians provide to them.

OVERVIEW OF RACIAL AND ETHNIC DISPARITIES IN MENTAL HEALTH AND ITS IMPACT ON CAREGIVERS AND WORK ROLES

Disparities in mental illness in adulthood must be seen from three perspectives: disparities in the prevalence of a mental illness, disparities in the diagnosis and treatment of the mental illness, and disparities in the outcomes of treatment. If we look first at the prevalence of mental illness in adults across racial and ethnic groups we find little difference as compared with various physical illnesses. It is well known that there is an increased incidence of hypertension in African Americans, diabetes in specific Latino populations, and severe heart disease in Southeast Asians. However, a recent large national survey of the prevalence of mental illness found an unexpected result: adult minorities in the United States report better mental health than whites. In a recent survey, data do not show poorer reported mental health than whites among racial and ethnic minorities in the United States. The recent NIMH-sponsored Consortium on Psychiatric Epidemiology Studies sampled a wide range of ethnic groups including multiple Hispanic groups, African Americans, Caribbean blacks, Asians including Chinese, Filipino, and Vietnamese, and found that except for Puerto Rican respondents, all reported lower rates of lifetime mental disorders than whites (1). There were some exceptions to prevalence in that American Indians had a higher prevalence of alcoholism and posttraumatic stress disorder and blacks may have a slightly higher prevalence of schizophrenia (although overdiagnosis may be a factor). Questions could be raised regarding whether minorities even in an anonymous reporting system still were more reluctant to report mental illness or symptoms, or perhaps their coping skills were superior to whites. The reason for the unusual finding is still unclear. Yet it does set the stage: disparities are more related to access and treatment issues than to prevalence of mental illness.

The picture is very different for disparities in adult's access to mental healthcare and outcomes of treatment. Here the disparities between whites and racial and ethnic minorities have been well demonstrated. When healthcare disparities prevent an individual from accessing and receiving quality mental healthcare, there is an impact on their ability to be effective caregivers and productive workers, to successfully fulfill their role as adults. McGuire applied the Institute of Medicine definition of health service disparities, "population group differences in treatment or access not justified by difference in health status or preferences," and found significant disparities between whites and both African Americans and Latinos in mental health service use (2). If we remove the common obstacle of insurance, we still see disparities. Schneider, Zaslavsky, and Epstein assessed more than 300,000 managed Medicare beneficiaries and found significant disparities in quality care, with blacks receiving poorer quality healthcare than whites, including follow-up care after hospitalization for a mental illness (3). Blanco et al. looked at trends in a large national survey of office based treatment of mental disorders for adults between 1993 and 2002 and found a consistent decrease in mental health services for Hispanics, whereas most services for non-Hispanics increased (4). Gilmer et al. (5) looked at access to care as affected by limited English proficiency in San Diego County and found a higher intensity of outpatient mental health services for minorities in clinics that specialized in working with limited English proficiency patients. Blanco et al. (4) further propose that patient preferences and culture may affect access. Hispanics may prefer psychotherapy over medication, and this has been shown to be the case for Hispanics with depression. Also, practical issues interfere with access for lower income groups such as transportation, child care, and inflexible work hours.

As adults, the roles of productive employment, participating in intimate relationships, bearing and raising children, and caring for loved ones are critical. Disparities in access and treatment for illnesses that occur in adulthood clearly affect these roles. In addition, stresses on these roles may vary in different racial and ethnic groups.

Because unemployment is higher in minority groups and worsens in difficult economic times, it follows that this increased stress on groups with less access to care will have negative outcomes. Alegria et al. (6) attempt to look at the complex issue of poverty, race, ethnicity, and social position as it affects access to mental health services. Utilizing data from the national comorbidity survey 1990 to 1992, they found disparities among Latinos, African Americans, and whites linked to economic and social factors as well as race and ethnicity. Poor Latinos had lower access to specialty care than equally poor whites, whereas poor African Americans had access comparable to whites. However, African Americans who were not poor had less access than whites. Alegria et al. (6) conclude that minority status, poverty, and regional location combine in various ways to affect access to specialty mental health services.

In addition to the work role, adults must navigate a variety of intimate and caregiving roles for decades. Intimate relationships in adulthood often provide support and growth but can also be a source of major stress and emotional risk. Intimate partner violence, from mild to severe, is estimated to victimize as many as 1.9 million women ages 18 to 49 in the United States. Women in clinically abusive relationships have a high incidence of developing depression, posttraumatic stress disorder, and anxiety disorders. Victims of intimate partner violence are twice as likely to report unmet need for mental health services as nonvictims, with Hispanic women reporting the highest unmet need. Minority women are less likely to access sources of formal or informal support and are at increased risk of depression or post traumatic stress disorder. Abusive relationships in families often lead to future generations of abusive relationships and require proactive ethnically and culturally sensitive treatment services to break the cycle. Disparities in access to services is a major issue for this vulnerable population.

Motherhood is a major caretaking role in the adult years. Although there are no exact data on the number of mentally ill mothers caring for children, Nicholson et al. (7) estimate from the national comorbidity survey that of the approximately one third of women in the United States with a diagnosable mental illness in the past 12 months, 65% are mothers. Mothers with serious mental illness are more likely to be single, have unplanned pregnancies, and have high likelihood of past victimization (7). It follows that disparities in access to care and treatment for serious mental illness affect the ability of mentally ill parents to care for and successfully raise their children. Practical parenting skills are critical for these mothers, and best practices in teaching and coaching mothers with the additional stress of mental illness must be developed.

Adults caring for adults is a major life role. We see marked disparities in caretaking needs and resources for elder adults that contribute to mid-life adults' stressors. Mid-life adults are euphemistically characterized as the "sandwich generation," layered between caretaking of their children and caretaking of their aging parents. As the U.S. population ages and there are an increasing percentage of the adult population older than 65 years, the volume of such caretaking grows.

To fully grasp the impact disparities of access and care in mental illness have on adulthood, we will now look in detail at three illnesses that affect large numbers of adults. By discussing disparities in depression, schizophrenia, and substance abuse access and treatment, we can see a picture of what is needed to ensure that all adults can benefit from the quality care they need.

MAJOR DEPRESSION

Any discussion of depression in adulthood should begin by describing its tremendous toll on individuals and society. The World Health Organization cites depression as the leading cause of life years lived with disability. Within 20 years it is expected to be second only to cardiac disease as a leading cause of disability adjusted life-years. The financial cost to society in lost productive work time per year is enormous, estimated at 44 billion dollars per year for the United States alone. Thirty-two to 35 million adult Americans will suffer from major depression in the course of their lifetime, and 13 to 14 million Americans each year will have an episode of major depression (8). Of the 14 million Americans who have a depressive episode each year, 59% will have severe role impairment that will interfere seriously with their daily functioning. It is estimated that 90% of the 32,000 suicides in the United States each year occur in individuals with depression. Families of depressed individuals also bear the burden of the illness and need support and assistance as caregivers. The toll on society of this illness during adulthood is enormous. Despite these statistics, depression is still woefully underdiagnosed and undertreated in the United States.

Because of this enormous impact of depression in adulthood, we have chosen to use depression as a prototype to first examine the disparities in the access to mental healthcare and treatment in adults. Since most adults in the United States present with depression not to specialty mental health clinics but to their primary care physician, it is appropriate to look in primary care clinics for disparities. By looking at the literature on the disparities in diagnosis, treatment and outcomes for depression in primary care clinics we have a useful snapshot of depression care on the front lines in the United States. Next we will examine disparities in the treatment of depression and their impact on the roles of work and caregiver.

Clearly, the diagnosis and treatment of depression in adult primary care is a major public health priority and recent screening and treatment protocols instituted in primary care clinics have increasingly shown successful outcomes. Therefore assessing whether there are significant racial and ethnic disparities in the diagnosis and treatment of depression in primary care might serve as a proxy for investigating real access for adults to care. However, disparities in the treatment of depression are found fairly consistently and imply issues of inadequate engagement in treatment, lack of sensitivity to minority treatment expectations and choices, and language and cultural barriers. Even though primary care physicians have improved in diagnosing depression among minorities, Latino and African American patients are still less likely to receive appropriate care. African American and Latino patients were less likely to receive and take antidepressant medications than were whites. Latinos were less likely to receive specialty mental health services than were whites or African Americans. Physicians of different ethnicities than the patient may be less collaborative with the patient and less likely to involve the patient in shared decision making. Language barriers may also be an issue for Latino patients. Harman and colleagues (9) looked at medical claims expenditures of 2000 patients and found that African Americans and Latinos were less likely to fill an antidepressant prescription, but if they did fill one, they were as likely as Caucasians to complete an adequate course of treatment, again pointing to the importance of engagement of the patient with the physician in treatment decisions. African Americans were more likely to complete a course of psychotherapy than whites or Latinos, again showing a preference for treatment without medication (10). A recent indirect approach to looking at disparities in treatment for patient groups most in need of treatment looked at Medicaid prescriptions filled for antidepressants in the year preceding a successful suicide. The findings showed that 51% of whites but only 29% of African Americans filled prescriptions for antidepressants (11). Engagement in care is critical for a successful outcome, and engagement involves sensitivity to ethnic and racial differences in attitudes and beliefs toward mental illness and the treatments we recommend.

Cooper et al. (12) looked at treatment preferences among different ethnic and racial groups in primary care offices and found that African Americans and Hispanics are less likely than whites to find antidepressant medication acceptable, and that more Hispanics preferred counseling than whites. African American patients with an affective disorder are less likely to receive ECT treatment that Caucasians. In a retrospective study of more than 1000 patients treated with ECT, this difference could not be explained by demographic or socioeconomic variables. Possible explanations to be investigated include physician preferences, cultural differences in patient's acceptance, or differences in clinical presentation (13). Adults are free to choose whether or not to accept a treatment recommendation. Providers' sensitivity to the treatment preferences of different racial and ethnic groups may influence patient's follow-through with treatment.

Despite these differences, an interesting study that looked at a diverse group of white, Hispanic, and African American patients over a 5-year period found that improvement in health outcomes and a decrease in disparities did occur as result of a 5-year quality improvement project that focused on a an enhanced model of care for depression (14). The model included supporting teams that received specialized training in the treatment of depression, patient education, and resources to support medication management or psychotherapy for up to 6 to 12 months after diagnosis for a depressive episode. After 5 years, 991 primary care patients who were assigned to usual care or enhanced treatment were interviewed. The results showed an improvement in health outcomes for the enhanced treatment group that was caused by an improvement in outcomes for the Hispanic and African American participants, with whites remaining unchanged. This poses the interesting question regarding whether some of the disparities in treatment that we see are indirectly the result of a lack of appropriate supports and best practices being systematically implemented in our daily practice. This project clearly showed a way to decrease disparities that is both practical and effective.

Now that it has been established that there are disparities in the treatment of depression, we will look at the impact of disparities more directly on the adult roles of work and caregiver. Work is a major role of adulthood. Disruptions in ability to work or to be productive in a way that society recognizes has a significant impact on an adult. Depression is known to adversely affect work and productivity and its adequate treatment to have a positive effect. Appropriate treatment of depression in adults in a primary care clinic at 6 months not only showed a decrease in depression but a higher quality of life and higher rates of employment.

Lack of insurance clearly limits access to care. Persons without insurance were less likely to initiate treatment for depression, although if initiated outcomes were similar. However, access is not limited only by insurance, as shown by numerous studies, but also by other factors that we still need to learn much about. A study by Schneider et al. (3) showed that minority use of mental health services was less than whites in a Medicare managed care plan where all were insured. When socioeconomic factors, illness, age, and so forth were removed, there was still less use. The conclusion was that "factors" in the provider patient relationship were at play.

Caretaking is the second major role of adulthood and spans the generations from childbearing and rearing to caring for elder parents. A major vulnerability for mothers is prenatal and postpartum depression, which can adversely affect the mother in her ability to care for her children and on her relationships with family and friends. Rich-Edwards et al. (15) studied 1662 women and the association of race, ethnicity, age, finances, and partnership status being associated with antenatal and postpartum symptoms. There were no differences among black and Hispanic and white mothers. There was an increase in depressive symptoms found if the woman had financial hardship, lower income, an unwanted pregnancy, and a prior history of depression. Race and ethnicity were less powerful than socioeconomic factors. Once again, social and economic disparities are major stressors and clearly increase depressive symptoms and decrease functioning.

The question of the interrelationship between racial and ethnic variables and a wide variety of other variables such as socioeconomic factors, education, gender, and age are a significant issue when trying to tease out reasons for apparent differences in access to care and outcomes. In the current limited prenatal and postpartum literature, economic factors play a major role in depressive symptoms postpartum. The impact on low-income families of now being responsible for the care and growth of a child are significant and may outweigh many other factors. This is a cautionary example of the power of socioeconomic factors in disparities in healthcare.

Adults are also caretakers of adults. In a large California survey of families of adults with major mental illness in the public sector, Snowden (16) found that 72% of Asian American clients, 62% of Latino clients, 35% of African American clients, and 22% of white clients lived with their families. Although the intensity of support varied, more intensive support generally followed the same pattern. The emotional and financial stress placed on these family caregivers often leads to symptoms of anxiety and depression.

Pinquart and Sorensen (17) completed in 2005 a comprehensive metaanalysis of the literature of ethnic differences in stressors, resources and psychological outcomes of caregiving for adult family members. Some of their major findings included that African American adult caregivers had lower levels of caregiver burden and depression than white caregivers. It has been suggested that African Americans' close family ties, spirituality, and value of the caregiver role decrease the emotional burden. This is despite the findings that in families with loved ones suffering from dementia, African American families wait longer for placement, and their family members with dementia have a larger number of dementia related behaviors than white patients. Pinquart and Sorensen also found that Hispanic and Asian American caregivers were more depressed than white non-Hispanic caregivers. Here it has been shown that although Hispanic caregivers may have informal supports, they have less access to formal resources, with resulting financial and social burdens. It is suggested that for Asian caregivers, the daughter-in-law is expected to assume the caretaker role for the aging parent with dementia, and to the degree there is conflict in the relationship, this contributes to the emotional burden and depression. Once again, Hispanic caregivers of patients with dementia wait longer for nursing home placement than whites, and again their loved ones have a higher number of dementia related behaviors than white patients. It is critical when working therapeutically with adult patients to take into account the stress and at times significant burden of the caregiver role and to be aware of the ethnic and racial differences in that role.

SCHIZOPHRENIA

Schizophrenia is a serious, debilitating, lifelong mental illness primarily affecting the entire adult life cycle. The effect of schizophrenia on a person's life can present a significant burden to those affected with the disease, but also to their families and to society in general. Schizophrenia is one of the leading causes of disability among adults, and especially young adults. The onset of schizophrenia is usually in young adulthood and persists throughout their life. Schizophrenia causes significant disability hindering the individual's ability to work, to attend school, to develop intimate relationships or social support network, or to act effectively in the roles of providers and caregivers to their families. In a study by the World Health Organization and the World Bank, schizophrenia ranked as the ninth leading cause of disability in people ages 15 to 44 years worldwide and the fourth leading cause of disability in developed countries (18).

Disparities are found among adults with schizophrenia. Disparities exist related to age, gender, race or ethnicity, cultural factors, socioeconomic factors, and insurance status. These disparities cross the continuum of healthcare of these individuals and are seen in both general healthcare and specialty mental healthcare settings. Affected areas include assessment and diagnosis, access to health and mental health treatment, types and modalities of treatment received, and differences in levels of care and treatment provided. Schizophrenia is a severe and persistent mental disease with profound disabling effects on individuals and families. The disparities that affect the schizophrenic patient negatively affect positive outcomes for the patient.

A cultural disparity has been found related to the role of family. Studies suggest that family may enhance ones ability to resist or adapt to stressors. In cultures in which the role and responsibility of the family is primary rather than a strong focus on individualism, the schizophrenic patient often is protected from some of the effects of stress and less optimal treatment (19). The emphasis of the role of the family may promote better outcomes than for patients where their culture emphasizes the role of the individual. The role and responsibility of the family help the patient to adapt and provide a level of structure and support within the family unit. The role of the family as the primary unit is frequently seen in the Asian cultures of Chinese, Japanese, and other Asian Americans (19).

Studies have demonstrated various disparities in diagnosis, symptom profiles, access to care, and the treatment of schizophrenia related to race, ethnicity, and socioeconomic status. Early studies in the United States found a higher rate of schizophrenia in African Americans and Hispanics than in Caucasians. This finding was the result of bias to overdiagnose schizophrenia in African Americans and Hispanics (20). Studies indicate mixed results that delusions and/or hallucinations are more common among African American patients. Auditory hallucinations were strongly correlated with a misdiagnosis of schizophrenia and American psychiatrists tend to give a diagnosis of schizophrenia with the presence of auditory hallucinations during an episode (20). Ethnicity was also found to be a factor in the misdiagnosis of bipolar patients as schizophrenic, even if treated by an African American, Hispanic, or Spanish-speaking psychiatrist (20).

The disparities in the mental healthcare of schizophrenics begin with the assessment and diagnosis. Issues related to disparity in the diagnosis of schizophrenia include service utilization differences, the stage of illness and intensity of symptoms at the time of presentation, sociocultural issues, and cross-cultural competence of clinicians. Several studies have indicated that African Americans may be more likely to be misdiagnosed as schizophrenic than Caucasians (20).

When compared with Caucasians with schizophrenia, non-Caucasians are less likely to be diagnosed with a co-occurring affective disorder but more likely to be diagnosed with a psychotic disorder. Possible explanations for this disparity include several theories. Diversity of symptom presentation is one idea. Non-Caucasian schizophrenics may seek care or gain access to care later in the illness and present with more severe psychotic symptoms that mask symptoms of depression. Non-Caucasian patients more frequently access care through emergency services rather than use clinics and individual practitioners. Clinicians may also lack training for cross-cultural competence and fail to recognize depressive symptoms. Sociocultural differences in treatment-seeking behavior among patients can also be a factor in the difference in diagnosis of comorbid depression.

Disparities exist in the rate at which second-generation antipsychotics are prescribed for African American, Hispanic, and Caucasian patients with schizophrenia. Studies show that Caucasians are six times more likely to receive second-generation antipsychotic medications than are African Americans or Hispanics. The finding that African American and Hispanic patients are less likely to receive a second-generation antipsychotic is a consistent finding in both academic and community-based treatment programs (21). Caucasian patients are more than twice as likely as African American patients to receive clozapine and are less likely to have clozapine therapy discontinued. Studies suggest that the differential use of clozapine with African American patients may result from a greater perceived risk of clozapine-induced diabetes and agranulocytosis among African American patients. Pharmacological evidence has suggested that African Americans may have lower baseline white blood cell and neutrophil counts and that benign leukopenia in African Americans may not be indicative of a higher risk of agranulocytosis. Further investigation of this fact is certainly indicated and may lead to the development of guidelines for the use of clozapine among African Americans and may increase access to clozapine, currently one of the most effective antipsychotics available (21).

Although evidence is inconclusive, some studies indicate that African Americans metabolize antipsychotics more slowly than Caucasians. The difference in metabolism can result in a faster and higher rate of response and an increase in side effects when African Americans are treated with the same dosages as Caucasians (22). Other studies have indicated that African Americans require the same dosages and have the same rate of response as Caucasians but that Hispanics and Asians require lower dosages than Caucasian or African American patients. Other studies indicate that racial differences are caused by clinician's biases rather than pharmacokinetic or pharmacodynamic factors (22).

Variability in the use of second-generation antipsychotics among different racial or ethnic groups may also be related to financial barriers. African American and Hispanics are less likely to have health insurance or to have private insurance and are more likely to be publicly insured. African Americans and Hispanics also rely more on the use of emergency services for treatment rather than on clinics or individual psychiatrists (22). The second-generation antipsychotics are frequently associated with higher costs. As a result, some public treatment systems and health plans require trials of conventional antipsychotics prior to the use of any second-generation antipsychotic. This factor may limit the use and availability of second-generation antipsychotics, especially in minority groups with public insurance plans. African American patients with schizophrenia are more likely to receive depot medications than are Caucasian and Hispanic patients with schizophrenia (23). The increased use of depot medications was found across treatment settings, including emergency services and inpatient and outpatient settings. These prescribing disparities were noted in studies even after demographic characteristics, education level, and source of payment were controlled (23).

In addition to pharmacological differences, other differential service use patterns are found between ethnic groups. Caucasian patients with schizophrenia are more likely to receive a variety of mental health services than are non-Caucasian patients.

Studies have found that African American patients were less likely than Caucasian patients to receive intensive case management or partial hospitalization and are more likely to have emergency services contacts. This indicates that African American patients are not as engaged in the more continuous and intensive type of treatment services associated with persistent mental health disorders (23).

Prescription practices as well as other treatment practices should be guided by various factors of a patient's need determined through the assessment and treatment process. These treatment practices and decisions are also influenced by the skill and investment of the clinician in engaging patients in the assessment and treatment process. Race, ethnicity, and culture can influence communication and the ability of the clinician to effectively engage the patient in the process of treatment. Studies have found that when clinicians made efforts to engage non-Caucasian patients in the evaluation and treatment process, fewer differences were found in both pharmacological and other treatment practices (24).

In summary, schizophrenic patients are profoundly affected by the symptoms and natural course of the disease. Disparities may also have a negative effect on many suffering from schizophrenia. Access to care is more limited for some, whereas others receive a varying level of care depending on their ethnicity, race, culture, and even age. Often the schizophrenic patient may receive what could be considered less than an optimal level of care or certainly not what is currently the best or standard of care. Outcomes are therefore less than optimal. The schizophrenic's functional and cognitive abilities are compromised not only by the disease of schizophrenia but also from the influences and outcomes of the disparities of care and treatment. Further study may influence the understanding of the origin and effect of the disparities. Cross-cultural education, use of standardized assessment tools, and use of evidenced based practices can decrease the disparities seen in the treatment of the schizophrenic patient.

SUBSTANCE ABUSE

Alcohol and substance abuse–related problems affect numerous roles and responsibilities of adult life. Excessive substance and alcohol use may lead to social issues including loss of job, intimate partner violence, divorce, legal involvement from intoxication and driving, and physical factors of dependence, including tremors, neurological impairment, cirrhosis, and mortality. Disparities related to race, ethnicity, and culture are known to exist related to alcohol and substance use and abuse.

During the period of 1985 to 1995, studies demonstrated a shift in drinking patterns among ethnic groups, with a decrease in drinking among Caucasians but not among African Americans or Hispanics. When studies looked at substance and alcohol use–related problems, Hispanics reported twice the rate of problems of Caucasians and African Americans. Among Hispanics, Mexican Americans were found to have more alcohol-related problems than Cuban Americans and Puerto Ricans. African Americans were found to have a higher rate of intimate partner violence related to alcohol and substance use compared with Caucasians (25).

When treatment is considered, disparities exist across cultural groups as well as within subgroups of a culture. African Americans were found to use both primary care substance abuse treatment as well as specialty care substance abuse treatment services less than for Caucasians and Hispanics. Minority groups consistently reported less access to care, poor quality of care, and greater unmet need for alcoholism and substance abuse treatment.

Health insurance status represents an important barrier in accessing substance abuse treatment services. Adults in the lower income levels, especially Hispanics and Asians, and less educated adults are more likely to be underinsured. Lower income levels usually correlate with being uninsured or underinsured. Many insurance plans do not have parity related to substance abuse treatment. Minorities, especially Hispanics, African Americans, and Asians, have lower rates of insurance or are have public insurance plans that affect the access to treatment services for these groups.

Co-occurrence of substance abuse and psychiatric disorders increase the need for the access to appropriate treatment services. Untreated psychiatric disorders usually indicate poor outcomes of substance abuse treatment. Some of the most common types of coexisting psychiatric disorder are mood disorders. Studies have shown that the SSRI antidepressants improve the outcome of patients with comorbid affective and substance abuse disorders. Analysis of prescription practices in this population revealed lower access to SSRI medications among racial and ethnic minority groups, especially African Americans and Hispanics. These disparities result from characteristics of patients, including insurance coverage, socioeconomic status, and cultural differences in treatment seeking. The differences also result from biases of medical providers.

Native Americans have high rates of mental health and substance abuse disorders (26). Within the Native American culture, there are significant tribal differences in the prevalence of substance abuse disorders. Studies including the National Comorbidity Study show a higher rate of substance abuse in both men and women of various Native American Tribes. Southwest men had the highest rate of substance abuse, but not the Northern Plains men. Women in the Northern Plains tribe were at higher risk than subjects in the NCS study (26). Although not conclusive, disparities related to substance abuse risk exist in several Native American groups by tribe and gender. Other treatment services for both mental health and substance abuse are not as easily available as with other minority groups and settings. However, studies have found a high rate of treatment seeking behavior in Native Americans related to substance abuse disorders (26).

The effects of substance abuse on the adult encompass physical, psychological, and functional aspects of one's life. Substance abuse can lead to loss of family, job, income, and physical health. Disparities in access to treatment and in treatment modalities have a direct effect on the individual's ability to carry out the roles of the adult life cycle. The effects of the disparities in care increase the negative effects experienced by the individual and on their roles as an adult. A better understanding of disparities in relation to substance abuse can improve outcomes for those with this disorder.

CONCLUSION

Adulthood is characterized by the key roles of work and caregiving. Mental illness, if it is not recognized and treated appropriately, will have a negative impact on these roles. If treatment is not accessible and accepted by the patient and family, it will not be successful. Disparities exist in all these variables across race and ethnicity in the care system in the United States.

This chapter has presented these disparities in psychiatric care for three major mental illnesses of adulthood: major depression, schizophrenia, and substance abuse, and how these disparities affect an individual's ability to successfully navigate the decades of adulthood. Much more must be learned about how to prevent these disparities, how to design a system of care to meet the needs of multiple races and ethnicities, and how to help clinicians to treat our diverse patients more effectively.

References

1. McGuire TG, Miranda J. New evidence regarding racial and ethnic disparities in mental health: Policy implications. *Health Affairs* 2008;27:393–403.
2. McGuire TG, Alegria M, Cook BL, et al. Implementing the Institute of Medicine definition of disparities: An application to mental health care. *Health Serv Res* 2006;41: 1979–2005.
3. Schneider EC, Zaslavsky AM, Epstein AM. Racial disparities in the quality of care for enrollees in Medicare managed care. *JAMA* 2002;287:1288–1294.
4. Blanco C, Patel SR, Liu L, et al. National trends in ethnic disparities in mental health care. *Med Care* 2007;45:1012–1019.
5. Gilmer TP, Ojeda VD, Folsom DP, et al. Initiation and use of public mental health services by persons with severe mental illness and limited English proficiency. *Psychiatr Serv* 2007;58:1555–1562.
6. Alegria M, Canino G, Rios R, et al. Mental health care for Latinos: Inequalities in the use of specialty mental health services among Latinos, African Americans and non-Latino whites. *Psychiatr Serv* 2002;53:1547–1555.
7. Nicholson J, Biebel K, Hinden B, et al. *Critical Issues for Parents with Mental Illness and Their Families.* Center for Mental Health Services Substance Abuse and Mental Health Services Administration. July 2001.
8. Kessler RC, Beglund P, Demler O, et al. The epidemiology of major depressive: Results from the National Comorbidity Survey Replication (NCS-R). *JAMA* 2003;289: 3095–3105.
9. Harman JS, Edlund MJ, Fortney JC. Disparities in the adequacy of depression treatment in the United States. *Psychiatr Serv* 2004;55:1379–1385.
10. Simpson SM, Krishman LL, Kunik ME, et al. Racial disparities in diagnosis and treatment of depression: A literature review. *Psychiatr Q* 2007;78:3–14.
11. Ray WA, Hall K, Meador KG. Racial differences in antidepressant treatment preceding suicide in a Medicaid population. *Psychiatr Serv* 2007;58:1317–1327.
12. Cooper LA, Gonzalez JJ, Gallo JJ, et al. The acceptability of treatment for depression among African American, Hispanic, and white primary care patients. *Med Care* 2003;41: 479–489.
13. Breakey WR, Dunn GJ. Racial disparity in the use of ECT for affective disorders. *Am J Psychiatry* 2004;161:1635–1641.
14. Wells K, Sherbourne C, Schoenbaum M, et al. Five-year impact of quality improvement for depression: Results of a group-level randomized trial. *Arch Gen Psychiatry* 2004;61: 378–386.
15. Rich-Edwards JW, Kleinman K, Abrams A, et al. Sociodemographic predictors of antenatal and postpartum depressive symptoms among women in a medical practice group. *J Epidemiol Comm Health* 2006;60:221–227.
16. Snowden LR. Explaining mental health treatment disparities: Ethnic and cultural differences in family involvement. *Cult Med Psychiatry* 2007;31:389–402.
17. Pinquart M, Sorensen S. Ethnic differences in stressors, resources, and psychological outcomes of family caregiving: A meta-analysis. *Gerontologist* 2005;45:90–106.
18. Murray CJL, Lopez AD, eds. *The Global Burden of Disease: A Comprehensive Assessment of Mortality and Disability from Diseases, Injuries, and Risk Factors in 1990 and Projected to 2020.* Cambridge, MA: Harvard University Press, 1996.
19. Sue S, Chu JY. The mental health of ethnic minority groups: Challenges posed by the supplement to the Surgeon General's report on mental health. *Cult Med Psychiatry* 2003;27: 447–465.
20. Mukherjee S, Shukla S, Woodle J, et al. Misdiagnosis of schizophrenia in bipolar patients: A multiethnic comparison. *Am J Psychiatry* 1983;140:1571–1574.

21. Mallinger JB, Fisher SG, Brown T, et al. Racial disparities in the use of second-generation antipsychotics for the treatment of schizophrenia. *Psychiatr Serv* 2006;57:133–136.

22. Herbeck DM, West JC, Ruditis I, et al. Variations in use of second-generation antipsychotic medication by race among adult psychiatric patients. *Psychiatr Serv* 2004;55: 677–684.

23. Kuno E, Rothbard AB. Racial disparities in antipsychotic prescription patterns for patients with schizophrenia. *Am J Psychiatry* 2002;159:567–572.

24. Segal SP, Bola JR, Watson MA. Race, quality of care, and antipsychotic prescribing practices in psychiatric emergency services. *Psychiatr Serv* 1996;47:282–286.

25. Caetano R. Alcohol-related health disparities and treatment-related epidemiological findings among whites, blacks, and Hispanics in the United States. *Alcohol Clin Exp Res* 2003;27:1337–1339.

26. Beals J, Novins DK, Whitesell NR. Prevalence of mental disorders and utilization of mental health services in two American Indian reservation populations: Mental health disparities in a national context. *Am J Psychiatry* 2005;162:1723–1732.

14 Older Adults

Maria D. Llorente, Vernon I. Nathaniel, and Shunda McGahee

INTRODUCTION

Practically all healthcare providers will work with older adults at some point in their career, and are likely to do so in ever-growing numbers. In the United States, with improved access to healthcare, today's elderly are healthier, more active, and in better financial circumstances than previous generations of seniors. The majority of elderly consider themselves to be in good to excellent health, and 75% report minor, if any, limitation in activities of daily living (1). Despite these successes, older adults have more complex conditions and greater healthcare needs than do younger persons. Many barriers persist in access to mental healthcare for older adults. Additionally, there is a dangerous shortage of providers with specialty training in geriatrics generally, and geriatric mental health specifically, at a time when the population is aging. This chapter will describe some of the challenges that currently exist in meeting the vast mental health needs of our older adult population, and some of the anticipated future needs.

DEMOGRAPHIC TRANSITION

The world is currently undergoing an unprecedented demographic transition. Although fertility rates have declined worldwide, life expectancy has significantly increased. By 2045 to 2050, average life expectancy is projected to reach 76 years for the world as a whole, 80 years in the more developed regions and 71 years in less developed areas (2). In 2007, almost 40 million Americans were 65 years or older (12.6% of the U.S. population). By 2030, the number of older adults is expected to increase to more than 71 million persons (almost 20% of the total population), and the majority of these older adults are women because of their lower overall mortality rates.

Not only are people reaching older age, but having achieved this, they tend to live longer. The average annual growth rate of persons aged 80 years and older (nearly 4%) is twice as high as the growth rate of those older than 60 years (1.9%). More than half of the population older than 80 years reside in just six countries: China (12 million), the United States (9 million), India (6 million), Japan (5million), Germany (3 million), and Russia (3 million).

The diversity of the U.S. aging population is also changing. From 2000 to 2030, the proportion of persons aged greater than 65 years who are members of racial minority groups (i.e., black, Native American, Asian/Pacific Islander) is expected to increase from 11.3% to 16.5% and the proportion of older Hispanics are expected to nearly double, from 5.6% to 10.9% (3). By 2050, the percentage of the non-Hispanic white older group is expected to decline from 84% to 64%. Hispanics are projected to account for 16% of the older population; 12% of the population is projected to be non-Hispanic black; and 7% of the population is projected to be non-Hispanic Asian and Pacific Islander. In fact, the Hispanic older population is projected to grow the fastest, from about 2 million in 2000 to over 13 million by 2050.

EPIDEMIOLOGIC TRANSITION

Simultaneously, and partly as a result of this demographic transition, there has been a parallel epidemiologic transition. In the developed world, chronic diseases and degenerative illnesses now surpass infectious agents as the leading causes of death and disability. This epidemiologic transition, in conjunction with the growing number of older adults, represents a tremendous public health challenge. In the United States, for example, nearly 80% of adults aged 65+ years have at least one chronic illness and half have at least two (4). The incidence and prevalence of cardiovascular diseases and diabetes mellitus, both which cause excess morbidity and higher healthcare costs, and are associated with depression and cognitive impairment, are expected to increase. Similarly, the prevalence of progressive dementias increases with age. The prevalence of Alzheimer's disease, for example, approaches 50% in those aged 85 and older and is currently the major cause of functional dependence among U.S. elderly. Women are more likely to be affected, but this is mainly because of their longer life expectancies. Lower levels of education are associated with Alzheimer's disease, presenting unique concerns for disparities among ethnic minority elderly (5). Despite the incremental advances in educational attainment among older Americans, substantial educational differences among racial and ethnic elderly remain. In 1998, among elderly aged 65 and older, about 72% of non-Hispanic whites had finished high school, compared with only 65% of Asian and Pacific Islanders, 44% of non-Hispanic blacks, and 29% of Hispanics.

Chronic medical conditions are also associated with an increased risk for major depression, which is associated with nonadherence to treatment of co-occurring medical conditions, poorer medical outcomes, increased healthcare utilization, and significant disability (6,7). As a result, adults with chronic conditions tend to use far more health services, resulting in the increased Medicare expenditures seen during the past two decades (8) and a significant cause for concern for the next several decades.

GERIATRIC SPECIALTY SHORTAGES

Adequate workforce numbers and training has long been a concern for geriatric providers, older adults, and policy makers concerned about meeting the healthcare needs of older adults. A recent Institute of Medicine report (9) concluded that without significant national changes, older Americans will lack access to affordable, quality healthcare, including mental health services. Currently, there is only one geriatric psychiatrist for every 10,000 Americans older than 75 years. Estimates are that 5000 geriatric psychiatrists are needed, but there are fewer than 1600 board-certified specialists in this area. Of concern is that only 65% of psychiatrists currently accept Medicare, the primary third-party payer for older adults.

This problem extends to other disciplines as well. Only about 5% of social workers and 3% of psychologists self-identify their primary area of practice as aging, with fewer than 28% of psychologists having graduate geriatric training. The National Institute of Aging has estimated that by 2020, more than 60,000 gerontological social workers and about 6000 geriatric psychologists will be needed. Most geriatric mental health services are thus delivered by generalists who often have had minimal, if any, specialty training in geriatrics, and report feeling ill-equipped to address the complex medical and psychosocial needs of older patients.

Several reasons have been cited for this severe shortage: lack of parity in reimbursement that makes mental health a generally less desirable area to pursue, lack of recognition of the impending geriatric imperative and inadequate training of the general healthcare workforce, costs associated with additional years of specialty training that do not translate into added income, and generally, lower income for geriatric specialists than either other specialists, or generalists in their own disciplines. Additionally, a significant proportion of geriatric psychiatrists and mental healthcare providers are Baby Boomers themselves, and are expected to retire or reduce their workloads in the near future. To add these concerns, Baby Boomers have used mental health services to a greater extent than their parents and were more likely to have used recreational substances of abuse. It is likely that there will be a greater demand for geriatric mental healthcare services than current estimates might suggest.

PREVALENCE OF MENTAL ILLNESS AND ACCESS DISPARITIES IN THE ELDERLY

Older adults are more likely to seek mental health treatment in primary care settings, however, than in specialty mental health. Mental health disorders are, unfortunately, often unrecognized or inadequately treated. The prevalence of primary psychotic disorders, such as schizophrenia and delusional disorders, decreases with age to about 0.5% of older adults. The prevalence of alcohol use disorders varies by gender (men have higher rates than women) and setting, with rates varying from 2% to 3% in community-dwelling men, to 15% to 20% in medical settings. Older problem drinkers are identified less often by clinicians and are less often referred for treatment than their younger counterparts for several reasons. The older retired person, who drinks at home, alone, is less likely to become involved in fights, get arrested, or drive while intoxicated, so that applying DSM criteria becomes problematic. Providers may easily overlook the physical effects of alcohol use, attributing them instead to common disorders of late life. Some older adults increase drinking as the result of excess free time, available disposable income, and psychiatric disorders, particularly depression. Mood and cognitive disorders, however, are most commonly seen in this age group and will be the primary disorders covered in this chapter.

Ethnic and racial minority adults are even less likely than Caucasian elderly to seek specialty mental healthcare (10), and there are within-group differences. Among Latinos, for example, Mexican American elders are less likely to visit physicians than are Cuban American seniors. Because of the stigma associated with having a mental illness, minority elderly are more likely to express psychological distress through somatic symptoms and are thus more likely to go to primary care providers for help with mental health problems. Additional reasons for these findings include lack of health insurance, stigma, language barriers, lack of transportation and geographic distance, costs, long waits for appointments, clinician-patient cultural distance, and mistrust. Last, among ethnic minority elderly, spiritual leaders, complementary or alternative medicine providers, or traditional healers may be used preferentially, as are the use of folk medicine and herbs, plants, roots, and teas for medicinal purposes (11).

DISPARITIES IN DEPRESSION CARE

Lack of identification of depressive symptoms and resultant lack of treatment is a significant disparity that disproportionately affects older adults. Both prevalence and incidence studies consistently report that DSM-based diagnoses of major depression decline with age, but symptom-based assessment studies demonstrate increased rates of depressive symptoms in older adults. Mood disorders meeting full DSM criteria affect 2% to 4% of community-dwelling seniors. Minor depression, however, is much more prevalent, with as many as another 10% to 37% exhibiting subsyndromal symptoms that significantly interfere with daily functioning and are of clinical significance. Only 29% of depressed older patients in primary care receive adequate antidepressant treatment (dose and duration), and, although most preferred psychotherapy over medications, only 8% had received such treatment (12).

There are many reasons for this. First, older adults often present with vague somatic symptoms and loss of interest, without a sad mood per se. Second, their symptoms are more likely to be attributed to chronic medical conditions rather than being recognized as depression. Third, providers often overidentify with patients or falsely believe the widely held myth that depression is a "normal" part of aging. Complex psychosocial factors, such as losses of significant others or decline in physical functioning can further divert attention from consideration of a depression diagnosis. Last, both patients and healthcare providers may be concerned about the stigma associated with having a mental health disorder and/or receiving treatment.

There are additional disparities associated with lack of appropriate depression management when one considers the consequences of untreated depression. Worldwide, by 2020, untreated depression is projected to be the second leading cause of Disability Adjusted Life Years (DALYS) for all ages and both genders. DALYS are the sum of years of potential life lost as the result of premature mortality and the years of productive life lost as the result of disability (13). Untreated depression is also associated with poorer adherence to medical treatment recommendations, poorer medical outcomes, and increased health services utilization. For example, when depression co-occurs with diabetes, studies have consistently demonstrated poorer glycemic control, less adherence to oral hypoglycemic medications, decreased physical activity, poorer adherence to dietary recommendations, higher obesity, and more diabetes end-organ complications (14–17).

Similarly, untreated depression is associated with greater mortality from co-occurring medical causes. The most consistent evidence comes from patient populations who have had myocardial infarctions (MI). Depression commonly occurs following an MI in older patients. Among older primary care patients, depression has been found to contribute as much to mortality as did MI or diabetes (18). Older post-MI patients with depression have almost a fourfold increased risk of dying with the first 4 months after discharge (19). This risk persists with depression being a significant predictor of 18-month post-MI cardiac mortality (20). The risk associated with depression was found to be greatest among patients with 10 or more premature ventricular contractions per hour, suggesting an arrhythmic mechanism as the link between psychological factors and sudden cardiac death. Other possible mechanisms underlying this association include a higher number of comorbidities among older post-MI patients with depression; sicker patients who are older and depressed may be prescribed medications known to reduce post-MI mortality less often; and these patients may be less adherent to recommendations to reduce cardiac risk.

An added cause for increased mortality among older adults is the association between depression and suicide, with the largest disparity occurring in elderly white men. In 2005, the average rate of suicide for the United States was 11 per 100,000. The rate for adults 65 or older was 14.7 per 100,000, but for elderly white men was 32 per 100,000. Risk factors for suicide among older persons differ from those among the young. Older persons who commit suicide have a much higher prevalence of depression and alcohol abuse, are more likely to use highly lethal methods, especially firearms, and are more likely to be socially isolated. They also make fewer attempts per completed suicide and have a higher male-to-female ratio than other groups. They are more likely to have a larger number of co-occurring chronic medical conditions and have often visited a healthcare provider in the month before their suicide. Among individuals with suicidal ideation, one large study of diverse elderly primary care patients found that the highest rates of suicidal ideation occurred in persons with comorbid anxiety and major depression (21). Asians report the highest proportion of suicidal or death ideation, and African Americans, the lowest reports. Fewer social supports and greater severity of mood and anxiety symptoms were associated with greater ideation. Although much research has investigated the risk factors, very little research has examined the protective factors associated with lower suicide rates in some minority elderly groups.

Among minority elderly, African Americans have lower lifetime prevalence of depression with less reported dysphoric mood or anhedonia compared with whites, and, not surprisingly, as a result, antidepressants are less likely to be prescribed for African Americans. Interestingly, when structured interviews are used, prevalence rates are similar to those of Caucasians (22), suggesting the possibility that raising the index of suspicion for the presence of a depressive disorder among healthcare providers working with minority elderly may enhance detection and treatment rates. Latinos, as a group, have a large number of risk factors associated with depression. Lack of immigration documentation creates added barriers to seeking mental healthcare and can make Latino elderly more susceptible to discrimination, poor housing and poor work conditions, and increased fears of being reported to law enforcement officials. Length of time residing in the United States may be associated with increased prevalence of depressive disorders among Mexican Americans, although ability to speak English has been associated with improved well-being among Latino elders.

MODELS TO ADDRESS DEPRESSION CARE DISPARITIES

The most effective models to date that enhance detection and treatment adherence for depression are those that use collaborative care. These models typically embed a mental health depression specialist within primary care, where most elderly seek assistance. In addition, these models provide structured collaboration between primary care and mental healthcare providers, utilize active monitoring of antidepressant adherence, implement disease self-management education, and in some cases deliver time-limited and structured psychotherapy within primary care. A basic component of these models is the use of standardized tools to screen all patients for depression. The most commonly used instruments include the Beck Depression Inventory (23) and the Patient Health Questionnaire (24).

Studies have consistently demonstrated efficacy of this approach and acceptability to older adults (25,26). Of interest is that when this model is implemented, quality of depression care improves for all patients in the primary care setting, regardless of race or ethnicity. This suggests that a standardized approach, provided to all patients can significantly impact healthcare disparities, even among minority elderly. This model may be particularly effective for elderly Latino patients who tend to prefer treatments that include giving advice, having a concrete focus, and using a problem-centered approach. Additionally, in working with minority elderly, involvement of family members provides added psychosocial support and acceptance for the affected person, and facilitates reintegration of the older person within his or her family system.

The implementation of guideline-based depression interventions in primary care settings worldwide has the potential to reduce the disease burden of depression by 10% to 30% (27). Outreach and maintenance strategies that recognize depression as a recurrent disease, and proactively follow patients on an ongoing basis yield greater health gains, than episodic treatment. Further, collaborative care models for depression are associated with lower total healthcare costs during long-term (4-year) follow-up compared with usual care (mean total costs of $29,422 vs. $32,785) (28). There are fewer data currently available regarding medical outcomes and treatment of depression, and the available data are unclear. For example, in patients with depression and co-occurring diabetes, collaborative care models have improved depression outcomes but not glycemic control. Some have suggested that collaborative care model programs that are targeting co-occurring medical illnesses and depression are most likely to be effective if guideline-based interventions are implemented to address both conditions simultaneously (17). With respect to mortality outcomes, depressed diabetic patients in depression care management practices were less likely to die over the course of a 5-year interval than depressed diabetic patients in usual care practices (29).

Regarding suicide prevention among the elderly, one recent study screened older primary care patients for depression and suicidal ideation and then randomized patients to receive usual care or a guideline-based depression care management intervention (30). Rates of suicidal ideation significantly declined faster in intervention patients compared with usual care patients. At 4 months, rates of suicidal ideation declined from 29.4% to 16.5% in the intervention group compared with a 3.0% decline in the usual care. Among patients reporting suicidal ideation, resolution of ideation was faster among intervention patients ($p = .03$) and intervention patients had a more favorable course of depression.

DISPARITIES IN DEMENTIA CARE

The prevalence of dementia continues to increase with the aging of the population. The most common dementia is Alzheimer's disease, followed by Lewy body dementia and vascular dementia, which collectively account for 20% to 25% of cases. A DSM diagnosis of dementia is made by the presence of memory impairment and disturbance in at least one area of cognitive function, such as the presence of aphasia, apraxia, agnosia, or executive dysfunction. There are currently more than 5 million people affected by Alzheimer's disease in the United States, and this is expected to reach 16 million by 2030. Several studies have found that dementia is significantly more prevalent among African Americans than among whites: 5% versus 3.9% in a recent study (31). The percentage of minority elderly with Alzheimer's disease is projected to increase from 16% to 34% by 2050. It is important to note that there are overall differences in the prevalence of types of dementias among ethnic groups, with a higher prevalence of vascular dementia noted in blacks compared with whites (32). The APOE-4 allele, a recognized genetic risk factor for Alzheimer's disease, occurs with increased frequency in African Americans and Caribbean Hispanics, compared with whites. Individuals with the APOE-4 allele have lower baseline cognitive scores and increased odds of cognitive decline by 59%, but there were no overall racial differences noted (33).

Like detection of depression, recognition of dementia can be challenging, as the differential diagnosis is broad. Reversible factors, such as thyroid disease and vitamin deficiencies, must be considered. Overcoming healthcare provider barriers, however, is a significant problem. In a survey of more than 8000 primary care providers in England, only 60% agreed that it was important to diagnose dementia early (34). One recent study found that 65% of older primary care patients with dementia did not have the diagnosis documented in their medical records, and 67% were not thought to have dementia by their primary care provider (35). In the United States, only 60% of those with significant cognitive impairment are recognized as such by their primary care physician (36). Proposed reasons for this poor recognition include lack of knowledge or skills in suspecting or identifying dementia, attribution of symptoms to other causes, lack of time, and lack of access to specialty geriatric services. An additional barrier is the widely held myth, even among healthcare providers, that memory loss is a normal part of aging.

Additional disparities exist for racial and ethnic minority elderly. In many Asian and Latino communities, for example, there is limited understanding of the diagnosis of dementia. Asian caregivers are more likely to endorse folk explanations, such as stress, as a cause for memory loss. Persons with dementia have higher rates of health service utilization, with African Americans with dementia having the highest levels of service use, compared with Caucasian and Hispanics. Inpatient service utilization and outpatient psychiatric visits were higher for African-Americans with a diagnosis of dementia (37). Persons with hypertension or hypercholesterolemia are 4 times more likely to develop dementia than individuals without these conditions. Since these conditions are more prevalent among African Americans and Latinos, this relationship may be particularly relevant. Minority elderly with moderate to severe dementia residing in the community, have a higher prevalence of dementia-related behavioral disturbances than whites (38),

The legacy of the Tuskegee experiment has had long-lasting detrimental effects on the ability of many clinicians to recruit minority subjects for clinical trials. Elderly minorities are less likely to participate in clinical trials evaluating pharmacologic treatments for dementia. For example, of the more than 10,000 study subjects who participated in the clinical trials for donepezil, galantamine, sabeluzole, and rivastigmine, only 1.9% were African American, 0.9% were Asian, and 0.4% were Hispanic (39). Therefore, current dosing recommendations and side effect education and monitoring are occurring for minority elderly based on very limited information. This may partially explain the finding that minority patients had 40% lower odds of acetylcholinesterase inhibitor use compared with white patients (40). The implementation of culturally sensitive recruitment strategies is likely to improve future recruitment of minority subjects.

ADDRESSING DISPARITIES IN DEMENTIA CARE

Two methods are immediately available to address disparities in dementia care. The first is to aggressively manage those conditions that increase the risk for dementia, namely hypertension, diabetes, and hypercholesterolemia. The second is to improve early detection. There are multiple advantages to early diagnosis. Treatable causes of dementia may be identified and provided early interventions. Patients can be given the diagnosis with enough time to make informed medical, personal, and financial decisions while maintaining the cognitive capacity to do so and to provide input into their preferences for care. Families can also have more time to adjust to the changes that will occur in relatives and engage in longer-term planning without having to make crisis decisions. Additionally, treatments can be offered to patients that may delay disease progression, thus prolonging independence and functionality as long as possible. As such, providing education to healthcare providers and the lay community on recognition of the warning signs of dementia is likely to improve early diagnosis and decrease the normalization of memory problems.

It is important to be cognizant of the presence of caregiver burden. This burden can be exacerbated by several factors, such as the presence of social isolation, resentment toward the family member and resulting feelings of guilt, and lack of understanding of the overall disease process. Multiple psychosocial interventions have been demonstrated to improve outcomes in dementia and decrease caregiver burden, including collaborative care models. Behavioral techniques that target family caregivers can help them identify, plan, and engage in pleasant activities for the patient. Both patients and caregivers have been shown to significantly improve their quality of care and behavioral and psychological symptoms of dementia through a collaborative care model (41). Psychosocial interventions have also been shown to reduce caregiver distress and can delay institutionalization. Those programs that involved patients and caregivers were more intensive and were adapted to the caregiver's specific needs were more likely to be successful (42). In a study that assessed the effects of a structured multicomponent intervention, which addressed caregiver depression, burden, self-care, and social support on caregivers of varying ethnicities, Hispanics and blacks in the intervention group reported significant improvement in quality of life (43). However, psychosocial interventions are not wholly cross-cultural. For instance, within the African American Diaspora, there are many different cultures, including those of Caribbean, African, and Afro-Hispanic descent. Clinicians must be aware of the heterogeneity of people of color. The assignment of a caregiver who has a similar cultural background, if family members are unable to provide primary support, is one method of facilitating improved communication, as well as the formulation of treatment plans that is mindful of the patient's cultural background, incorporating ethnic and sociocultural factors. Caregiver education, increasing in-home support, and expanding community-based resources are likely to be particularly helpful to minority caregivers and patients.

CONCLUSION

Today's elderly are healthier and better prepared financially to cope with aging. As a result of the ongoing unprecedented demographic and epidemiologic transitions, however, healthcare needs as the population ages will present a tremendous public health challenge. Coupled with the shortage in geriatric mental health specialists, models of mental health service delivery direct to primary care settings or even community educational efforts will be needed to address disparities in identification and treatment of commonly encountered psychiatric illnesses in older adults. Research efforts will also be needed to increase the numbers of minority elderly participants, to respond to the growing diversity of the senior population.

References

1. Kennedy GJ. *Geriatric Mental Health Care: A Treatment Guide for Health Professionals.* New York: The Guilford Press, 2000.
2. *Department of Economic & Social Affairs: Population Division. World Population Ageing: 1950–2050.* New York: United Nations Publications, 2002.
3. U.S. Census Bureau. *State and National Population Projections.* Available at http://www.census.gov/population/www/projections/popproj.html. Accessed June 2, 2008.
4. National Center for Chronic Disease Prevention and Health Promotion, CDC. Chronic disease notes and reports: Special focus. *Healthy Aging* 1999;12:3.
5. Ngandu R, vonStrauss E, Helkala L, et al. Education and dementia: What lies behind the association? *Neurology* 2007;69:1442–1450.
6. Moussavi S, Chatterji S, Verdes E, et al. Depression, chronic diseases, and decrements in health: Results from the World Health Surveys. *Lancet* 2007;370(9590):851–858.
7. Simon GE, Katon WJ, Lin EH, et al. Diabetes complications and depression as predictors of health service costs. *Gen Hosp Psychiatry* 2005;27(5):344–351.
8. Medicare Payment Advisory Committee. *Report to the Congress: Promoting Greater Efficiency in Medicare.* June 2007. Available at http://www.medpac.gov.
9. Institute of Medicine. *Retooling for an Aging America: Building the Health Care Workforce.* 2008. Available at http://www.iom.edu.
10. Cohen CI, Magai C, Yaffee R, et al. Comparison of users and non-users of mental health services among depressed, older, African Americans *Am J Geriatr Psychiatry* 2005;13(7):545–553.
11. APA Committee on Ethnic Minority Elderly Curriculum on Cultural Competency. In: Ahmed I, Kramer E, eds. 2006. Available at http://www.psych.org.
12. Unutzer J, Katon W, Callahan CM, et al. Depression treatment in a sample of 1801 depressed older adults in primary care. *JAGS* 2003;51(4):505–514.
13. Ustun TB, Ayuso-Mateos JL, Chatterji S, et al. Global burden of depressive disorders in the year 2000. *BJP* 2004;184:386–392.
14. de Groot M, Anderson R, Freedland KE, et al. Association of depression and diabetes complications: A meta-analysis. *Psychosom Med* 2001;63:619–630.
15. Lustman PJ, Anderson RJ, Freedland KE, et al. Depression and poor glycemic control: A meta-analytic review of the literature. *Diabetes Care* 2000;23:934–942.
16. Ciechanowski PS, Katon WJ, Russo JE. Depression and diabetes: Impact of depressive symptoms on adherence, function, and costs. *Arch Intern Med* 2000;160:3278–3285.
17. Llorente M, Malphurs J, eds. *Psychiatric Disorders and Diabetes Mellitus.* London: Informa Healthcare, 2007.
18. Gallo JJ, Bogner HR, Morales KH, et al. Depression, cardiovascular disease, diabetes and two-year mortality among older, primary care patients. *Am J Geriatr Psychiatry* 2005;13(9):748–755.
19. Romanelli J, Fauerbach JA, Bush DE, et al. The significance of depression in older patients after myocardial infarction. *JAGS* 2002;50(5):817–822.
20. Frasure-Smith N, Lesperance F, Talajic M. Depression and 18-month prognosis after myocardial infarction. *Circulation* 1995;91(4):999–1005.
21. Bartels SJ, Coakley E, Oxman TE, et al. Suicidal and death ideation in older primary care patients with depression, anxiety, and at-risk alcohol use. *Am J Geriatr Psychiatry* 2002;10(4):417–427.

22. Harralson TL, White TM, Regenberg AC, et al. Similarities and differences in depression among black and white nursing home residents. *Am J Geriatr Psychiatry* 2002;10(2): 175–184.

23. Beck AT, Ward CH, Mendelson M, et al. An inventory for measuring depression. *Arch Gen Psychiatry* 1961;4:561–571.

24. Kroenke K, Spitzer RL, Williams JBW. The patient health questionnaire, 2: Validity of a two-item depression screener. *Med Care* 2003;41(11):1284–1292.

25. Bartels SJ, Coakley EH, Zubritsky C, et al. Improving access to geriatric mental health services: A randomized trial comparing treatment engagement with integrated versus enhanced referral care for depression, anxiety, and at-risk alcohol use. *Am J Psychiatry* 2004;161(8):1455–1462.

26. Hunkeler EM, Katon W, Tang L, et al. Long term outcomes from the IMPACT randomised trial for depressed elderly patients in primary care. *BMJ* 2006;332: 259–262.

27. Chisholm D, Sanderson K, Ayuso-Mateos JL, et al. Reducing the global burden of depression: Population-level analysis of intervention cost-effectiveness in 14 world regions. *Br J Psychiatry* 2004;184:393–403.

28. Unutzer J, Katon WJ, Fan MY, et al. Long-term cost effects of collaborative care for late-life depression. *Am J Managed Care* 2008;14(2):95–100.

29. Bogner HR, Morales KH, Post EP, et al. Diabetes, depression, and death: A randomized controlled trial of a depression treatment program for older adults based in primary care (PROSPECT). *Diabetes Care* 2007;30(12):3005–3010.

30. Bruce ML, Ten Have TR, Reynolds CF 3rd, et al. Reducing suicidal ideation and depressive symptoms in depressed older primary care patients: A randomized controlled trial. *JAMA* 2004;291(3):1081–1091.

31. Husaini BA, Sherkat DE, Moonis M, et al. Racial differences in the diagnosis of dementia and its effects on the use and costs of health care services. *Psychiatr Serv* 2003;54:92–96.

32. APA Work Group on Alzheimer's Disease and Other Dementias, Rabins PV, Blacker D, et al. *American Psychiatric Association practice guideline for the treatment of patients with Alzheimer's disease and other dementias. Second Edition. Am J Psychiatry* 2007;164:5–56.

33. Gerda G, Fillenbaum L, Landerman R, et al. The relationship of *APOE* genotype to cognitive functioning in older African American and Caucasian community residents. *JAGS* 2001;49:1148–1155.

34. Renshaw J, Scurfield P, Cloke L, et al. General practitioners' views on the early diagnosis of dementia. *Br J Gen Pract* 2001;51:37–38.

35. Valcour VG, Masaki KH, Curb D, et al. The detection of dementia in the primary care setting. *Arch Int Med* 2000;160:2964–2968.

36. Chodosh J, Petitti DB, Elliott M, et al. Physician recognition of cognitive impairment: Evaluating the need for improvement. *JAGS* 2004;52(7):1051–1059.

37. Krishnan LL, Petersen NJ, Snow AL, et al. Prevalence of dementia among VA Medical care system users. *Dement Geriatr Cogn Disord* 2005;20:245–253.

38. Sink KM, Covinsky KE, Newcomer R, et al. Ethnic difference in the prevalence and pattern of dementia-related behaviors. *JAGS* 2004;52(8):1277–1283.

39. Faison WE, Mintzer JE. The growing, ethnically diverse aging population: Is our field advancing with it? *Am J Geriatr Psychiatry* 2005;13:541–544.

40. Mehta KM, Yin M, Resendez C, et al. Ethnic difference in acetylcholinesterase inhibitor use of Alzheimer disease. *Neurology* 2005;65:159–162.

41. Callahan CM, Boustani MA, Unverzaqt FW, et al. Effectiveness of collaborative care for older adults with Alzheimer disease in primary care: A randomized controlled trial. *JAMA* 2006;295(18):2148–2157.

42. Brodaty H, Green A, Koschera A. Meta-analysis of psychosocial interventions for caregivers of people with dementia. *JAGS* 2003;51:657–664.

43. Belle S, Burgio L, Buras R, et al. Enhancing the quality of life of dementia caregivers from different ethnic or racial groups: A randomized, controlled trial. *Ann Intern Med* 2006;145:727–738.

Disparities Among Special Populations

15 Migrant and Refugee Populations

Joseph J. Westermeyer, Michael Hollifeld, and José Cañive

INTRODUCTION

Minority and migrant people have identified four topical areas as barriers to mental health services that give rise to disparities in care. We obtained these categories in a qualitative study of Hispanic and American Indian community members, many of whom were intranational and international first or second generation migrants (1), and mental health professionals who worked with these two ethnic groups (2). The causes for disparity in healthcare services identified by these two groups (community members and clinicians), as well as the frequency of reporting these barriers, were virtually identical. Refugees experienced the same barriers experienced by migrants and immigrants, in addition to other obstacles that have been identified in previous research (3).

The qualitative study noted above utilized an open-ended question regarding barriers to mental healthcare. Participant responses were collected by audiotape and then transcribed. The several thousand transcribed responses then yielded 139 general *barrier statements*. From these 139 items, a list was made of 25 *barrier items*, with which each of the barrier statements could be coded. Although these data were collected among veterans, with reference to care in the Veterans Administration healthcare system, these categories are relevant to other healthcare systems. In addition to these four barrier categories, we subsequently added another category that is relevant to disparities in healthcare for migrants and refugees, that is, "Barriers Associated With Disasters."

DEFINITION OF MIGRANTS AND REFUGEES

Intranational and international migration both involve change and stress that can precipitate postmigration mental disorder in some people. At times, migration within a country can be more disruptive than migration to another country. Variables that contribute to greater or lesser stress include climate, topography, food, clothing, language, transportation, mass media, utilities (or lack thereof), available occupations, and subsequent social status.

Berry and coworkers have devised a typology of migration based on motivation for migration (voluntary versus involuntary) and duration (temporary versus permanent) (4). This typology is useful in considering the nature of a presenting clinical problem, as well as the course, prognosis, and treatment approaches.

Voluntary temporary migrants consist of diverse people who move away from their home temporarily, usually for education or work. Other rationales include a prolonged vacation, personal development, religious purpose, or escape from some personal exigency (e.g., addiction, legal problems, inability to pay back loans, family discord). The nature of their problems may be related to the culture-of-origin, the migration, or the new tasks being pursued. Some people plan to temporarily live in another place, but then decide to remain permanently. This occurred among many migrants from China to the United States and other countries of Asia. Despite their original intents to return to China, many remained in the country-of-immigration. Some veterans, Foreign Service workers, business people, and others return to the foreign country in which they worked as permanent residents.

Mental health problems in this group can be the result of chronic preexisting problems or crises incident to the travel or migration. The nature of the problem may be related to the life in the country-of-origin, the migration itself, or the new life in the country-of-relocation (5). In the current U.S. system, access to care can pose problems for this group, who often do not have health insurance. Even with insurance, migrants may not be able to access mental health services easily because of "carved out" services, lack of knowledge about the indigenous care systems, or cultural and stigma factors. Consequently, they often surface in emergency rooms, police stations, and emergency medical services. In larger cities with large numbers of visitors, some psychiatrists and other clinicians have specialized in the care of these migrants, but these resources provide adequate care for only a minority of migrants in need of care.

Voluntary permanent migrants typically decide prior to migration that they will relocate permanently (or at least for many years) to a new setting. Around the world, hundreds of millions of people have migrated from rural to urban areas over the last century. Smaller numbers have migrated in the reverse direction, from cities to rural or suburban areas. International migrants are called emigrants vis-à-vis their country-of-origin, and immigrants vis-à-vis their country-of-relocation. In some cases, many of most migrants in a cohort return to the place of origin; in other cases, most remain in the new country or location. On retirement, some migrants to urban areas return to their rural home communities. If people from this group encounter a mental health problem early on, they can experience the same obstacles to care as the temporary migrants.

Involuntary temporary migrants are forced to leave their home community for some period of time before they are allowed to return. Historical examples include American Indian children forced into boarding schools, men drafted into military service, or Japanese American citizens and immigrants interred during World War II.

Paradoxically, this group often has better access to mental healthcare than voluntary migrants, at least for a period of time.

Involuntary permanent migrants and refugees have been forced to relocate away from their homes, with little or no chance of returning home. Within-country migrations have included people forced to abandon their homes on a flood plain, or in the path of a highway or an urban renewal project, and in an area of be flooded by a dam. International flight typically follows persecution of a group because of their national origin, political beliefs, religious preference, education, or other identity. Many of this group have experienced or witnessed horrific violence including murder of relatives, separation from friends and family, traumatic brain injury, and other experiences increasing the risk for psychiatric disorders (6).

Refugee status definitions vary across international associations, national governments, foundations, and various clinical centers and investigators (3). Among international groups such as the World Health Organization (WHO), the definitions are general and describe groups who flee because of persecution, religion, ethnicity, class, or other demographic characteristics. National governments are far more specific in their definitions than WHO, typically designating specific countries. Foundations, clinics, and helping professionals may focus on individuals, personal histories, and individual experiences, rather than particular countries or time frames. Predictably, a patient or client may be considered a refugee by one or two of these criteria, but not necessarily by all of them. "Asylum seekers" are often illegal migrants who are trying to change their status to that of legal immigrants or refugees.

This group—probably the most needy of the four groups—typically has the greatest difficulty accessing care. Patient factors obstructing care include lack of familiarity with mental health concepts, ignorance regarding mental health resources, distrust of clinicians and government-sponsored health resources, and various concomitants of posttraumatic stress disorder. Brain injury, nutritional deficiencies, and other neuropsychiatric problems are also prevalent in this group and impair judgment to seek help.

PATIENT-CENTERED FACTORS CONTRIBUTING TO DISPARITIES

According to both community members and clinicians, people with psychiatric disorder are themselves a major source of disparities in mental healthcare (1,2).

Stigma creates disparity most powerfully at the level of the individual in need of services. The person who views mental health problems as a sign of personal weakness, moral inferiority, or individual choice is not apt to seek services for these problems. On the other hand, the person surrounded by biases against clinical care but desiring help may eventually find a way to obtain it.

The inability to conceptualize cognition, emotions, and behavior as being a part of health component lies at the heart of much stigma. Many historical concepts regarding mental health have moral, religious, and political overtones. Although it is relevant for people to assess their thoughts, feelings, and actions in a moral context, holding on to emblems of past eras or applying overly simplistic moral models to human experience can be dysfunctional. Past symbols of mental healthcare, such as lifetime institutionalization in state hospitals, also promote stigma.

Ignorance regarding the manifestations of psychiatric disorder can reduce a person's likelihood of seeking care (7). In the United States, many people learn the signs and symptoms of many common mental disorders in school, from family and peers, and from TV and cinema. This is not the case in many areas of the world or in some isolated communities in the United States.

Education of migrant and refugee communities can help in eliminating ignorance as an obstacle to care. Such education need not focus on particular diagnostic entities, but rather on signs and symptoms of psychiatric disorder. Even among highly literate Americans, psychiatric disorders are often understood in a "folk" sense, rather than in a syndrome-oriented sense of "diagnostic criteria." These "folk" entities also appear in mass media as well as in peoples' daily conversations. These entities include "nervous break down," "nerves," "strung out," "alcoholism," "schizo," or "being paranoid." One might consider them as "idioms of distress," which can facilitate care-seeking. "Folk" entities do not always bear a close relationship to our diagnostic nomenclature.

Somatization, the expression of psychosocial distress as somatic symptoms, can complicate and delay mental healthcare in migrants and refugees (8). The neurobiology of anxiety and posttraumatic stress disorder can give rise to somatic symptoms involving the autonomic nervous system (9), which may delay the recognition and treatment of mental, emotional, or behavioral disorders. Somatic expression of distress can evolve from one or more of the following:

- Cultural taboos against the expression of emotional distress or cognitive distortions;
- Posttrauma effects, which can dampen insight into emotional self-perception while emphasizing the focus on somatic symptoms;
- Brain injury from combat, hypotension caused by hemorrhage or infectious disease, torture, malnutrition, refugee flight, and other causes;
- Substance use disorder, which appears in many migrant and refugee groups, especially beginning several years following relocation.

Stereotypic thinking regarding psychiatric disorder and care can also pose an obstacle to care. Many migrants and refugees know about psychiatric disorders and treatment, but their experience tells them that psychiatric disorder consists only of "madness" or "craziness," leading to involuntary hospitalization and treatment. Many people would prefer constant misery to these perceived alternatives (exemplified in the popular book and movie *One Flew Over the Cuckoo's Nest*, in which an eccentric but not mentally ill man is first hospitalized involuntarily, then given electroconvulsive treatments, and finally a frontal lobotomy). Such thinking can be overcome, although often not easily.

Distrust of clinicians and healthcare systems can arise from ignorance and stereotypic thinking. Lacking knowledge about psychiatric methods, clinicians, or facilities, the patient or family might not want to trust an unfamiliar institution at a time of personal distress or family crisis. The notion of bringing someone with disturbed thoughts, feelings, or actions to the clinician may be strange indeed to some migrants and refugees. In addition, distrust can arise from other sources as well.

Another factor potentially undermining the clinician-patient relationship is paranoid symptoms, which have been observed more frequently in several types of migrants. The latter include refugees, economic migrants, and immigrants. Social isolation of migrants may contribute to the evolution of paranoid symptoms.

Paradoxically, the individual or family who wants to take charge and act responsibly may be the most reluctant to allow intrusion from clinicians. Countering this reluctance is the universal role of healers who supplement the actions of family members when the latter are not longer effective, or when the patient worsens despite family care.

Survivors of war or political oppression are especially apt to mistrust authority figures, including clinicians. Since some regimes have viewed anxiety or depression as a criticism of the government, with possible arrest and punishment, patients may be reluctant to express psychological symptoms.

Lack of knowledge regarding healthcare entitlement can lead to failure to utilize mental health services. Even if they are aware of their right to mental healthcare, they may not know how to access it. Or, they want try to access care but not know how to do so. For example, they might call for an appointment in a crisis, but then be given an unacceptable appointment in 2 weeks or 2 months.

Failure to cooperate with evaluation may arise out of distrust. As with most patient-induced behaviors described here, this approach may be a rationale decision under the circumstances. Some clinicians may view this as a reason to deny care rather than to seek the source of the distrust and find ways to establish trust. Turned away or denied care, the migrant patient then feels rejected, which may flower into a communal belief with the retelling of having been rebuffed.

Preference for care in other venues besides professional mental healthcare occurs among many migrants and refugees. The person may decide to seek the services of a primary health clinician, since psychosocial distress often gives rise to somatic symptoms (which may become the focus for help-seeking). Or, if the problem is viewed as moral or spiritual, the individual may seek a member of the clergy or a spiritual healer. Overwhelmed and adrift, the sufferer may seek counsel from a clan elder, a community leader, or a social agency worker, with medical consultation occurring only as a last resort.

The resolution to this problem lies not in dissuading the migrant from utilizing these resources, but in helping clinicians and healers address the mental health problem as it presents. In clinical settings, this can occur via integrated mental healthcare in the primary care setting—an increasingly available model of care. This "one-stop shopping" approach reduces stigma, brings care to the patient on a timely basis, and treats psychiatric illness as one might manage a migraine headache or allergic reaction (10). The challenge to colocate care in the offices of clergy or community leaders is more daunting. However, first responders can be trained to provide support and to recognize the need for further evaluation.

Lack of resources to be able to access professional care can pose a major obstacle. These may include the lack of a stable address or telephone number, since appointments (and appointment changes as well as reminders) depend on these resources. The inability to get to an appointment via public or private transportation can impede care or lead to delayed care and expensive transportation in an ambulance. In today's environment, work-related insurance may be a critical component to care-seeking.

CLINICIAN FACTORS

Both community members and clinicians reported that mental health clinicians themselves were a frequent barrier to mental health services (1,2). Although this category was third most frequent rather than second most frequent, we have chosen to list it following patient factors to point up possible pitfalls in the physician-patient relationship.

Stereotyped thinking about the patient's culture was the most frequent complaint about clinicians. Mental health clinicians generally draw their concepts from their limited memories and experiences with the patient's culture. These stereotypes may have been drawn from the mass media, ethnic jokes, historical recounts, and other sources. Some concepts about others' cultures may even come from factual sources such as ethnographic accounts, socioeconomic analyses, or governmental reports. The source or truth of the information is always the issue as much as how the cultural information is used. Patients mostly protest the application of group data to themselves as individuals.

This protest is highly appropriate. No one possesses all elements of their culture and its history. Each person manifests some of these characteristics, or some of them to a partial extent, but does not fit the stereotype in all its respects. The clinician's task is to know and understand the individual as he or she lives and copes with their particular sociocultural milieu (or, as often occurs in the United States, "milieus"). Since no one manifests all aspects of their culture, clinicians must inquire regarding each individual's beliefs and practices.

Curiosity about the culture of others can result in a clinician becoming curious about his or her individual culture, or as a bearer of the cultures that he/she manifests. This insight-producing foray can be enlightening or threatening, or both. Although we are all prone to idealize cultures, especially our own, all cultures incorporate attitudes and behaviors that may be ethnocentric, prejudicial, irrational, or unhygienic from a mental health perspective. Often a given characteristic is hygienic in one context and pathogenic in another. Despite elements of narcissism in understanding ourselves as bearers and practitioners of our own cultures—including our psychiatric "culture"—this pursuit can inform and guide our work in the care of migrants and refugees from other cultural backgrounds (11).

Ignorance about the patient's culture is the second most common complaint regarding mental health clinicians. This may seem paradoxical in light of the complaint about cultural stereotyping, just reviewed above. One might assume that patients would prefer that clinicians be "blank tablets" on which they, the patients, can write their cultural preferences and characteristics. However, there is strong justification for the clinician to have a modicum of knowledge about the patient's culture.

Knowing something of the patient's culture can guide the clinician toward those areas of the patient's life or beliefs that might be contributing to stress and/or to psychiatric disorder. Patients may not be aware of their own cultural conflicts.

Understanding something of our patients' cultures does not require thorough ethnographic and historical expertise. It is impossible to fully comprehend the hundreds of cultures represented in patients. Fortunately, a few of the most important cultural variables (such as the cultural alternatives for deciding on kinship, the range of cultural norms and values, the ways of acquiring roles and manifesting status, gender- and age-assigned expectations, etc.) are not infinite. Thus, a discerning, curious, culturally informed clinician could readily understand these basics.

Communicating poorly with people of the migrant's culture encompasses the third clinician barrier. This is a profound criticism if one considers the time and effort, training, and supervision spent by psychiatrists and others in learning effective means of communicating. It has taken years to understand this common complaint and what we might do about it.

Much of the communication skills and styles taught to mental health professionals include conventions that, unknowingly, contain elements of European Judeo-Christian communication styles (12). These include shaking hands, maintaining eye contact, showing sensitivity about certain topics (e.g., sexuality, finances) and not about others (e.g., physiological functions, family illnesses), not subjecting patients to overly long silences, keeping at least arms-length distance from the patient, and so forth. Depending on the cultural group of the patient, any one of these (and other) prescribed communication behaviors might be offensive (13).

General principles of communication apply to cross-cultural work in the clinical setting. For example, establishing trust or "rapport" before entering into a clinical relationship remains key to working with patients from all cultural backgrounds. Core skills include when and how to ask (i) an open-ended question (to not force a response) or (ii) a closed-ended question (to obtain extremely important information). Understanding what questions or comments are facilitative, supportive, clarifying, probing, confronting, suggestive, interpretive, and when to use each approach, also applies to our providing care across cultures.

Cultural insensitivity by the clinician toward migrant or refugee patients is the fourth clinician barrier. The common theme is the patient's feeling demeaned, not understood, or not valued by the clinician. This perception has arisen from the interaction between the clinician and the migrant patient.

What causes such outcomes? It is not entirely clear from reviewing the complaints in the original reporting. The people reporting cultural insensitivity were angered, or even insulted at the clinician's communications and/or behavior.

Although the least frequent of the four barriers ascribed to clinicians, this barrier is both the most nebulous and the most troubling. Clinicians are drawn to their work for many reasons, but sensitivity to fellow human beings is usually a major value. They provide care for the prisoner, the homeless, and the alienated when others have abandoned them. In wartime, they render medical and surgical care to our nation's enemies. Accusations regarding lack of sensitivity cut deeply but need to be elaborated, understood, and altered.

SYSTEM FACTORS

The second most frequently reported barriers occurred in this category, following patient-centered barriers. This category includes the numerous contexts within which clinicians render care and patients obtain care.

Difficult, even foreboding access to available services posed the primary obstacle to mental healthcare, reported by more than half of people who reported any barrier (1).

The lack of a mental healthcare system that is integrated with other care (the prevailing model in most communities of the United States) contributes to this problem, even among people who understand the nuances of American society. For some patients, an appointment in a few weeks is appropriate and meets their lower level of acuity. For other patients, the acuity is such that they need to be seen in the next few hours or less. An initial crisis intervention and brief assessment is usually all that is needed in the moment of acuity. Follow-up assessment and care can begin tomorrow or next week, once the patient has had the chance to tell his or her story, enlisted the clinician's help in resolution of the acute problem, and developed a game plan for proceeding to solve, remediate, or accept the problem at hand.

Failure of outreach to those needing services or those who might benefit from new services or treatment modalities was reported second most often of all barrier items, again in more than half of cases (1). The complaints themselves, and accompanying affect, tell the story:

> *"At the state fair every summer, they set up a booth and take blood pressures. That's good, but our community has way bigger problems with depression, trauma problems, and lying around getting high every weekend. No one even mentions those things or asks about them. What are they thinking? Is it a screening or just an advertisement? Why don't they set up a breathalyzer?"*

Absence of convenient access in the study participant's community, reported by one-fourth of those who reported any barrier, challenges our system (1). Half of the people in the study were from rural areas, with no mental health access in the region. Others were from poor urban areas or suburbs without access. Migrants and refugees often must leave their familiar community to access care.

Creative solutions to the community access problems are becoming available. For example, telepsychiatry assessment and care are coming on-line in many rural and even urban community clinics (14). Some medical centers are permitting in-community registration, so that a chart can be started and people can access services through the phone at home or telemedicine at the clinic.

Absence of in-community access often leads to inappropriate (and expensive) use of emergency first-responder care. The emergency medical technician (EMT) may offer support, help a person get an ambulance to get to an emergency room, or make recommendations about available resources. However, the EMT may then become the known access point and the helper-of-choice, who is called again for the next crisis, compounding the expense and inappropriate use of the emergency system of care. Access to mental health services can avert inappropriate use of (and drain on) EMT services.

Absence of ethnic peers in the mental healthcare system conveys the impression of an "ethnic enclave" in which migrant or refugee people are not welcome. Respondents stated that they felt more comfortable coming into the clinic if someone from their group was visibly working at the clinic; then they felt as though they "belonged" in that clinic, or "had a right to be there," or wouldn't run into a rejection problem because of their ethnic identity. Knowing that someone from his or her community might be available as an advocate, if a problem arose, was reassuring. Or, they assumed that the staff would be sensitive to people of their ethnic background because they were working shoulder-to-shoulder with others from of their ethnic group.

A study in a community clinic found that hiring two people from the community had the following dramatic and highly significant consequences. There were fewer emergency visits, more scheduled visits, fewer follow-up "no shows," and fewer complications (such as otitis media following pharyngitis) (15). One of the hired staff was a clerk who registered patients; the other was a health aid who helped clinicians with vital signs, taking people to the laboratory, and performing similar supportive tasks. The significant effects on patients' behaviors and their medical outcomes were not to the result of more physicians and nurses but rather because of community-dwelling staff members visible to patients.

Accusations of cultural insensitivity by healthcare systems, as well as by clinicians, involved broadly mixed complaints, ranging from where facilities were placed geographically, to lack of familiar décor, to hiring-and-firing practices, to requirements for registration (such as having an address or a telephone number). As with insensitivity reports about clinicians, the term "insensitivity" connoted a perception of disrespect for the patient because of his or her ethnic identity.

Healthcare systems tended to be rigid and rule-bound, at times when flexibility and openness were required. The intake and registration process conveyed this impression to community members. They complained that the healthcare system seemed to operate for its own internal reasons rather than for the patients and their problems. It also was a process fraught with potential rejection for patients and their families. Complaints indicated that the processes for efficiently obtaining care were not clear or evident but were a secret or "in-group" set of facts and principles to which they were not privy. The purpose of the rigid rules was not evident to these community members. In the absence of data to the contrary, it seemed another means of excluding them.

Healthcare systems are not aware of the pressing health and other needs in the migrant or refugee community. Without such knowledge, how can the system develop programs and resources to meet the needs of the people? These criticisms, although expressed by a smaller percentage of people, reflected the awareness that clinical facilities need to be aware of community health needs (and to some extent, other socioeconomic needs as well).

How health facilities manifest awareness of health needs requires thought and planning. First, it requires some epidemiological information regarding the healthcare needs of groups of patients, analyzed by community and ethnic group. This goal, recognized perhaps better by patients than by healthcare administrators, requires a synthesis of epidemiological knowledge with clinical knowledge and expertise. This expectation, which is simple and conceptually obvious, ignores the reality that epidemiologists, facility administrators, patient representatives, and clinicians rarely discourse together, much less work together to devise healthcare programs that meet communal needs.

Healthcare systems may not support those clinicians who are concerned about and effective in providing services for patients from migrant communities. Many of these reports were more graphic, indicating that systems "undercut" or "ignore" those clinicians who have patient interests at heart. This report was considerably more common among clinicians (2) as compared with community members. The latter findings suggest that many community members may not perceive this problem, or view it as important as other barriers.

Awareness of this barrier among mental health staff members conveys a message to new or uninvolved staff members. The perceived absence of system support for those caring for migrants and minorities indicates that involvement with these patients is undesirable and should be avoided.

FAMILY-COMMUNITY FACTORS

Family and community factors may be grouped together for two reasons. First, for some people in remote rural areas or recent migrants, the family (or extended family) may encompass the individual's total social network. Second, many patient complaints about the human environment could relate to either family or community, or both.

Both community participants and mental health clinicians reported family-community barriers least often. We doubt this ranking reflects the importance of these barriers from an operational perspective.

Stereotypic thinking and lack of awareness regarding psychiatric disorder may affect families and communities, just as it affects prospective patients. The following case illustrates this barrier:

> A 16-year-old Vietnamese refugee began to hear voices threatening his life and that of his family. His family hired a healer who informed them that a deceased aunt had cursed the family because they had neglected to honor her after death. A school social worker visited the home to learn why he had dropped out from school. She found him living in a large cardboard box in a back room. The family refused psychiatric consultation, fearing that their only son would be taken from them and put into an institution for his lifetime. They also feared that the psychiatrist could not counter a malignant spirit and might even agitate the spirit, causing it to persecute their son even more. When a judge ordered an evaluation for the minor child, the family fled to another state. ■

Family and communities may ignore their members with mental health problems. Certain factors appear to be associated with stigma and abandonment of this kind: poverty, nuclear family (rather than extended family), social organization, embarrassment, shame, guilt, and/or alienation. In some societies, families may perceive that they pay taxes for society to provide services to dysfunctional family members.

Noninvolvement by the family can affect access to care, especially in today's complex and nonintegrated healthcare systems. Family members can help by serving as advocates in a setting where the "squeaky wheel gets the oil." Advocacy requires a thorough knowledge and assertive attitude nowadays, in systems of care that often realize greatest profits or least cost (over the short term) by providing no services, or as little as possible.

DISASTERS AS A CAUSE OF DISPARITY

Disasters can precipitate migration and contribute to disparities in care, while also increasing the prevalence of psychiatric disorders (16). Recent disasters include refugee flight, forced migration from an area (such as a governmental decision to build a dam or move people out of flood plain), and various natural disasters, hurricanes, tornados, volcanoes, earthquakes, and fires (17). Disasters can wreak havoc on mental health in several ways.

First, disasters can destabilize people with psychiatric disorders who are functioning well with a relative minimum of care. The disaster affects those people and institutions providing maintenance care, as everyone takes flight, so that care becomes unavailable. Medications may no longer be available to those whose continued function requires them.

Second, disasters can create new psychiatric patients among people who had never required psychiatric services. Common new problems include major depressive disorder, simple phobia related to the disaster or stressor, generalized anxiety disorder, posttraumatic stress disorder, and substance use disorder (18). Some disasters may produce high rates of brain injury through accidents involving the head, malnutrition including avitaminosis and protein deficiency, severe dehydration, and infectious disease following disasters. Even adjustment disorders, often benign in more stable settings, can (in the absence of indigenous resources) lead to irreversible consequences, such as family separation, alienation from friends and community, assault, or suicide.

Third, disasters can undermine the natural resources that people use to cope with loss and stress. Extended family and friends may not be at hand to provide intervention and support. Loss of meaningful work and important social roles can create crises in identify and self-esteem. Community associations, churches, recreational outlets, ethnic ceremonies, and groups may be lost or unavailable.

Fourth, systems of mental healthcare are lost. Mental healthcare exists in wide panoply across society. It exists not only in hospitals and mental health clinics, but also in the primary care clinic, school counselor's offices, social agencies, visiting nurses, emergency responders, drug courts, policy, and other security services. The complex community-specific mental health network that addresses personal crises are not functioning or may not even exist.

Fifth, the consequences of disaster are seldom distributed equally across a population. Those with the least personal and financial resources are least able to remedy their situation. They may not have been able to flee in a timely fashion, or they may not have advocates who can assist them, or they may not know people or institutions that can help them in crisis.

References

1. Westermeyer J, Canive J, Thuras P, et al. Perceived barriers to VA mental health care among Upper Midwest American Indian veterans: Description and associations. *Med Care* 2002;40(Suppl 1):I-62–I-71.
2. Westermeyer J, Canive J, Garrard J, et al. Perceived barriers to mental health care for American Indian and Hispanic veterans: Reports by 100 VA staff. *Transcultur Psychiatry* 2002;39(4):516–530.
3. Williams C, Westermeyer J. *Refugee Mental Health in Resettlement Countries.* New York: Hemisphere, 1986.
4. Berry JW, Kim U, Minde T, et al. Comparative studies of acculturative stress. *Internl Migration Rev* 1987;21:491–511.
5. Cheng D, Leong FT, Geist R. Cultural differences in psychological distress between Asian and Caucasian American college students. *J Multicultur Counsel Dev* 1993;21(3): 182–190.
6. Aaron A. Testimonio, a bridge between psychotherapy and sociotherapy. *Women Therap* 1992;13(3):173–189.
7. Westermeyer J. A case of koro in a refugee family: association with depression and folie a deux (see comments). *J Clin Psychiatry* 1989;50(5):181–183.
8. Westermeyer J, Bouafuely M, Neider J. Somatization among refugees: An epidemiological study. *Psychosomatics* 1989;30:34–43.
9. Cannistraro PA, Rauch DL. Neural circuitry of anxiety: Evidence that structural and functional neuroimaging studies. *Psychopharmacol Bull* 2003;37:8–25.
10. Katon W, Vitalliano PP, Russo J, et al. Panic disorder: Spectrum of severity and somatization. *J Nerv Ment Dis* 1987;175(1):12–19.
11. Hollifield M, Geppert C, Johnson Y, et al. A Vietnamese man with selective mutism: The relevance of multiple interacting cultures in clinical psychiatry. *Transcultur Psychiatry* 2003;40:329–341.
12. Enelow AJ, Swisher SN. *Interviewing and Patient Care.* New York: Oxford University Press, 1972.
13. Collins TC, Clark JA, Petersen LA, et al. Racial differences in how patients perceive physician communication regarding cardiac testing. *Med Care* 2002;40(Suppl 1):I-27–I-34.
14. Shore JH, Manson SM. The American Indian veteran and post-traumatic stress disorder: A telehealth assessment and formulation. *Culture Med Psychiatry* 2004;28:231–243.
15. Westermeyer J, Tanner R, Smelker J. Staff integration at a neighborhood health center. *Urban Health* 1976;5:43–48.
16. Green BL, Grace MC, Vary MG, et al. Children of disaster in the second decade: A 17-year follow-up of Buffalo Creek survivors. *J Am Acad Child Adolesc Psychiatry* 1994; 33(1):71–79.
17. Lima BR, Pai S, Santacruz II, et al. Psychiatric disorders among poor victims following a major disaster: Armero, Colombia. *J Nerv Ment Dis* 1991;179(7):420–427.
18. Smith E, North CS, McCool RE, et al. Acute postdisaster psychiatric disorders: Identification of persons at risk. *Am J Psychiatry* 1990;147(2):202–206.

16 Rural Populations

Suzanne Vogel-Scibilia

INTRODUCTION

Currently, 25% of the United States population lives in rural America (1). Rural America in comparison to urban America has higher rates of poverty, greater numbers of elderly persons, and poorer overall health. There is also pervasive difficulty in accessing all medical services—partially as a result of fewer doctors and hospitals and the distances required to obtain care.

Within the realm of mental health services, individuals in these areas experience a marked degree of disparities that effect not only quality of life but life expectancy. These quality of life disparities result from complications of both psychiatric illness and comorbid medical conditions.

The disparities of care for those in rural areas include marked infrastructure service deficits, lack of access to adequate crisis and emergency services, increased challenges for diverting consumers from inpatient or criminal justice systems, problems with transportation to local services, greater distance to more intensive services, greater challenges in workforce recruitment and retention, inadequate support programs including supportive housing, supported education and employment opportunities and a lack of adequate population density to support specialized services, group programs, or comprehensive psychiatric rehabilitation services. This chapter will review the extent of these disparities and then discuss options for remedies within the current mental healthcare system.

MARKED INFRASTRUCTURE DEFICITS CREATE A SYSTEM THAT IS OFTEN UNABLE TO MEET THE NEEDS OF SEVERELY ILL CONSUMERS OR TO RAMP UP INTENSITY OF CARE WHEN NEEDED

A previous chapter explored marked disparities in care that all consumers face. For rural clients, these problems are even greater. Rural psychiatry systems suffer from more marked provider shortages, lack of specialty services, lack of crisis and hospitalization diversion programs, and limited choices of agencies that provide care. Often, services are more limited, and dispersed over a wider geographic area with poor communication between agencies.

Medical care in rural areas is equally affected. Many rural medical hospitals have turned away from the traditional inpatient medical focus toward more outpatient care because of economic pressures. Despite the fact that one in three rural United States adults is in poor to fair health (1), the number of rural primary care practitioners is decreasing. Some inpatient psychiatry units as well as smaller rural hospitals have closed as other hospitals struggle with significant financial challenges. A study of rural hospital CEOs (2) identified a physician shortage in the community 86% of the time, whereas the shortage of family practitioners was specifically mentioned 64% of the time. This same study identified deficiencies of other providers including registered nurses (91%), pharmacists (64%), and nurses' aides (46%). These shortages impact hospital bed capacity, flexibility of service hours, and availability of emergency care.

In many rural areas, a single public mental health program is the only viable option for severely ill consumers. Often for extended periods, these programs have existed without competition and without adequate service capacity. This combination often creates a treatment environment that is neither flexible nor innovative.

Rural mental health providers often have greater difficulty recruiting clinicians so programs often function with chronic staff shortages especially involving psychiatrist positions. Rural mental health systems grapple with not only how to attract psychiatric providers but also how to retain them. Clients have negative clinical outcomes from having a rotating cadre of clinicians—none of whom learned the subtitles of his illness or have provided care over an adequate time duration to consider addressing long-term treatment issues. Many psychiatrists in rural areas cite the lack of collaboration and feelings of isolation as huge barriers to long-term practice in rural areas.

Besides programs being chronically understaffed, these shortages also create an environment where services cannot expand to meet individual needs. The never-ending number of clients to be served stresses rural mental health centers because it may be the only place for locals to receive care. When a client requires more intensive outpatient services, the system is unable to accommodate the extra appointments. Providers may slowly begin to feel "burnout" or fatigue from the constant demands of clients and their pressing social service needs. Clinicians may feel pressured to work extra hours or accept clients with needs that are beyond the treatment facility's capabilities. Providers and administrators hare great clinical demands from these unmet community needs. Personnel in charge may be unable to problem-solve a long-term solution to the service deficits because of the daily struggle to address urgent clinical issues at understaffed, rural clinic.

Example:

"A client needs more frequent medication adjustments, and is unable to be seen more intensively on an outpatient basis. After a 10-day wait for an intake appointment at the only local partial over 45-minute drive from her home, she begins the program where she is seen once a week for medication changes because of a limited amount of psychiatrist time. When the consumer has further progression of symptoms, no crisis or inpatient diversion system exists. She has to travel an even greater distance to an inpatient unit which has little contact or knowledge about providers and services in her home area. Her family cannot travel regularly to participate in the family-specific therapy and even has difficulty picking her up at time of discharge. She is transferred back to the same local system which 'squeezes her in' for an outpatient follow-up appointment with her psychiatrist in three and a half weeks." ■

This reliance on safety net services such as inpatient hospitalization or emergency rooms when outpatient capacity is inadequate causes more money to be directed toward inpatient and crisis services at the expense of outpatient care. Rural areas are greatly affected by managed care's cost containments. Any strategy in rural areas to decrease the inpatient bed utilization rate must support outpatient infrastructure capacity especially the availability of psychiatrists that do medication monitoring and crisis assessments.

Psychiatrists recruited from other areas may not desire to work in a rural area for the long term and may leave after their contracted period has finished. This causes a steady turnover of providers further stifling flexibility and innovation because newer providers' early focus is often mastering the intricacies of the job placement and learning the local service system. The lack of competition and the constant replacement of clients who leave the system with newer clients may remove many external pressures for flexibility or innovation.

From a financial perspective, insurance companies deal with a single contractor who may have little incentive to change problematic policies. Some clinics are well aware that they have a service monopoly in the area. Additionally a closure of a rural health clinic can cause catastrophic problems for the area's often impoverished clients who have limited transportation options. These comments are not meant to infer that all rural programs are inflexible and stagnant. But, the impetus for flexibility of service and programming innovation often needs to come from motivated individuals within the program as opposed to external pressure from outside.

RURAL SYSTEMS LACK ADEQUATE CRISIS AND INPATIENT CARE SERVICES AS WELL AS NOT HAVING CAPACITY TO TREAT CONSUMERS WHO NEED LONGER PERIODS OF RESIDENTIALLY-BASED CARE

Both crisis and inpatient services are costly and complex services that are impossible to obtain in many rural areas of the United States. Even if inpatient services are available, the distance may discourage many clients from utilizing needed services. Often child and adolescent, substance dependence treatment, or detoxification services have even greater shortages. Specialty inpatient programs such as geriatric or eating disorder programs may be unable to be obtained or occur at such a distance that family involvement is impossible. Likewise, if clients need state hospital placement, the facility is often located far from the client's family.

In rural areas, emergency rooms often take the brunt of providing safety for consumers who are in need of crisis care. Rural emergency room physicians often lack experience with psychiatric emergencies and have overloaded departments that do not have the staff capacity to address consumers' complex needs. When inpatient facilities are located a distance away, the waiting time for a bed may be lengthy. This may require patients to wait in the emergency facility, potentially in some type of seclusion or restraint before transfer is arraigned. Many rural providers feel that improved assessment and treatment capacity for emergency care is an urgent priority (3).

DIVERTING CONSUMERS FROM MORE RESTRICTIVE AND COSTLY LEVELS OF MENTAL HEALTHCARE AS WELL AS AVOIDING CRIMINAL JUSTICE INTERVENTIONS FOR CONSUMERS IS MORE DIFFICULT IN RURAL AMERICA

The recent attempts by managed insurance plans to shift consumer care away from more costly services and the recent public focus on obtaining services in the least restrictive environment provide a partnership between cost containment and civil liberties. These two forces focus on inpatient diversion. Since the mid-20th century, state governments have prioritized deinstitutionalization from long-term psychiatric care for the same two reasons. The consequence of downsizing state hospitals is the lack of longer-term care and resultant homelessness for consumers who are disruptive within society and need periods of longer-term care to function. In rural areas, jail diversion programs such as mental health courts and postincarceration support programs are vital to preventing criminalization of persons with mental illness. The potential positive impact is diminished if the mental health court does not accept clients with felony crimes or when jail-to-community transition programs are of limited scope. Jail diversion programs may also utilize a large percentage of existing intensive community treatment slots. Therefore, the institution of jail diversion should only occur with an increase in intensive outpatient infrastructure including supportive housing and intensive case management to prevent shortages for others in the community. Some rural areas are trying to adapt programs such as Assertive Community Treatment, Continuous Treatment Teams, Peer Support Programs, and Mobile Crisis Teams that have been successful in more populated areas. Lack of start-up funding and personnel shortages are significant barriers to implementation of these important programs.

CONSUMERS IN RURAL AREAS FACE MORE COMPLEX TRANSPORTATION CHALLENGES BOTH FOR LOCAL SERVICES AS WELL AS GREATER DISTANCES TO TRAVEL FOR MORE INTENSIVE SERVICES

In rural areas, programs that require frequent participation for successful care or reimbursement often provide free transportation with an agency van. Although urban programs can reimburse participants with transportation coupons or vouchers, the lack of public transportation is a further barrier to adherence for rural consumers. Insurance companies or rural welfare programs may need to transport clients who need a distant, locally unavailable intensive service such as an inpatient unit to encourage adherence. But clients diverted to a distant area may find that they are responsible for transportation home after discharge. The provider of intensive services may be unaware of local follow-up providers, or unable to arrange face-to-face collateral contacts with significant others. These issues are commonly reported factors in rural consumers' refusal of services far away from the local area.

WORKFORCE RECRUITMENT AND RETENTION OF CLINICIANS IS MORE CHALLENGING IN RURAL AREAS

Although workforce shortages occur commonly throughout the United States, rural areas suffer the greatest disparities. The lack of an adequate number of providers not only burdens the current psychiatrists with a greater case load but also discourages new providers from joining. Many providers relocate because of clinical burdens, isolation, problems with cultural adaption to the area or lack of mentorship. One rural psychiatric care system in Australia (4) had an acute crisis with only one psychiatrist retained in 1994. Between 1994 and 2006, their staff psychiatrists increased to eleven. The article cited changes such as working to build individual rapport with entering doctors, meeting the individual and family needs of the provider, ongoing educational support, linkages to city-based psychiatrists and services, focusing on cultural adaption and improved professional supervision with the improved statistics.

SUPPORTIVE HOUSING AND SUPPORTED EMPLOYMENT PROGRAMS ARE LESS COMPREHENSIVE AND LESS AVAILABLE IN RURAL AMERICA

Rural supported housing programs have little research data to base decisions since the preponderance of research in supported housing is done in urban areas. Clearly, the research shows that supported housing allows consumers to live independently in these urban studies, but rural consumers face a host of further challenges. Housing in rural areas tends to be less available and often of poorer quality. Rural housing programs tend to be smaller and lack a broad continuum of housing options or support services (5).

Although supported employment is especially effective when integrated into mental health services in urban models (6), rural areas often have less available and fewer diverse job opportunities than their urban neighbors. One study (6) that compared rural populations that integrated ACT services with individual consumer work placement and support showed similar results to urban supported employment results suggesting that overcoming system fragmentation, staff shortages and poor interagency communication would advance ACT goals.

For more than 40 years, a grassroots consumer-empowered and consumer-driven, mixed supported employment, supported housing model, Fairweather Lodges have found roots in communities including rural areas. These lodges are independent, self-supporting and ideally suited to rural American culture. Despite their clinical success and cost effectiveness, Fairweather Lodges receive little research attention or programmatic notice. This is probably because the model functions without mental health professional support and is financially self-sustaining.

THE LACK OF ADEQUATE POPULATION DENSITY CREATES DIFFICULTY IN PROVIDING SERVICES THAT NEED AN ADHERENT REGULAR GROUP OF CLIENTS TO MAINTAIN FINANCIAL VIABILITY—THIS INCLUDES SPECIALTY SERVICES, GROUP TREATMENT, OR PARTIAL PROGRAMMING

The dispersed nature of population in rural areas along with the presence of smaller agencies with limited communication and barriers to easy collaboration creates a tremendous barrier on collaborative models that allow specialty psychiatric care programs to survive. Currently children and adolescents, dual diagnosis clients, and elderly populations are markedly underserved in most areas. Often group models and partial programming also fail to maintain adequate numbers unless referrals arrive from other providers. Models that encourage collaborative care between agencies are the only way to destroy clinical silos that impair any agency from providing specialized services because of population size.

WHAT ARE SUGGESTIONS TO RECTIFY MENTAL HEALTH DISPARITIES IN RURAL AREAS?

Establishing Evidence-Based Practices Will Help Use Limited Mental Healthcare Dollars More Wisely

Using limited resources in a manner that is more cost effective and associated with good clinical outcomes is a wise first step. Unfortunately, many areas of treatment have limited amounts of evidence based data. This highlights the importance of research on rural populations in addressing best practices for mental healthcare services.

Designating Specific Programs to Be Centers of Excellence in Specialized Clinical Areas Will Increase the Variety of Programs in a Given Region

Having multiple smaller providers in rural areas means that no one program will have the expertise or an adequate clinical population to provide certain specialty services. Encouraging each clinic to develop an exclusive subspecialty service such as child/adolescent care, geriatric group therapy, eating disorder counseling or dual diagnosis treatment may allow rural areas to address specialty service needs. Lastly, greater governmental support of diversity in providers of critical support and treatment programs would improve access to care for all consumers.

Promoting Universal Education in Co-occurring Mental Health/ Substance Abuse Treatment and Culturally Competent Services Will Improve Quality for Rural, Typically Underserved Populations

The importance of having a competent clinician to understand the cultural dynamics of an individual of minority race/ethnicity or assist in designing an evidence-based addiction recovery program should not be underestimated. In areas where providers are more scattered and turnover of trained clinicians is high, universal education in co-occurring disorders and culturally competent care is vital.

Many rural communities are seeing a greater influx of recent immigrants, individuals of racial and ethnic minorities and people transplanted from other parts of the country. Addressing the new citizens' needs and providing culturally competent care for persons with minority racial, ethnic, religious or sexual orientation status is a vital part of behavioral healthcare.

Clients with gay, lesbian, bisexual, or transgender (GLBT) orientation often have difficulty finding culturally competent care in rural areas and because of greater risk of adverse outcomes should be considered a priority population. Rural GLBT consumers cite great reluctance to seek care especially psychotherapy and inpatient services because of a lack of a supportive treatment environment. Fostering even one small agency or private therapist in rural areas to specifically focus on providing culturally sensitive counseling to GLBT clients would help access and treatment for this at-risk population by providing a gateway intake into the mental healthcare system.

Using Telepsychiatry for Provider Shortages and Care Needs That Are Chronically Inadequate or Difficult to Establish

Telepsychiatry, interactive videoconferencing that provides psychiatric services, holds promise to address rural staffing deficiencies that are unable to be rectified by traditional recruitment techniques. Several studies endorse the feasibility of telepsychiatry by describing model programs such as eastern Oregon's RodeoNet or the telemedicine program at Kansas University Center (7) or citing randomized, controlled data that finds telepsychiatry is as effective as face to face contacts when used for psychiatric consultation and short term follow-up (8). Longer term models of care such as the e-Mental Health Consultation Service at University of California, Davis Medical Center provide primary outpatient mental healthcare to rural consumers (9). Further study should evaluate the possible broader application of the David Medical Center program because it also offers clinicians provider-to-provider consultations and provider education.

Telepsychiatry could also address the lack of specialty services in less densely populated areas. A growing body of research reports telepsychiatry programs that specifically address pediatric populations (10), care in rural county jails (11,12), or focused care for victims of domestic violence (13).

Despite these optimistic reports, there is still much controversy over telepsychiatry's role in rural healthcare. Older consumers are a demographic that most often voices hesitancy about talking to a clinician on a monitor screen, while children and young adults are probably the most receptive. Some providers have concerns about reimbursement issues that may limit feasibility. Many ethical questions including the mechanics of involuntary commitment or vital sign/medical monitoring via remote monitor require further investigation.

Recruiting and Retaining Providers to Establish Personal and Professional Roles in the Rural Community

Providers in rural areas must contend with clinical isolation, stress from a greater amount of on-call time, limited access to tertiary care services and decreased economic status.

Rural clinicians are most effective and most likely to remain in under-served areas when they establish valued roots and ties in their communities. Part of this process includes cultivating both personal and professional roles which not only lead to individual fulfillment but enhance the health of the community at large.

One natural opportunity to increase local providers is to recruit individuals who were raised in the local area. Programs that expose "hometown" students-in-training to future practice in their community of origin often report anecdotal success and should be studied more rigorously. Another idea would be increase the amount of residency training curricula in rural psychiatry to foster a greater appreciation of the value of rural behavioral healthcare and encourage more rural practice choices in graduates (14).

One issue about practicing in a rural area that is very different than in a more urban areas involve boundary issues of overlapping personal-professional roles. There is research documenting the greater likelihood that rural providers compared with urban clinicians know and interact with clients in nonprofessional roles within their communities (15,16). Often a provider may be the only available clinician to individuals in the local area and therefore have to address the prospect of treating people whom he sees regularly in his personal life, or treating multiple members of the same family. Clients and clinicians may belong to the same church council or be opposing youth baseball coaches. Because of confidentiality, a provider may have to feign lack of recognition when one client comes home with his wife to sort Girl Scout cookies in his garage. Confidentiality issues are often more prominent in rural communities and need to be vigilantly maintained.

Another difference in small closely connected rural communities is that a psychiatrist's "failures" become common knowledge within hometown social circles.

Providing a support system for rural providers to discuss treatment failures or poor outcomes would be a first step in addressing provider isolation and lack of clinical peer support.

Additionally, providers who have medical or psychiatric illness themselves may find that there is little ability to seek private treatment or recover in small town America. Rural consumer-providers often need to travel greater distances to receive their own psychiatric treatment. This distance and the increased time commitment it entails is often a factor in rural practitioners with mental illness not seeking treatment and having adverse clinical outcomes.

Training and Enabling Medical Practitioners to Provide Mental Healthcare to Clients Who Have Low Complexity, Common Illnesses

Primary care providers (PCPs) continue to provide the majority of behavioral health-care throughout our country, yet the percentage of consumers obtaining care from PCPs is even higher in rural areas. Increasing the training for primary practitioners and providing mentorship and supervision by behavioral health specialists are crucial steps to increasing primary practitioners' comfort levels with psychiatric clients. One paper (17) that describes a specific framework for formal supervision of rural general practitioners (GP) in Victoria, Australia, focuses on how essential a formal system is in providing access for GPs. Another Australian group has utilized GPs in a peer support network utilizing small groups which discuss treating clients with behavioral health needs (18). The project, Better Outcomes in Mental Health Care Initiative, utilizes a GP facilitator training program and manual.

The American Academy of Pediatrics has developed a specific educational toolkit for its members to manage treatment of children with attention deficit disorders. This decision comes at a time when pediatricians have more requests for care from their patients because of chronic service infrastructure deficits throughout the majority of the United States. Rural PCPs could benefit from a similar strategy designed for internists, family practitioners and obstetrician-gynecologists to treat uncomplicated depression, anxiety, or dementia within the medical office setting.

Address the Shortage of Emergency Physicians Who Are Knowledgeable About Mental Health Assessments by Fostering the Education of Specialized Nurses, Physician Extenders, or a Telepsychiatry Model

While the ideal model would be to post psychiatrists in emergency rooms that serve persons with mental illness, current provider shortages make this unreasonable outside of academic treatment centers or highly urbanized areas. The use of physician extenders such as physician assistants and nurse practitioners or registered nurses with advanced practice training, Advanced Practice Psychiatric Nurses, may help to address the current use of undertrained behavioral health nurses who currently advise emergency room physicians in some rural emergency rooms.

Emergency rooms are inherently ill-suited to provide crisis care to clients with mental illnesses. Yet, these facilities currently provide one of the few safety nets for rural consumers in crisis. Telepsychiatry may have potential to address these concerns in rural emergency rooms. Despite the literature being fairly limited, Jay Shore and associates in General Hospital Psychiatry discuss this issue in great detail and provide useful emergency management guidelines (19).

Providing a Practical Transportation and Housing Schema for Rural Consumers

The need for viable housing and transportation for consumers makes the difference between treatment adherence and recovery versus clinical drop-outs and disabling psychiatric conditions. In rural America when supported housing options exist, there may be only one provider. Some clients report being "permanently" discharged from this sole provider during a more disruptive phase of illness. When no other options exist, clients may be unable to receive housing support that will aid in their recovery. The concept of choices in rural psychiatric care is a much touted goal from public funding administrations, but the reality of limited capacity in low-population areas often collides with this goal. Programs such as Housing First (20), which provides housing without tying sobriety or treatment adherence to the service, would be an excellent first step for rural areas. Another option is to encourage grassroots nonprofit organizations such as Our Own Home in Western Pennsylvania to promote recovery-based Fairweather Lodge housing. Consumer-driven Fairweather Lodges are blended housing and employment programs that could empower and rehabilitate larger numbers of consumers in rural America.

Adequate transportation is necessary to maintain access to behavioral healthcare in rural areas. Placing more funding and infrastructure support for programs that get consumers and their advocates to treatment as well as to psychosocial rehabilitation sessions and social service appointments will be cost effective in the long run. One crisis contact in an emergency room caused by failure to provide for transportation negates any cost savings from slashing transportation budgets. Following the old adage "an ounce of prevention is worth a pound of cure," creating transportation programs will aid adherence and improve clinical outcomes while helping to reign in increased crisis and inpatient costs.

Focusing on Establishing Electronic Medical Records to Allow Communication Between Agencies Over a Larger Geographical Area

One viable solution to the fragmentation of services, communication barriers and the large geographic area over which service providers practice involves the institution of electronic medical records. Although electronic medical records are underutilized in the broader medical community, behavioral health systems have voiced additional concerns about matters of confidentiality and cost. Rural providers could be more adversely dissuaded by the financial outlay to start a system with no guarantee that other similarly organized, local clinicians would participate. One solution suggests that financial support from a local hospital or government system may assist smaller, more rural programs with the ethical issues involved and promoting "coming on line."

Encouraging the Use of Mental Health Courts in the Criminal Justice System So That Consumers Who Commit Crimes Because of Mental Illness Are Not Incarcerated and Are Able to Access Services or Secure Needed Support Programs

Rural consumers whose illness manifestations disrupt the community's social order are at great risk to be criminalized. Fred Markowitz (21) has eloquently shown that despite the presence of extended acute inpatient hospital capacity, criminalization remains related to homelessness throughout America. The criminal justice system providers are well aware of the increasing numbers of persons with severe mental illness who languish in our jails and prisons. Unfortunately, the options for intervention are perceived as less likely in rural health centers than in urban areas because of the geographic issues, lower population density and lack of both intensive and diversionary services. The opportunity to have mental health courts, jail diversion and re-entry programs would be an important component in any rural mental health plan. Some mental health court designs diminish these programs' utility by only accepting clients who have low acuity offenses. Clients who have more serious charges directly caused by their illnesses would in fact be the most promising candidates. Some diversion criteria may exclude individuals from participation if they have certain types of felony charges. The importance of expanding outpatient services that will be mental health court-mandated is crucial to prevent other individuals not in these programs from having decreased access because of the finite number of rural intensive care slots.

Prioritizing Web-Based Psychiatric Education Programs and Grassroots Mutual Support Groups to Help Address Feelings of Isolation and Improve Opportunities for Education

Using distance and web-based education and support options creatively in low population density areas is another important suggestion to help individuals with mental illness in America's grassroots. Education programs and support programs can be made readily available in the 21st century to consumers who tend to be more internet savvy than older generations. Rural consumers are increasingly able to obtain free internet access in public libraries, community centers, fire halls, granges and psychiatric support programs such as drop-in centers, clubhouses and supported workshops.

Traditional mental health advocacy organizations such as the National Alliance on Mental Illness (NAMI), CHADD (Attention Deficit Disorder Support), the Depressive Bipolar Support Alliance (DBSA), and the Mental Health Association (MHA) all offer Internet-based educational materials and on-line member services. NAMI has over 1000 local affiliates in many rural areas that provide education and peer support for both consumers and family members of people with mental illnesses.

Other internet list-serves such as KNOWHOW (consumers within NAMI) and Two-hats (mental health providers who are consumers) also exist independent of a bricks-and-mortar organization to provide education, support, and advocacy to consumers in rural areas who struggle with isolation or have difficulty obtaining face-to-face assistance. Often the founder-creator obtains a host site and serves as the initial list monitor. Over time, the list may have an existence of its own with established leaders and group norms that define safety, etiquette, and confidentiality. These list-serves often function as cyber-support systems and can survive despite the departure of the founder-creator through delegation of a new leader.

In summary, rural mental healthcare presents both challenges and opportunities to re-define how mental healthcare with be obtained in the 21st century. With the current priority to transform mental healthcare to a more community-based, recovery-oriented system of care, hope exists to mold rural areas into progressive treatment communities that foster modern mental health ideals.

References

1. *Improving Health Care for Rural Populations. Research in Action Fact Sheet.* AHCPR Publication No. 96-P040, March 1996. Agency for Health Care Policy and Research, Rockville MD. Available at http://www.ahrg.gov/research/rural.htm.
2. Glasser M, Peters K, Macdowell M. Rural Illinois hospital chief executive officers' perceptions of provider shortages and issues in rural recruitment and retention. *J Rural Health* 2006;22(1):59–62.

3. Mehl-Madrona LE. Prevalence of psychiatric diagnoses among frequent users of rural emergency medical services. *Can J Rural Med* 2008;13(1):22–30.

4. Wilks CM, Oakley Brown M, et al. Attracting Psychiatrists to a Rural Area: 10 years on. *Rural Remote Health* 2008;8(1):824.

5. Montgomery P, Forchuk C, Duncan C, et al. Supported housing programs for persons with serious mental illness in rural northern communities: A mixed method evaluation. *BMC Health Servs Res* 2008;24(8):156.

6. Gold PB, Meisler N, Santos AB, et al. Randomized trail of supported employment integrated with assertive community treatment for rural adults with severe mental illness. *Schizophrenia Bull* 2006;32(2):378–395.

7. Brown FW. Rural telepsychiatry. *Psychiatr Servs* 1998;49(7):963–964.

8. O'Reilly R, Bishop J, Maddox K, et al. Is telepsychiatry equivalent to face to face psychiatry? Results from a randomized, controlled, equivalence trial. *Psychiatr Servs* 2007;58:836–843.

9. Neufeld JD, Yellowlees PM, Hilty DM, et al. The e-Mental Health Consultation Service: Providing enhanced primary-care mental health services through telemedicine. *Psychosomatics* 2007;48(2):135–141.

10. Sulzbacher S, Vallin T, Weatzig EZ. Telepsychiatry improves paediatric behavioral health care in rural communities. *J Telemed Telecare* 2006;12(6):285–288.

11. Manfedi L, Shupe J, Batki SL. Rural jail telepsychiatry: A pilot feasibility project. *Telemed J E Health* 2005;11(5):574–577.

12. Zaylor C, Whitten P, Kingsley C. Telemedicine services to a country jail. *J Telemed Telecare* 2000;6(Suppl 1):S93–S95.

13. Thomas CR, Miller G, Hartshorn JC, et al. Telepsychiatry program for rural victims of domestic violence. *Telemed J E Telecare* 2005;11(5):567–573.

14. Nelson WA, Pomerantz A, Schwartz J. Putting "rural" into psychiatry residency programs. *Acad Psychiatry* 2007;31(6):423–429.

15. Purtilo R, Sorrell J. The ethical dilemmas of a rural physician. *Hasting Center Report* 1986;16(4):24–28.

16. Mutel C, Donham K, eds. *Medical Practices in Rural Communities*. New York: Springer-Verlag, 1983.

17. Hodgins G, Judd F, Kyrios M, et al. A model of supervision in mental health for general practitioners. *Australas Psychiatry* 2005;13(2):185–189.

18. Wilson I, Howell C. Small group peer support for GPs treating mental health problems. *Aust Fam Physician* 2004;33(5):362–364.

19. Shore JH, Hilty DM, Yellowlees P, et al. Emergency management guidelines for telepsychiatry. *Gen Hosp Psychiatry* 2007;29(3):199–206.

20. Stefancic S, Tsemberis S: Housing first for long term shelter dwellers with psychiatric disabilities in a suburban county. *J Primary Prev* 2007;28(3–4):265–279.

21. Markowitz FE. Psychiatric hospital capacity, homelessness, and crime and arrest rates. *Criminology* 2006;44(1):45–47.

17 Addicted Populations

Beny J. Primm, Warren W. Hewitt, Jr., Annelle B. Primm, and Marisela B. Gomez

INTRODUCTION

This chapter will present the current data regarding disparities in substance use disorders, utilization, and treatment among African Americans. Although it is evident that health disparities exist for African Americans in the United States, it is only recently that direct targeting of these disparities has become a part of the national agenda. Specifically, disparities in substance use disorder and treatment have yet to be highlighted. The reason for choosing African Americans is that they are the predominant subject of the limited studies on ethnic and racial disparities in the substance abuse literature. Furthermore, selecting one group to focus on within the scope of a single chapter in this volume will facilitate comprehensive coverage of the topic.

Substance use disorders encompass the use, abuse and dependence on alcohol and illicit drugs (1). Abuse relates to problems at work, home, and school; problems with family or friends; physical danger; and trouble with the law because of substance use. Dependence pertains to health and emotional problems associated with substance use, unsuccessful attempts to cut down on use, tolerance, withdrawal, and reducing other activities to use substances, spending a lot of time engaging in activities related to substance use, or using the substance in greater quantities or for a longer time than intended. Dependence defines a more severe substance use problem than abuse characterized by the involvement of psychological and physiological effects of tolerance and withdrawal (2).

EPIDEMIOLOGY OF SUBSTANCE USE DISORDERS

Based on data from the 2007 National Survey on Drug Use and Health (NSDUH), an estimated 19.9 million people used illicit drugs in the past month. More than half of all Americans over age 12 (126.8 million) considered themselves current alcohol drinkers, 57.8 million people participated in binge drinking at least once in the 30 days prior to the survey, and 17 million reported heavy drinking (1). Among African Americans the prevalence of illicit drug use was 9.5% among those ages 12 and older. Past-month consumption of alcohol among African Americans was 39.3% (including 20.2% who were current alcohol users, 15% who were binge, but not heavy users, and 4.1% who were heavy users). Overall, the prevalence of substance use disorders (alcohol and drug use) is greater in African Americans than in whites (3). These data represent reports for past year use and lifetime use.

Substance use disorders typically exist in the presence of multiple co-occurring psychiatric disorders that warrant treatment. Based on current data, nearly 5.4 adults age 18 and over are estimated to have both serious psychological distress (SPD) and substance use disorder (1). Past-year illicit drug use was higher for adults 18 years and older with SPD (20%) compared with those without SPD (12.2%) (1). The National Epidemiologic Survey on Alcohol and Related Conditions (NESARC) found that nearly 20% of the respondents with any 12-month mood disorder also had at least one substance use disorder, whereas 15% with a 12-month anxiety disorder had at least one substance use disorder. In contrast, 20% of the respondents with any substance use disorder also had at least one independent mood disorder and 18% of respondents had at least one independent anxiety disorder (4).

DISPARITIES IN CARE FOR SUBSTANCE USE DISORDER: UTILIZATION AND QUALITY

NSDUH data indicated that an estimated 23.2 million people age 12 and older required treatment for an illicit drug or alcohol use problem. However, only 2.4 million received treatment at a specialty facility leaving 20.8 million people who needed treatment but did not receive it (1). Several research studies have offered important insights about the extent of disparities in service utilization and treatment of substance use disorders. Wu and colleagues, using data from the 1998 Household Survey on Drug Use, reported that whites were three times more likely to utilize substance abuse services and that uninsured African Americans appeared to have a greater unmet need for services (5). Among those substance users with co-occurring mental illness, one study reported that while African Americans were less likely to receive treatment for their mood and anxiety disorders, there were no significant racial differences in their utilization of drug treatment services (3). In a study examining access to antidepressants in drug treatment programs, Knudsen et al. found evidence of an inverse relationship between the proportion of African American and Hispanic clients in drug treatment and the availability of SSRIs (6). They also reported that integrated drug treatment programs designed to treat co-occurring disorders tended to be affiliated with hospitals or mental health centers but were less likely to have African Americans represented among their clients (6). Other findings suggest that even where there is access to care, there are disparities in the quality of care provided (7). Reports suggest that increased problems (legal problems, intimate partner violence, higher unemployment rates, lower incomes, extensive family history of alcohol use, co-occurring drug use) associated with alcohol use exist for African Americans and other people of color, yet they are less likely to receive specialty or recurring care (8).

CAUSES AND CONSEQUENCES OF RACIAL AND ETHNIC DISPARITIES IN SUBSTANCE USE

This section will focus on current data regarding disparities in substance use disorders and treatment in African Americans and some of the potential causes and consequences of these disparities. We will use a "health determinants" framework to review how each determinant individually or together may affect the health outcome of substance use disorder in African Americans. Continuing within this framework, a discussion of how prevention practices can be designed to match population-specific health determinants is presented, along with challenges and recommendations.

The determinants of an individual's or a collective's health status or outcome were delineated by The Surgeon General's Report of Healthy People 2010, for the U.S. population (9). These were (a) social environment; (b) access to quality health-care; (c) policies and interventions; (d) physical environment; (e) individual behavior; and (f) individual biology. Together, these factors combine to determine wellness or contribute to the manifestation of symptoms that are labeled as a specific illness. Health status does not simply reflect the current condition a person exhibits via symptoms, but the factors and subsequent processes leading up to and maintaining a health status or outcome. We will highlight two key determinants of health, *social environment,* and *access to quality healthcare* because of their particular salience as contributors to disparities in substance use disorders and care for these conditions in African Americans.

The *social environment* includes interactions with family, friends, coworkers, and others in the community, social institutions (law enforcement, workplace, place of worship, school), housing, and public transportation. The role of the individual or population in the society has a significant impact on their health outcome or status. Membership in diverse racial and ethnic groups such as U.S.-born African Americans or non–U.S.-born Africans and Afro-Caribbeans is a central factor that determines the potential interactions that occur between such groups and social, economic and health systems. These interactions are vital because they delimit the scope, texture and quality of that interaction which may subsequently affect health policy choices and outcomes.

Numerous data show that after controlling for socioeconomic status, the quality of care and health and mental health outcomes of African Americans and other racially and ethnically diverse populations remain disparate (10,11). These disparities are ubiquitous and have existed for centuries bearing the manifestations of separate and unequal treatment, higher mortality, and with African Americans and other populations of color not receiving the benefits of advances in healthcare. These disparities continue to exist across multiple areas of service utilization, disease states and health outcomes including cardiovascular, infectious disease, kidney disease, mental illness or substance abuse, pediatric disorders, disorders of maternal and child health, rehabilitative and nursing home use, and surgical procedures.

Given the global disparities in disease prevalence and health outcomes among African Americans, it should not be surprising that substance use disorders commonly co-occur with other diseases. Hence, the clinician and the policymaker need to consider the multiple comorbidities in African Americans with substance use disorders. One common example of disorders co-occurring with substance use disorder is HIV/AIDS. African Americans are overrepresented (49%) among those in the United States who have HIV or AIDS and in 2006 they had the highest number of cases in 2006 (56.2/100,000 for women and 119.1/100,000, for men) (12). In 2005, HIV was a leading cause of death among African American adults. Throughout the HIV/AIDS epidemic, the use of illicit substances by injecting drug users (IDUs) has featured prominently as a major risk factor in parenteral transmission. However, alcohol and noninjecting illicit drugs (i.e., cocaine (crack), marijuana, methamphetamine), are also significant cofactors that affect the transmission of HIV as well as the course and outcome of the disease.

Evidence suggests that after accounting for access to care, unequal healthcare delivery based on racial and ethnic differences continues to be a major contributing factor in continuing disparate health outcomes (10). However, it is also important to remember that these disparities are not exclusively inequalities of care and services but fundamentally represent inequities based on practices and choices that have been intrinsically unjust and unfair since African Americans arrived on this continent as slaves several hundred years ago. Furthermore, the way healthcare is delivered hinges on individual and institutional discriminatory practices implemented through the healthcare system. This may occur at the provider, health system, and/or the regulatory and policy level (10).

Residential segregation has been instrumental in shaping the socioenvironmental context of African Americans and health disparities, especially with respect to substance use. More than 40 years since the enactment of the Civil Rights Act, residential segregation creates a toxic social environment, underpinning systematic attrition in employment opportunities, diminished economic business development, reduced educational attainment, limited access to all types of healthcare, precipitated increases in crime and incarceration and the creation of multiple generations of truly disadvantaged African Americans living in concentrated poverty among African Americans. Residential segregation has produced insidious damage to all facets of the African American socioenvironmental context, not the least of which has been the deployment of illicit drugs and unabridged access to alcohol irrespective of age (13).

Economic status is a key social determinant of health outcomes for African Americans (13). An assessment of the economic status (as an indicator of class) of African Americans in the year 2000 showed more than 20% of this population living in poverty. African Americans showed the highest rate of unemployment in 2003 (10.8%), the highest rate of wage loss (−2.4%) and the highest rate of poverty-level wages in 2003 (30.4%). African American women are more likely to earn poverty-level wages (33.9%), which, along with other low-wage employment, seldom provide health insurance to employees. Research shows that individuals living in poverty and economically strained status are at increased risk of mental health and physical disorders and are more likely to report substance use disorders (3).

When intact, the African American family serves as a strong social support network influencing behavior. However, in many poor urban neighborhoods, deteriorated housing and subsequent development has resulted in disenfranchised communities and decreasing social networks (14). As a potential risk factor for substance use and other unsafe health behaviors, addressing the social context of poverty and its effect on intact African American neighborhoods is significant in prevention and treatment.

A sobering study examining racial differences in etiology of substance abuse, observed that compared with whites, African Americans' use of drugs appeared to be in response to socioenvironmental conditions rather than to address emotional and psychological disturbances to alleviate dysphoria (15). This reminds us of the importance of assessing the social environment as a health determinant of substance use disorders in African Americans.

Access to quality healthcare includes services, education, and preventive measures received through healthcare providers as well as other venues (school, media, and religious institutions). Barriers to accessing substance abuse treatment programs reported by African Americans include child care, affordability, and identifying services; these differ from barriers reported by their white counterparts (stigma and perception of ineffectiveness of care) (16).

Access to care in the United States is tempered by three distinct factors. Foremost is the ability to pay the fee charged for the services rendered. For the larger employed population, this ability to pay is based on the type of insurance coverage offered by the employer. For those who have illness and enter the healthcare system at an entry point where a "wallet biopsy" is conducted or the individual's ability to pay is examined, a finding of "wallet necrosis" or an adverse ability to pay determination usually sets the tone for whatever care may or not may follow.

A major determinant of access to quality care is health insurance. In 2002, the percentage of African Americans with employer-provided health insurance was only 53.8%, while approximately 25% of African Americans remained uninsured. Compared with whites, African Americans had worse access to care for about 40% of access measures, including lacking health insurance or a source of ongoing health-care, having problems getting a referral to a specialist, and rating their healthcare poorly (17).

Although the government (state and federal) is the primary source of funding for public substance use treatment programs, there remain disparities in access to services. Uninsured African Americans are less likely to receive substance abuse treatment and alcohol treatment compared with their white counterparts (5). Based on a survey of the medical directors of a sample of Federally Qualified Community Health Centers (CHCs), referrals made to specialty mental health or substance abuse treatment services posed a major barrier to care for CHC patients with Medicaid or those who were uninsured (18). With the growing pharmacopeia for the treatment and medical maintenance of addictive disorders (from methadone to buprenorphine, acamprosate, naltrexone), medication choice is affected by insurance status, ability to pay out of pocket or local pharmacy availability (19).

The second factor relevant to insuring access to appropriate treatment is the availability of services in locations in proximity to the African American community. Many African American communities do not have local access to primary care, hospital services, or mental health and substance abuse treatment. Even in communities where these services still exist, the continuing challenges of high costs, low reimbursement, and uncompensated care have precipitated a major fiscal crisis in health and public health that has jeopardized the integrity of the community health safety net serving the African American community.

Finally, access to healthcare cannot occur in the absence of a supply of trained community health, mental health and drug treatment clinicians. Typically, African Americans reside in areas where there are insufficient culturally and linguistically competent health professionals to flexibly meet the treatment needs of diverse populations (20). Studies have reported that engaging and retaining African Americans and other diverse populations in alcohol treatment programs is more difficult compared with whites because of longer waiting times and greater dissatisfaction with treatments (16). The types of services offered in specialty settings and nonspecialty settings affect the extent of treatment-seeking in diverse populations. Recovery support programs such as Alcoholics Anonymous and Narcotics Anonymous play a vital role in the recovery process; however, there is some evidence that African Americans are less likely to use Alcoholics Anonymous (21).

Access to substance abuse care has another dimension related to comorbid issues, both in the medical and nonmedical realm. For example, data shows that African Americans with alcohol problems present with other nonclinical concerns such as unemployment, low income, and homelessness. A patient who presents with these comorbidities in a primary care setting may benefit from a provider with knowledge of these associated problems in African Americans with alcohol abuse. The provider should also recognize the importance of engaging the patient by offering screening, brief interventions, and appropriate referral in a culturally competent manner.

At the intersection of the service delivery system and high quality care is the connection between effective, evidenced-based practices and information that can be examined from the cultural context of the population to be served. The Institute of Medicine's Unequal Treatment report acknowledged the fundamental incongruity of the "one size fits all paradigm" that has not been enriched with a "cultural stamp of approval" (10). The achievement of higher retention in care and successful outcomes among African Americans is contingent on providers being able to adapt science-based treatment by acknowledging and integrating diverse values, beliefs, and behaviors that are tailored to meet the patient's social, cultural, and linguistic needs.

One example of a multisystem, comprehensive, culturally appropriate treatment approach to substance use disorders exists currently in the New York City-based, Addiction Research and Treatment Corporation (ARTC). ARTC provides illicit substance abuse and alcoholism treatment as well as comprehensive medical and social services targeted to primarily African Americans. It has a staff of substance abuse treatment, primary care, HIV care, mental health and social service providers, and care managers who are largely of African American, Afro-Caribbean and Latino descent, a reflection of the patient population served. ARTC works closely with the nonprofit, Urban Resource Institute (URI), which offers non–addiction-related services: residences, vocational training, shelter and jobs for victims of intimate partner violence; training for developmentally disabled youth; and intermediate care facilities for developmentally disabled and mentally ill adults. This constellation of services reflects a one-stop shop, "supermarket of services" approach that is regarded as an indicator of quality substance abuse treatment (22).

A survey of people in the correctional system (parole, jails, state prisons) revealed alcohol (40%) and drug use (20%) at the time of offense with two-thirds of the jail population actively involved with drugs prior to admission to jail (23). Among these two-thirds jail inmates, only 20% reported that they had received treatment or participated in any type of substance abuse treatment program since admission. While non-whites constitute approximately 25% of the general U.S. population, they represent the majority of the prison (62%) and the jail population (57%); African Americans represent 47% of the prison population (24). African Americans arrested for drug possession are more likely to be incarcerated than their white counterparts. Programs that include training and services to address these co-occurring factors, with culturally competent providers and mechanisms for follow up and financial support could be a valuable way to give access to this population of substance users. Instead of an unjust punitive process, a rehabilitative process could be the outcome for African Americans and others arrested and identified as substance users. These interventions could begin at the point of arrest and continue throughout the period of incarceration with follow up on release back into communities. Follow up may include referral for all co-occurring conditions that existed on release into the community (job training, education, medical care, parenting skills).

Policies addressing substance use disorder disparities in African Americans must include other systems associated with these disorders that can interfere with recovery. In the African American substance user, the co-occurrence of social factors such as low income and education, poor neighborhoods, legal problems, and medical illnesses suggest their involvement as potential risk factors for substance use, dependence, and abuse. Therefore policies targeting prevention and treatment of substance use disorders must be linked to policies addressing these social environment factors and access causing disparities in African American health outcomes. Housing, employment, health, education, and legal systems must all be targeted to address the disparities reflected in the African American population. Only when the co-occurring conditions and determinants that likely increase the risk of substance use in the African American population are addressed can real change be realized in preventing substance abuse and treating an affected person.

PREVENTION PRACTICES INFORMED BY HEALTH DETERMINANTS

Effective prevention practices begin with a deep understanding of the underlying causes and conditions leading to presenting signs and symptoms of a targeted illness. Disparities in substance use disorders and treatment in African Americans are the signs and symptoms, or outcome. Using the framework of health determinants of illness presented above helps in better understanding the causes and conditions that may individually and collectively interact to result in these identified signs and symptoms.

The demographics of the United States continue to show disproportionately low levels of socioeconomic status, employment, education, general health outcomes and various social indicators in African Americans and other populations of color. Addressing all the potential causes and conditions would begin to break this cycle of interdependence that leads to substance use disorders and disparities in treatment in African Americans. Indeed, a concerted effort to target any one of the conditions unilaterally would only slow down the cycle as the other identified risk factors continue to be present and contribute to disease outcome. A greater awareness of these underlying causes and conditions, and how they potentially act individually or together to result in disparate substance use disorders and treatment in African Americans will aid future policies and interventions in addressing these signs and symptoms. This type of prevention will require collaboration from all areas: education, justice, social services, economic, housing and health. Within the health arena, all specialties of health must be involved in planning prevention practices.

A focus on health determinants as risk or resiliency factors provides a comprehensive planning process whether for policy, community-level interventions, or clinical services that target existing or potential health outcomes. This model of building prevention practices also allows for incorporation of different health determinants to achieve a specific outcome. While treatment targeted to existing conditions would constitute tertiary prevention, secondary and primary prevention must be offered for the known determinants in this affected population. For example, substance abuse treatment programs for African American clients must be prepared to offer direct treatment which is informed by service utilization research for this population (tertiary prevention) as well as screening (secondary) and direct services or reliable and affordable referral with follow up, for all the potential determinants of the targeted outcome. Education (primary prevention) on the potential determinants of substance use disorder should also be available, such as comorbid medical and nonmedical conditions and how they interact to outcome in the targeted disease. Knowing that this population has increased rates of HIV, programs must be prepared to offer HIV screening and services. In designing this type of community-level prevention program and clinical preventive services targeted to African Americans with substance use disorders, policies that incorporate a health determinant framework offer guidance in implementation and evaluation.

Last, resiliency factors must be incorporated into prevention practices. Promoting policies and interventions which highlight the historical context of the wisdom and strength of the intact family and community in overcoming challenges of the African American population in the United States is important. These strategies introduce changes that begin to buffer the negative interdependent determinants leading to substance use disorders in African Americans.

CONCLUSION

Substance use disorders are brain disorders characterized by chronic relapse and uncontrolled craving, seeking, and use that persist even in the face of extremely negative consequences. However, in the African American community, substance use and abuse may not only be associated with low income, interrupted, or abridged education, or some predilection to use despite all negative consequences, rather, it is more likely a response to the toxicity of the socioenvironmental circumstance, allostatic overload, reactions to discrimination or racial profiling, or the conflict associated with internalized racism. Clearly, addiction is much more than just a brain disease.

Like so many of the disease conditions that are considered health disparities, substance use disorders are in some measure artifacts of the long term effect that residential segregation has had in shaping all facets of the socioenvironmental context of the African American. Therefore, in approaching African Americans affected by chronic substance use, a systems approach must be utilized, informed by the history of this population.

With this understanding, our approach to prevention and treatment of substance use in the African American population must be diligent in addressing the inherent risk factors that have and continue to increase vulnerability to addiction. The interplay between these existing risk factors and their effect on initiating substance use, accessing care, and following through with treatment is necessary to break the cycle.

The enactment of the Paul Wellstone-Pete Domenici Mental Health Parity and Addiction Equity Act of 2008 has eliminated the arbitrary practices of group plans to impose arbitrary limits, unreasonable consumer cost participation and deductibles for mental health or addiction treatment. This law has unparalleled significance for both the substance abuse and mental health fields. For African Americans and other racial/ethnic minorities, the significance of this law as a force to mitigate mental health and substance use care disparities has yet to be determined. However, the removal of this major barrier will have resounding implications for Federal, state, and local expenditures which support the substance abuse and mental healthcare delivery system.

RECOMMENDATIONS

The research on mental health and substance abuse treatment is meager in comparison to acute and chronic illness. Clearly, a much more systematic investment is warranted in psychiatric and substance use epidemiology and as well in mental health and substance use services research.

High-quality services for mental health and substance use are dependent on the recruitment and retention of well-trained clinicians including psychiatrists, social workers, psychologists, psychiatric nurses, counselors, and others who play a role in these service systems. There is a clear need for a new legislative authorization for clinical training fellowships, specialized practice start up loans and loan forgiveness programs for students seeking Masters, PhD, and MD level training in the substance use and mental health fields.

The "cookie cutter" methodology applied in mental health and substance abuse assessment is imprecise and overly biased toward normative views of substance use and abuse that may be inappropriate in assessing African Americans. A greater emphasis must be placed on improving psychometric screening and assessment instruments that lead to a symptom and diagnosis outcome that is driven by the sociological connection of the client/patient to their socioenvironmental context.

A culture-driven response to substance use and mental health disparities cannot occur where all the programs and the providers are not part of the community. Efforts must be made to support the development of indigenous community-based providers of substance abuse and mental health services.

The substance user is no longer viewed as having a unitary substance use disorder. Most substance users present for treatment with mixed morbidities that require clinical intervention and continuous case management from a program that can provide multimodality treatment services including: pharmacotherapy; mental health treatment; primary care; HIV/AIDS services, including HIV testing and management of HIV/AIDS treatment; and a wide range of services such as housing, vocational counseling and education, employment counseling and assistance, support groups (Alcoholics Anonymous and Narcotics Anonymous), transportation, and child care that enable recovery. Comprehensive, recovery-oriented treatment systems, like ARTC, represent the new standard of care for substance users with multiple, simultaneously occurring health and mental health disorders and social, educational and vocational needs.

Substance users from African American and other diverse racial/ethnic communities, irrespective of the types of drugs they use (illicit drugs or alcohol) or the delivery system (injecting or oral/nasal), all have a substantial and continuing risk of HIV infection. Culturally capable, comprehensive, integrated, substance use treatment and recovery support systems of care represent the best platform to reduce HIV risk associated with drug use or sexual contact with a drug user (injecting, noninjecting, and alcohol users).

Finally, research to practice or best practice innovations should not be considered treatment-ready for a diverse racial/ethnic population unless there is significant clinical evidence that they have been adapted for use and are compatible with cultural and linguistic conventions for the diverse racial/ethnic community of focus.

References

1. SAMHSA. *Results from the 2007 National Survey on Drug Use and Health: National findings. NSDUH Series H-34. Office of Applied Studies.* Rockville, MD: DHHS, 2008.
2. American Psychiatric Association. *DSM-IV-TR, Diagnostic and Statistical Manual of Mental Disorders, Fourth Edition, Text Revision.* Washington, DC: American Psychiatric Association, 2000.
3. Keyes KM, Hatzenbuehler ML, Alberti P, et al. Service utilization differences for axis I psychiatric and substance use disorders between white and black adults. *Psychiatr Serv* 2008;59(8):893–901.
4. Grant BF, Stinson FS, Dawson DA, et al. Prevalence and co-occurrence of substance use disorders and independent mood and anxiety disorders. *Arch Gen Psychiatry* 2004;61(8): 807–816.

5. Wu LT, Kouzis AC, Schlenger WE, et al. Substance use, dependence, and service utilization among the U.S. uninsured nonelderly population. *Am J Public Health* 2003;93(12): 2079–2085.

6. Knudsen HK, Ducharme LJ, Roman PM, et al. Racial and ethnic disparities in SSRI availability in substance abuse treatment. *Psychiatric Serv* 2007;58(1):55–62.

7. Schmidt L, Greenfield T, Mulia N, et al. Unequal treatment: Racial and ethnic disparities in alcoholism treatment services. *Alcohol Res Health* 2006;29(1):49–54.

8. Caetano R. Alcohol-related health disparities and treatment-related epidemiological findings among whites, blacks, and Hispanics in the United States. *Alcohol Clin Exp Res* 2003; 27(8):1337–1339.

9. Department of Health and Human Services. *Healthy People 2010: National Health Promotion and Disease Prevention Objectives.* Washington, DC: Department of Health and Human Services, 2000.

10. Smedley BD, Stith AY, et al., eds. *Unequal treatment: Confronting racial and ethnic disparities in health care.* Washington, DC.: National Academy Press, 2003.

11. Department of Health and Human Services. Mental health: Culture, race, and ethnicity a supplement to mental health: A report of the Surgeon General Washington, DC: Department of Health and Human Services, 2001.

12. Centers for Disease Control and Prevention. HIV/AIDS Surveillance Report, 2006. Vol. 18 Atlanta, GA: U.S. Department of Health and Human Services, Centers for Disease Control and Prevention, 2008.

13. Williams DR, Jackson PB. Social sources of racial disparities in health. *Health Affairs* 2005;24(2):325–334.

14. Gomez MB, Muntaner C. Urban redevelopment and health in East Baltimore, Maryland: The role of social capital. *Crit Public Health* 2005;15:83.

15. Roberts A. Psychiatric comorbidity in white and African American illicit substance abusers: Evidence for differential etiology. *Clin Psychol Rev* 2000;20(5):667–677.

16. Tonigan JS. Project Match treatment participation and outcome by self-reported ethnicity. *Alcohol Clin Exp Res* 2003;27(8):1340–1344.

17. Department of Health and Human Services). *Overview of the uninsured in the United States: Analysis of the 2005 Current Population Survey.* Washington, DC: Office of the Assistant Secretary for Planning and Evaluation, 2005.

18. Cook NL, Hicks LS, O'Malley AJ, et al. Access to specialty care and medical services in community health centers. *Health Affairs* 2007;26(5):1459–1468.

19. Green CR, Ndao-Brumblay SK, West B, et al. Differences in prescription opioid analgesic availability: Comparing minority and white pharmacies across Michigan. *J Pain* 2005; 6(10):689–699.

20. Collins SR, Kriss JL, Doty M, et al. *Losing Ground: How the Loss of Adequate Health Insurance Is Burdening Working Families Findings from the Commonwealth Fund Biennial Health Insurance Surveys, 2001–2007. The Commonwealth Fund Biennial Health Insurance Surveys.* T. C. Fund. New York: The Commonwealth Fund, 2008.

21. Tonigan JS, Connors GJ, Miller WR, et al. Special populations in Alcoholics Anonymous. *Alcohol Health Res World* 1998;22(4):281–285.

22. Ducharme LJ, Mello HL, Roman PM, et al. Service delivery in substance abuse treatment: Reexamining "comprehensive" care. *J Behav Health Serv Res* 2007;34(2):121–136.

23. Department of Justice. *Prison and Jail Inmates at Midyear 2001.* Washington, DC: Bureau of Justice Statistics, 2002.

24. Iguchi MY, Bell J, Ramchand RN, et al. "How criminal system racial disparities may translate into health disparities. *J Health Care Poor Underserved* 2005;16(4 Suppl B):4856.

18 Incarcerated Populations

Henry C. Weinstein

INTRODUCTION

From the station house, perhaps to a psychiatric emergency room, to arraignment before a judge (accompanied by a lawyer), to the Department of Correction for pretrial detention, or perhaps to be released on probation (under the aegis of the parole department) and then there is, perhaps, a plea bargain or a trial and then, perhaps, to "incarceration" in a jail or prison, to parole and then discharge back into the community.

Thus, "the incarcerated mentally ill person" in a jail or a prison is in the center of a much more extensive social control system—the criminal justice system—throughout which the seriously and persistently mentally ill patient faces formidable challenges and disparities and, in the mentally ill minority patient, even more so.

Figure 18.1 shows the progression of a mentally ill person through the criminal justice system and demonstrates the complexity of the system and the formidable difficulties the patient and his or her family have navigating the system.

This "Flow Chart of the Events That May Be Experienced by a Person with Mental Illness in the Criminal Justice System" (Fig. 18.1) before during and after "incarceration" is taken from one of the most important documents on the subject of this chapter: The Criminal Justice/Mental Heath Consensus Report of 2002 of the Criminal Justice/Mental Health Consensus Project (1).

At every point during the mentally ill person's contact with the criminal justice system he or she may experience multiple instances and multiple layers of disparities. These disparities are superimposed on what may be called the "free world" disparities, such as disrespect, racial bias and treatment disparities. In other words, the superimposition onto the disparities of the minority patient's everyday life with the overlay and added burden of specific disparities that are unique to the criminal justice system.

As contrasted to many other contexts of psychiatric treatment, the "eligibility" of a person with serious and persistent mental illness for psychiatric services in jails and prisons is not, itself, an issue because mental healthcare is constitutionally mandated in the jails and prisons of the United States—constitutionally guaranteed.

Under the Eighth Amendment of the U.S. Constitution, which prohibits "cruel and unusual punishment," whenever a state or the federal governmental entity takes custody of a person, it must provide for the necessities of life, which the person otherwise is unable to obtain. These include food, clothing, shelter, and medical care, which includes psychiatric care.

181

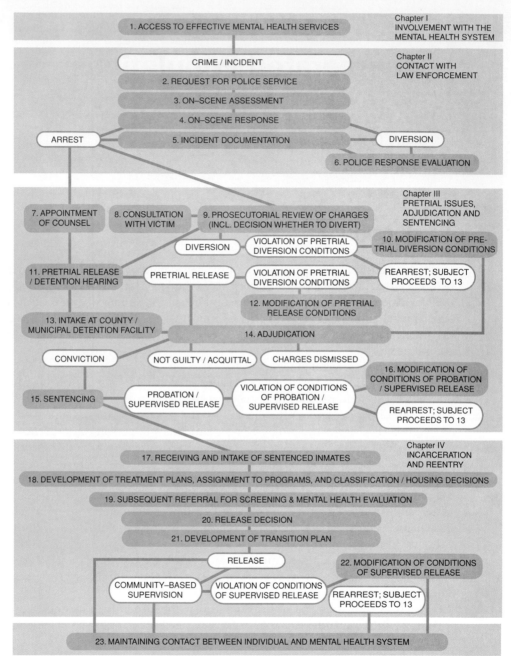

Figure 18-1. Flow chart of the events that may be experienced by a person with mental illness in the criminal justice system.

However, actually providing psychiatric treatment in a jail or a prison is an unusually complex undertaking. As contrasted to most other settings, the correctional psychiatrist is a "guest" in the domain of corrections—practicing psychiatry on the "turf" of corrections where security is the primary goal. This requires adjusting to the "culture" of corrections. And, although psychiatric treatment may be legally mandated, the correctional psychiatrist is not "in charge" of the jail or the prison in which care is provided.

To set the stage, there are, at present, more than 2.2 million inmates in our country's jails and prisons. Of these, an estimated 350,000 are severely and persistently mentally ill; i.e., carrying a diagnosis of a serious mental disorder such as schizophrenia, bipolar disorder, or severe depression.

The disparities are different in jails and in prisons. Jails are local city- or county-operated correctional facilities that confine individuals involved in the criminal justice system who are awaiting trial or serving short sentences for misdemeanors. There are approximately 3500 jails in the United States. A prison is a facility operated by state or federal government for the confinement of adults convicted of a felony whose sentences generally exceed 1 year. There are approximately 1300 state and federal prisons in the United States.

And, it is not hyperbole to state that each one of these almost 5000 facilities has its own unique "culture" (as is true of many such "facilities," such as state hospitals) and each differs in regard to the availability and access to psychiatric care and each may present a wide variety of barriers to care.

A consideration of the overarching barriers to psychiatric care in jails and prisons must begin with the historical perspective that jails and prisons existed almost solely for custody and psychiatric services were in no way regarded as a priority. Also, the public has always been reluctant to provide better conditions for those who have broken its laws or who have offended its sense of morality. In the correctional facility, correctional leadership is concerned that psychiatric services may jeopardize security. The correctional staff may resent what they perceive as better healthcare than they can provide for themselves and their families. The facility itself is often located in rural areas and so may be out of the medical mainstream, with limited access to psychiatric specialists. Correctional systems usually fail to allocate sufficient funds to attract and to retain qualified mental health professionals. Mental health professionals may find that correctional facilities are not satisfying places to work and offer little in the way of money, status, or prestige. For correctional psychiatrists the correctional milieu may subvert the trust that is necessary for the doctor-patient relationship, making many psychiatrists uncomfortable in a correctional environment. These correctional institutional barriers sometimes prevent the practice of good psychiatry or make professional psychiatric practice quite difficult.

Programmatically, there are major barriers to effective prevention, screening, and treatment. For the obvious reason that screening is critical to prevention and intervention and access to mental health treatment is assured by appropriate screening, the APA Guidelines for Psychiatric Services in Jails and Prisons call for a sequence of screenings that begins with a Receiving Mental Health Screening followed by an Intake Mental Health Screening which may result in a Referral for Mental Health Evaluation which would include a Brief Mental Health Assessment, then, if appropriate, a Comprehensive Mental Health Evaluation, and then, if necessary the Mental Health Intervention (2). Obviously these steps are important—interventions before the disparities causes its effects and to prevent further trauma—safely with understanding and without bias or prejudice.

However, in jails and prisons, there are often major logistical barriers, such as short periods of incarceration, security-conscious procedures for distributing medications, and difficulty coordinating discharge planning.

Since there are usually very limited resources difficult budgeting decisions must be made to meet the high cost of many healthcare services and some medications.

There are other correctional issues that are barriers to adequate psychiatric care such as the failure to specify minimum levels of such care in contracts with private healthcare vendors. There are the serious barriers of the delays caused by the need to escort inmates to medical treatment. There is often no communication or poor communication between public health agencies and prisons and jails and the lack of adequate clinical guidelines.

Of course, it hardly needs be emphasized that the environment of regimentation and perhaps violence and mistreatment is a barrier to treatment and prevention. Pagacz addresses the issue of "social invisibility," contrasting the considerable reaction to the Abu Ghraib revelations but noting that there is, regrettably, mistreatment of prisoners in the our correctional system that does not receive the same attention, even though similar humiliation and abuse are regular practices (3).

She cites as an example how in 1996, videotape from Brazoria Detention Center in Texas uncovered guards forcing dozens of prisoners to crawl naked along prison floors while the guards kicked and beat them, zapped their backs and genitals with stun guns, and had guard dogs bite prisoners. In 1997, an investigation found that guards at Corcoran State Prison staged gladiator fights between inmates and sometimes shot those who would not stop fighting.

Stating that "there are many more examples of cruel treatment" and that the list of abuses is long and, in addition to violence at hands of prison officials, includes rape both by other inmates and prison guards; inadequate medical and mental healthcare; overcrowding; lack of sanitation; and dangerous or otherwise inhuman and degrading conditions, "but unlike Abu Ghraib, there is no public outrage, pressure, or demands for investigation and reform."

As the Special Commission report stated after the 1971 Attica prison uprising: "We Americans have made our prisons disappear from sight as if by an act of will. We locate them mostly in places remote from view, and far removed from the homes of the inmates . . . and we manage to forget inmates . . . by pretending that [they] will not return to our cities and our villages and our farms."

Pagacz notes that scholars have argued that by portraying poor and minority communities as faceless individuals who perpetrate crimes, media, and political interest groups encourage the public to treat them as unimportant and dispensable.

Such societal disenfranchisement works to support use of violence as an oppressive force, including use of the death penalty and confinement of prisoners in inhuman conditions. Imagery of prisoners as disposable and undeserving of any compassion, let alone rights, gets reinforced in the context of warehouse prisons, the latest form of incarceration that offers inmates little to no constructive activities such as work, vocational instruction, or education.

THE OVERCROWDING BARRIER

The dramatic overcrowding that has resulted from the increase in the correctional population over the past three decades persists, and it has been noted that many large jails, such as the Cook County Jail in Chicago and the Los Angeles County Jail, have become the country's largest mental institutions.

Thus, in 2006, over 7.2 million people were on probation, in jail or prison, or on parole at year end 2006—3.2% of all U.S. adult residents or 1 in every 31 adults. State and federal prison authorities had jurisdiction over 1,570,861 inmates at year end 2006: 1,377,815 in state jurisdiction and 193,046 in federal jurisdiction. Local jails held 766,010 persons awaiting trial or serving a sentence at year end 2006. An additional 60,222 persons under jail supervision were serving their sentence in the community.

Along with this is another particularly thorny social policy issue has been the "criminalization" of the mentally ill (4). Some of the factors contributing to the high rates of people with serious mental illness in the criminal justice system include, as reasons for the increased entry; i.e., at the "front door" of correctional facilities, the process of deinstitutionalization and its accompanying phenomenon of "transinstitutionalization" the inadequate access of the seriously and persistently mentally ill to community treatment, the fact that these patients are arrested at disproportionately higher rates and often have co-occurring substance related disorders, the prejudice that the mental ill are more violent and the use of jails and prisons as housing of last resort.

At the "back door" there are problems of discharge planning and reentry into the community including that these patients spend longer periods of time incarcerated, the pathogenic nature of incarcerated environments, the lower rates of parole, and the higher rates of recidivism caused by inadequate community mental health services.

Finally, there are obvious overarching public policy issues that permeate the criminal justice/mental health realm. The United States has the largest percentage of its population incarcerated than any other country in the world. Since 1989, the National Drug Control Strategy, which called for a mandatory minimum sentence for drug crimes, caused the jail and prison populations to grow at a rapid rate. In 1985, the percentage of sentenced drug offenders was approximately 13%. Currently, it is more than 30%. The relationship between the increase in the number of inmates incarcerated for drug offenses and the disproportionate increases in the numbers of female, nonwhite, and foreign-born inmates cannot be overstated.

Most of the inmates in jails and prisons represent poor, nonwhite individuals. Many in jail are there for minor misdemeanors related to manifestations of chronic mental illness or homelessness, or both. Convicted felons in prison are unable to vote, have little control of their lives, and are believed to be the dregs of society. They have few advocates.

In this regard, there is the difficult and delicate but devastating problem of racism in the criminal justice system and in corrections—one of the greatest social scandals of our time. According to the Bureau of Justice Statistics in 2006, blacks were almost three times more likely than Hispanics and five times more likely than whites to be in jail (Fig. 18.2) (5).

THE BIAS BARRIER

In an American Bar Association publication, Robert M. A. Johnson, former president of the National District Attorneys Association and a former chair of the ABA Criminal Justice Sections, asks, "Is there racial bias, either conscious or subconscious, in the operation of the criminal justice system? (6).

"Even those who answer, 'No,'" he continues, "would likely concede that a perception of bias exists within communities of color. The community simply looks at the number of its members who are arrested and imprisoned, compared with the white community.

"Numerous research projects have demonstrated at least a prima facie case of racial bias in the criminal justice system. Statistics show significant disparity in jail and prison populations. Although African, Hispanic (Latino), and Asian Americans make up only 26% of the general population, they make up 58% of the prison population. In New York, where the state's adult minority population is less than 31.7%, 9 of

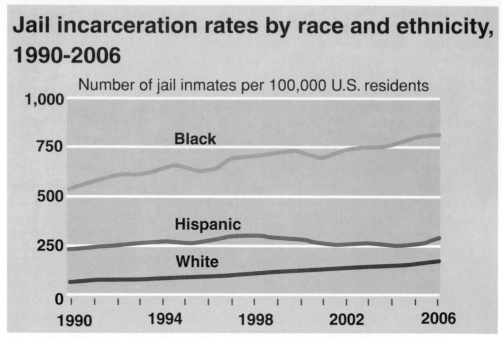

Figure 18-2. Jail incarceration rates by race and ethnicity, 1990–2006.

10 new prisoners are from an ethnic or racial minority. In 1997, the statewide population of Maryland, Illinois, North Carolina, Louisiana, and South Carolina was two thirds or more white, but for each, prison growth since 1985 was 80% nonwhite."

"Blacks are arrested, convicted, and incarcerated at far higher rates than whites or any other ethnic or racial group," Johnson continues. "Nationally, black Americans account for fewer than half of the arrests for violent crimes, but they account for just over half of the convictions, and approximately 60% of the prison admissions.

"Hispanics are the fastest growing group being imprisoned, increasing from 10.9% of all state and federal inmates in 1985 to 15.6% in 2001.

From 1985 to 1995, the number of Hispanics in federal and state prisons rose by 219%, with an average annual increase of 12.3%. Despite equal rates of drug use proportionate to their populations, Hispanics are twice as likely as whites, and equally as likely as blacks, to be admitted to state prison for a drug offense.

He concludes that "the overwhelming data contribute to a perception of bias. In a 1995 Gallup poll, more than half of black Americans said the justice system was biased against them. Moreover, two-thirds of black Americans in that same Gallup poll said that police racism against blacks is common across the country, and a majority of white Americans (52%) agreed."

A remarkable confirmation of the bias of the criminal justice system against minorities is the recent article "Cross-Racial Identification of Defendants in Criminal Cases: A Proposed Model Jury Instruction" by David E. Aaronson in the magazine of the ABA Section of Criminal Justice (7). Noting that erroneous eyewitness identification is the single leading cause of wrongful conviction in the United States, and that studies indicate most of the faulty identifications have a racial component, Aaronson proposes a model jury instruction that cautions jurors to consider the possibility of erroneous eyewitness identification, especially when the eyewitness and the defendant are of different races and when such identification is the primary evidence against the accused.

THE LANGUAGE BARRIER

One obvious example of a disparity for minorities in the criminal justice system is the language difficulties. So, while there are an estimated 10,000 Spanish-language-dominant speakers in the New York State prison system, there are very few Spanish-speaking healthcare professionals within the New York State Department of Correction. Spanish-speaking prisoners often seek the help of a bilingual prisoner to translate their needs to a prison healthcare provider. In the process their privacy and confidentiality are breached, there are omissions of information, and a potential for misdiagnosis exists. Although prisoners try to help one another, they are not trained in medical terminology and it is difficult for them to provide accurate translations (8).

The National Commission on Correctional Health Care's Standards for Mental Health Services in Correctional Facilities addresses the issues of privacy and confidentiality in regard to interpreters, stating that "the use of interpreters may be frequent mental health assessment process since psychological evaluation is more likely to be valid when language and culture are appropriately addressed (9). Interpreters need to be advised on how to protect the patient's privacy." However, the National Commission's standard goes on to say that "the use of inmates as interpreters should be discouraged and used only in urgent or emergency situations."

DEALING WITH DISPARITIES

The American Psychiatric Association has taken a leadership role in dealing with the pressing need for adequate psychiatric services in jails and prisons and the disparities in the criminal justice system. In 1974, before these issues had become of significant national concern, the APA published a Position Statement on Medical and Psychiatric Care in Correctional Institutions (10).

POSITION STATEMENT ON MEDICAL AND PSYCHIATRIC CARE IN CORRECTIONAL INSTITUTIONS

The American Psychiatric Association recognizes that so-called correctional institutions are established by various levels of government. Their ability to provide a full range of medical (including psychiatric) services varies according to a multitude of factors: e.g., public opinion, funding, and administrative structure in relation to the goals set for a particular institution, such as punishment, containment, deterrence, rehabilitation, and/or treatment.

An essential part of a minimum medical care delivery system consists of the early detection, diagnosis, treatment, and prevention of psychiatric illness. Many "correctional" facilities are not so structured to supply this care delivery system even minimally.

It is never part of the penalty imposed to deprive a prisoner of adequate medical (including psychiatric) care. Further, it is never proper to use medical (including psychiatric) care for punitive and coercive purposes or as an instrument of social repression. The fact of incarceration imposes on public authority the special duty to provide adequate medical services, including psychiatric services. Availability of such services is and should be a right of each incarcerated individual.

References

1. Council of State Governments. *Criminal Justice/Mental Health Consensus Project Report.* New York, Council of State Governments, 2002. Available at http://consensusproject.org/the_report/downloads (6/1/08).

2. American Psychiatric Association. *Psychiatric Services in Jails and Prisons,* 2nd ed. Washington, DC: American Psychiatric Association, 2000.

3. Pagacz E. Book review of Stanko S, Gillespie W, Crews GA. *Living in Prison: A History of the Correctional System with an Insider's View.* Westport, CT: Greenwood Press, 2004. Available at http://bad.eserver.org/reviews/2004/livinginprison.html (5/15/08).

4. Torrey EF, Stieber J, Ezekiel J, et al. *Criminalizing the Seriously Mentally Ill: The Abuse of Jails as Mental Hospitals.* Washington, DC: Public Citizen's Health Research Group and the National Alliance for the Mentally Ill, 1992.

5. United States Department of Justice, Office of Justice Programs, Bureau of Justice Statistics, Special Report, Revised, *Mental Health Problems of Prison and Jail Inmates,* September 2006, NCJ 213600.

6. Johnson RMA. Racial bias in the criminal justice system and why we should care. *Criminal Justice* 2007:Winter:1.

7. Aaronson DE. Cross-racial identification of defendants in criminal cases: A proposed model jury instruction. *Criminal Justice* 2008;23:4.

8. Sanchez R. *AIDS Community Research Initiative of America, Prison Health = Public Health: HIV Care in New York State Prisons. The Body, The Complete HIV/AIDS Resource, Fall 2005.* Available at: http://www.thebody.com/content/art14527.html (5/15/08).

9. National Commission on Correctional Health Care. *Standards for Mental Health Services in Correctional Facilities.* Chicago: National Commission on Correctional Health Care, 2008.

10. American Psychiatric Association. *Position Statement on Medical and Psychiatric Care in Correctional Institutions.* Washington, DC: American Psychiatric Association, 1974.

19 Chronic Mentally Ill Populations

Jacqueline Maus Feldman

INTRODUCTION

Special consideration must be given to a particularly vulnerable population, those with chronic mental illness; this is a population composed of individuals with serious and persistent mental illness (SPMI) who most often carry the diagnoses of schizophrenia or psychosis, bipolar disorder, or chronic severe (often treatment-resistant) depression. Their daily existence is replete with symptoms, manifested by a disease process that at best is relapsing and remitting, but at its most challenging, chronic and totally debilitating. For decades, these patients have faced the challenges of not only on-going symptoms, but lives complicated by systems of care that fail to meet even their most basic needs, such as housing, education, vocational support, substance abuse treatment, and medical care. Unique fiscal, societal, and clinical exigencies must be considered to begin to change the course of their illnesses and to assist those with SPMI in the process of recovery.

Patients with SPMI face a myriad of challenges. Their lives are often defined and limited by their mental illness and by the lack of commitment, expertise, and will of the systems of care that ostensibly offer treatment and support. While there have been haphazard attempts to provide systems of care that meet these challenges, historically multiple variables have conspired to ensure that disparities in care persist. Prevention and treatment recommendations are offered to ameliorate these disparities.

DEMOGRAPHICS

Those with SPMI constitute a small minority of a larger population who experience mental illness some time during their life. However, because of the special nature of their illness, they are much more likely to suffer serious and enduring sequelae. "Mental illness is the second leading cause of disability and premature mortality in the United States....collectively, mental disorders account for more than 15% of the overall burden of disease from all causes" (1). In the United States, these patients constitute more than 3.3 million people over the age of 18 in the last 12 months; of these, 2.6 million have sustained limits in their capacity to function in school and at work, and in their personal care, social functioning, and capacity to function cognitively; 1.4 million have been unable to work, 40% live with their family members, 24% attend some structured daily program, 11% attend school, and 14% are involved in volunteer work situations; 46% are involved in no part-time activities, spending most of their days in inactivity; 79% of this population have problems with concentration, 60% with social withdrawal; 37% will attempt suicide some time during their life, with 5% to 10% completing these actions. Although 23.2% of adults with SPMI receive SSDI, SSI, or Veteran's benefits, one-third to one-half of those with SPMI are at or near the federal poverty level, such that 80% are unemployed and have extraordinary difficulties with paying for transportation, attending appointments or paying for medications. More than one-half report problems with adherence with their treatment plans. Forty percent have been arrested. In 1999, 16% of all inmates in state and federal prisons carried some diagnosis of psychosis or affective disorder (2). Only half the persons with SPMI report seeing a regular physician or nurse practitioner for routine healthcare. Fifty percent to 90% of those with SPMI have at least one chronic health problem, and those with schizophrenia are likely to die 25 years earlier than the general population. Approximately one-third of those who are homeless are mentally ill, and depending on the source, 29% to 60% of those with SPMI are also abusing or dependent on substances (3).

A plethora of statistics, to be sure, all of which reflect a vulnerable population, debilitated not only by their symptom constellation, but by systems of care that fail to provide economic stability or sufficient supports that will not only sustain them, but allow them to choose adherence, participate in their healthcare decisions, and facilitate their recovery.

HISTORY

A brief historical review is imperative to understand the vast number of variables that complicate the lives of those with SPMI.

In the mid 1850s, Dorothea Dix and other advocates, having failed to convince the federal government of its responsibility to care for those with mental illness, sought to convince the existing states to provide asylum for those needing support and nurturing to cope with their mental illness. The basic tenets included embracing the concept of "moral treatment" (Phillip Pinel, early 1800s), which was predicated on anticipating and providing that which many of the ill patients lacked: stable housing, nutritious meals, and supportive care in kind and calming environments. Unfortunately, these institutions were overrun by society's less fortunate beyond those with mental illness, including those with chronic medical illness, orphans, and those laid low by poverty. Although several cycles of alternative care occurred, (analysis, "Mental Hygiene" Clifford Beers, early 1900s), use of ECT and insulin shock, Fountain House/peer support (1940s), by the mid-1950s state hospitals were crowded (more than 550,000 patients, or 339 patients/100,000 population) and rarely offered the kind of asylum envisioned by Dorothea Dix. Instead, many were mistreated, warehoused, and offered little treatment beyond endless days of inactivity. Unfortunately for those with SPMI, the systems of care have evolved slowly, and without significant progress toward recovery: "two generations ago a diagnosis of schizophrenia meant being locked away for life. One generation ago it began to mean homelessness or jail in the worst cases, and depending on parents or sibs, disability checks and odd jobs for the rest" (4).

The early 1960s were the beginning of a half century of extraordinary change for those with serious and persistent mental illness. It reflects a period of time where there were "efforts to transfer responsibility/costs (for the SPMI) between and among agencies, states, and the federal government, with persistent funding sources that were inadequate to meet the kind of resource and service needs of adults with serious mental illness," which "resulted in confusion, complexity in access to payment for services, created a burden on consumers and their families and disincentives from grass roots providers to meet service needs." What developed was a "lack of consistent national mental health policies . . . that led to a piecemeal financial system that diffused accountability, encouraged cost shifting, and obscured service responsibility resulting in vulnerable population being poorly served or abandoned" (1). Although cloaked in a philosophy of movement to a better life, deinstitutionalization (moving patients from state hospitals to communities) was more likely a strategy by the states (concerned about exorbitant costs of caring for hundreds of thousands of mentally ill) to reduce expenditures.

In 1963, the federal government passed several key legislative milestones, including the Mental Retardation Facilities and Community Mental Health Center Construction Act, and in 1965, the addition of staffing grants. The Community Mental Health Act offered funding for the building of community mental health centers to absorb patients as they were moved from the state hospitals to the community. Concomitantly, an increasing national awareness of and commitment to civil rights, and the use of antipsychotic medication, gave hope to patients and providers that improved living conditions were being created for those who segued out of state hospitals. In addition, the passage of Medicare, and the utilization of disability and Medicaid, offered funding for the provision of care and services. It must be noted, however, that Medicare and Medicaid were not conceptualized for patients with SPMI in mind. Those with serious and persistent mental illness were much less likely to have sustained continuous employment, and thereby would be unable to access SSDI (social security disability insurance). Medicare was regulated to offer a lower payment rate (and higher patient co-pay) for mental health services. Medicaid was helpful, but limited by the IMD exclusion, which prevented patients from being hospitalized at facilities that offered only psychiatric services.

Ultimately, the population of state hospitals dropped to 21/100,000. Despite these hoped-for supports after hospitalization, many of those with serious and persistent mental illness led dismal lives. The staffs of community mental health centers seemed terribly unprepared to care for these more challenging patients; despite promises, housing opportunities were negligible, and many patients ended up in transinstitutional settings (nursing homes, boarding homes, foster care, jails, prisons, or back with their unsuspecting families) with few psychiatric or social supports available (1). "As individuals with severe and persistent mental disorders spent more and more of their time in their communities, they found themselves in an ever-widening range of social institutions. They were involved in public housing, employment services and vocational rehabilitation programs, and schools (but) increasingly over time in the criminal justice system" (5). In addition, these times reflected the beginning of a philosophical shift in treatment; psychiatric predicated care fell to psychologists, and effective interventions were thought not to be medical or biologic in nature, but to be social or educational, and where it was proffered, that early intervention could *prevent* mental illness.

The ebb and flow of political will also played heavily on any progress toward shoring up those with serious and persistent mental illness. President Nixon tried to withdraw financial supports put in place by Presidents Kennedy and Johnson. However, President Carter established the first Commission on Mental Heath, which suggested a "National Plan for the Chronically Mentally Ill"; it identified fragmentation as a key problem with the mental health system and suggested that "service integration" along with organizational coordination and collaboration were the first steps of rehabilitating a chaotic system of care. It also recommended and facilitated the creation of the Community Support Program in 1977 through NIMH (National Institutes of Mental Health), which encouraged the establishment of integrated services at state levels and clarified lines of responsibility, and funded necessary supports to sustain individuals with serious and persistent mental health issues in the community.

The Mental Health Systems Act was passed and funded in 1980 during the latter part of President Carter's tenure; it was designed to provide additional monies to redirect community mental health centers to serve the needs of those who had been deinstitutionalized. Unfortunately, the Reagan administration repealed the law in 1981, reversing 30 years of federal leadership with the Omnibus Budget Reconciliation Act, instead diverting federal dollars (reduced by 25%) to the states through block grants (6). "The vision of an organized, community-based, and dedicated mental health system ended. The effect-intended or otherwise-was to thrust mental health policy making into the mainstream of health policy." The Reagan administration also changed the criteria for SSDI at that time. People with SPMI made up 11% of SSDI recipients, but represented 30% of those people losing program eligibility. A public hue and cry was raised and the criteria were revamped, but SSDI still took fewer persons with SPMI (7).

The 1980s and 1990s ushered in the concept of managed care, ostensibly designed to provide "quality services to an expanding number of clients while simultaneously controlling costs" (8). Themes of common assessments, monitoring (and limiting) enrollment rates and risk-based contracting, as well as a massive increase in external regulation (with accreditation standards, rules, and responsibility) placed enormous economic burdens on community mental health centers least able to sustain such demands. Hospital admissions were to be avoided at all costs, lengths of stay were vigorously scrutinized by utilization managers, and mental healthcare provision was subcontracted to non-psychiatry healthcare providers. Many proclaimed that access to mental healthcare was increased, but the reduced intensity of services often had a powerful negative effect on those with SPMI; managed care, which fostered a system in which choice was limited, care was managed to decrease costs, and continuity was threatened, was particularly troublesome for individuals with socially stigmatized, poorly understood illnesses that had traditionally been treated separately from standard medical practices (1).

The years of 1990 to 2000 were proclaimed by President George H. W. Bush as the "Decade of the Brain." New atypical antipsychotic medicine was developed and marketed, adding huge formulary costs and opening the door for massive influence by pharmaceutical companies (9). Enhanced accountability did help focus services on those who most needed them, and the change to the Medicaid rehabilitation option pushed for creating a funding mechanism for case management, influenced hiring practices, and the inventory of programs offered to consumers.

The type of programs offered and the quality of said programs vastly shifted over the 1990s. There were limited tool kits to guide clinical interventions, few effective medications, primitive evidence-based practices, no outcome measures and an increasing demand for services in the face of woefully insufficient numbers of psychiatrists competent in or enthusiastic about working with this patient population. In 1992 NIMH was reorganized under NIH (National Institutes of Health), and CMHS (Center for Mental Health Services) was moved under SAMHSA (Substance Abuse Mental Health Services Administration). Attempts at addressing issues of parity were made during the early Clinton years during the failed health-care reform process, (mental health parity was attempted and achieved on the federal level, but rarely at the state level) and the Mental Health Report of the Surgeon General in 1999 reflected the gap between psychiatric research and practice.

However, not until the administration of President George W. Bush was there again enormous attention paid to those with SPMI. The President's New Freedom Commission on Mental Health in 2005 offered observations on the fragmentation of mental health services and policies, and identified the need for small sequential steps to transition the system of care. "It reviewed the science of mental health, and mental health services, (and offered) an indictment of the mental health service system, which included fragmentation/gaps in care for children and adolescents, increased unemployment and disability (in those with SPMI) and noted that neither mental health nor suicide prevention were a national priority." There were six overarching premises and goals recommended by the commission:

1. It must be understood that mental health is essential to overall health;
2. Mental healthcare should be consumer/family driven;
3. Disparities had to be eliminated;
4. Early mental health screening assessments/referrals needed to be common;
5. Quality care should be delivered and research increased; and
6. Enhanced use of technology (5).

In addition, the MMA (Medicare Modernization Act, 2005) sought to stabilize and maximize the numbers of mentally ill who would be able to access their medication. Recent (2008) legislation related to mental health parity will hopefully end the financial discriminatory burden borne by those with and those who serve those with SPMI, and decrease the discrepancies (differential payment of those provided with mental healthcare) that had been in place for Medicare since its inception.

This brief historical review serves to underscore the painfully obvious. A person with serious and persistent mental illness, even to this date, is likely to be met with a system of care that is under funded, poorly regulated, inadequately organized, and insufficiently staffed (by practitioners not necessarily possessing the appropriate skills set to offer evidence based practices). "Financial and organizational policies lack an organized vision as well as the administration and resources to support them (there are insufficient) policies dictated by federal politics, state budgets, and local cultures that restrict access to care" (1).

UNIQUE BARRIERS TO CARE

At least 40% of individuals who suffer from severe mental illness in the United States do not receive the treatment they need. Barriers to care include difficulty: (i) gaining entrance to systems of care, (ii) receiving appropriate assessments, (iii) obtaining the highest quality of care and follow-up, and (iv) accessing additional supports that enhance recovery.

These barriers to care are predicated on several variables:

Stigma
There persists in today's society a stigma attached, particular to mental illness. The stigma of mental illness affects the ability of consumers and families to demand needed

services, for providers to adequately serve persons with SPMI and professionals from entering the field of service to those with mental illness. It is certainly reflected in the assumption by many providers and even leaders in planning and organizing systems of care, that recovery, however it is defined, cannot be attained by those with SPMI.

Financial (Including Medical Insurance Limitations)

Compared with the general population, individuals with mental health problems experience a deterioration of their health insurance status as time progresses. Their unemployment rate is 3 to 5 times higher than the general population for those who have a history of mental illness, and of those with SPMI, over 80% are unable to sustain significant employment. Systems of care for those with SPMI are chronically underfunded, with leaders and patients alike asked to do more and more with less and less. Healthcare insurance is difficult if impossible to purchase, and the cost of mental healthcare, like the rest of the field, in increasing asymptotically. Patients are unable to afford copays, lack insurance, are unemployed, often homeless, and lack transportation. For example, the Kaiser Commission found in FY 2002 to 2004 most states had reduced or restricted eligibility, decreased benefits, increased copayments, controlled drug costs in various ways, and reduced or frozen payments to providers or were planning to do so. For years, private insurers dropped the challenge of selection against high-use SPMI users, and refused to cover nonmedical services that included housing, rehabilitation and social services, to the detriment of this population (2).

Systems of Care That Are Unresponsive

It should be noted that today's systems of care have been particularly unresponsive to those homeless patients with SPMI. Homelessness among persons with SPMI is an invisible consequence of the current mental health system; several studies have documented a significant number of patients in state mental institutions, partial institutions, and local psychiatric hospitals were or have been homeless and that a large proportion of those discharged become homeless again. Many psychiatric admissions of persons who were homeless (52%) were for mental illness and substance abuse/dependence occurring concomitantly. Unfortunately, homeless patients with SPMI often do not access existing services. Limited and variable funding for specialized programs reflect inadequate resources and result in limited access to mainstream services, resulting in inadequate care to the poorest individuals in our communities.

Overall, systems also lack advocacy, evidence based practices, fidelity to practice models, adequate assessments or sufficient supplies of knowledgeable mental health professionals. "The challenge today is to somehow manage to deliver good care while maneuvering through a seemingly impenetrable maze of external laws, regulations and requirements governing behavioral healthcare: organizational risk management, fraud and abuse, antitrust, local/state/federal constraints, human resources, and HIPPA while balancing principle purpose and grounding beliefs of the organization" (1).

Stable housing, though crucial particularly for this population, is not yet well funded; there is minimal support from HUD (Housing and Urban Development), and multiple year waiting lists exist to access Section 8 housing. In terms of vocational rehabilitation, there has never been sufficient funding to serve more than a small portion of this population. There are also built-in disincentives to full time employment (patient are terrified they will lose their disability checks) although there have been some changes recently that allow for patients to work part-time, or even full-time earning up to a maximum amount without fear of losing their financial support.

Programs are also in place that allows patients with SPMI to work for a certain period of time without losing their check.

The Impact of Mental Illness on the Individual

The life of a person with serious and persistent mental illness is often defined by what he or she cannot do. Patients with SPMI often lack insight and judgment into their illness, which complicates their degree of motivation. They often have an impaired ability to recognize and interpret important medical symptoms and/or to communicate their concerns; it might make it difficult for them to remember recommendations and plan for future healthcare needs. Patients may fear physicians will not take their symptoms seriously because of stereotypes held by physicians of patients with mental illness. Patients may also have difficulty communicating the urgency of their medical health needs. In addition, as one-third of those who are homeless are SPMI, they are the most vulnerable, not only to multiple comorbidities including substance abuse, but also to stigmatization, exploitation and brutal victimization; consequently they are at highest risk for prolonged homelessness. Patients who are homeless may also have difficulty receiving and storing their medications.

In addition, patient populations with SPMI are plagued by chronic medical problems. Although persons with SPMI have a greater chronic disease burden than the general population, they receive primary care much less often. Only one-half of the people with SPMI report seeking regular healthcare. They have an increase rate of chronic illness, have medications with many adverse effects, have high rates of tobacco utilization, and unhealthy behavior (poor diet, low rates of exercise, limited awareness of the need to practice safe sex); they typically seek acute care (vs. prevention) and often lack coordinated healthcare (2).

UNIQUE TREATMENT CONSIDERATIONS/ RECOMMENDATIONS

To meet the needs of this unique and challenging population, philosophies need to be modified, stigma reduced, systems of care reorganized and adequately funded, and evidence based practices promulgated. Our understanding of the historical antecedents (abuse, neglect, subterfuge, cost-shifting, and politics) that led to the development of the present chaotic and inadequate system of care will also guide the development of solutions to best move those with SPMI along the spectrum of recovery.

(i) Reduce stigma; a national project must ensue that will educate the American public on the biologic nature of serious and persistent mental illness, the need for treatment, and the need to set aside blame or mischaracterization of mental illness, to be replaced by understanding and the acceptance that mental illness is real and treatment exists and can be successful. This includes embracing the concept that recovery is possible, as well as promulgation of models of care that are strengths based, consumer driven, and partnership oriented. A change to a recovery movement philosophy is imperative, one that shifts focus from deficits to capabilities, and from differences to shared aspirations and experiences.

(ii) Diligent and vigorous advocacy at all levels of care is imperative, which should always seek the inclusion of consumers and family members in decision- and policy-making processes.

(iii) Consistent, reliable funding which encourages innovation and accountability should be made available.

(iv) Early intervention: sentinels should be trained to observe children and adolescents for changes in premorbid functioning that might indicate the early onset of serious and persistent mental illness; once identified, access to a broad spectrum of treatment should be made available.

(v) Prevention of psychosocial stressors, including homelessness and criminalization of mental illness should be considered, and resources put in place to minimize variables that can exacerbate mental illness.

(vi) Evidence-based practice is imperative; this includes access to a broad spectrum of treatments (effective medications, case management, ACT [assertive community treatment] teams, substance abuse treatment, supported employment, illness management, integrated MI/SA treatment, recovery strategies, electronic technology, cognitive behavioral therapy, and dialectical behavioral therapy [programming that promotes self-competence, guiding consumers to reframe their thinking and learn calming strategies and emotion regulating techniques]) (see SAMHSA toolkits; 10).

(vii) Provision of supports including supported housing, vocational rehabilitation, social networks, and medical healthcare. Patients with SPMI need regular blood work and physical exams; they need to be counseled regarding health maintenance (smoking, lifestyle choices, diet, substance abuse), their care needs to be coordinated, they should be regularly assessed for symptoms of suicidality, and attention must be paid to the side effects experienced, all parameters related to enhancing adherence (11).

(viii) Development of an ample workforce that includes recovery oriented psychiatrists familiar with psychosocial rehabilitation models, peer support, and family-to-family education.

(ix) Support research in outcomes and supports that allow translation of proven evidence based practice into the community.

Perhaps by following these recommendations the lives of those with serious and persistent mental illness can surmount the extant disparities to futures headed for recovery. These hopes are best summarized (though certainly not mandated or funded) by the President's New Freedom Commission: "to achieve the promise of community living for everyone, new service delivery patterns and initiatives must ensure that every American has easy and consistent access to the most current treatment and best support services."

References

1. Grazier KL, Mowbray CT, Holter MC. Rationing psychosocial treatments in the United States. *Int J Law Psychiatry* 2005;28:545–560.
2. Gold KT, Kilbourne AM, Valenstein MV. Primary care of patients with serious mental illness: Your chance to make a difference: A primary care visit may lead to regular care of side effects and comorbidities, especially if you coordinate care. *J Fam Pract* 2008;57:515–525.
3. Rosenberg J, Rosenberg S, eds. *Community Mental Health: Challenges for the 21st Century.* New York: Routledge, 2006.
4. Sullivan WP. Mental health leadership in a turbulent world. In: Rosenberg J, Rosenberg S, eds. *Community Mental Health: Challenges for the 21st Century.* New York: Routledge, 2006.
5. Grob GN, Goldman HE. The dilemma of federal mental health policy: Radical reform or incremental change? New Brunswick, NJ: Rutgers University Press, 2007.

6. Mechanic D, Bilder S. Treatment of people with mental illness: A decade-long perspective. *Health Affairs* 2004;23: 84–95.

7. Frank RG, Glied SA. Mental health in the mainstream of health care. *Health Affairs* 2007; 26:1539–1541.

8. Sullivan WP. Mental health leadership in a turbulent world. In: Rosenberg, J, Rosenberg, S, eds. *Community Mental Health: Challenges for the 21st Century*. New York: Routledge, 2006.

9. Mechanic D. Mental health services then and now. *Health Affairs* 2007;26:1548–1550.

10. SAMHSA National Mental Health Information. About evidence-based practices: Shaping mental health services toward recovery. Available at http://mentalhealth.samhsa.gov/cmhs/communitysupport/toolkits/about.asp.

11. Kiraly B, Gunning K, Leiser J. Primary care issues in patients with mental illness. *Am Fam Practice* 2008;78:355–362.

20 Disabled Populations

Alex Kopelowicz, Steven R. Lopez, and William A. Vega

WHAT IS PSYCHIATRIC REHABILITATION?

The goal of psychiatric rehabilitation is to ensure that persons with a psychiatric disability can perform those cognitive, emotional, social, intellectual, and physical skills needed to live, learn, work, and function as normally and independently as possible in the community of their choice. To achieve this goal, symptoms and cognitive impairments associated with serious mental disorders need to be stabilized or compensated as they are obstacles to reaching optimal psychosocial functioning. A triad of treatment approaches promote rehabilitation: (i) pharmacotherapy, cognitive behavior therapy, and cognitive remediation to attenuate symptomatic and cognitive impairments; (ii) teaching disabled persons the specific skills required for independent functioning; and (iii) providing professional and natural community supports that counterbalance deficiencies in the skills repertoire of disabled persons, enabling them to participate in social, educational and vocational activities. When all three of these rehabilitation modalities are employed, individuals with mental disorders can make optimal progress in personally relevant areas of their lives.

The development of the field of psychiatric rehabilitation has been spurred by the growing recognition that many people with a major mental disorder experience long-term disability. Even with the best evidence-based treatments, individuals with psychotic, mood, anxiety, somatoform, and other serious disorders have suboptimal outcomes, with some level of symptoms persisting despite customary biological and psychotherapeutic treatment. Beyond persisting symptoms, social maladjustment in family, friendship, recreational, vocational, and educational roles interferes with the quality of life of a large number of those with mental disorders. Stigma, inadequate or inaccessible treatment services, unemployment, poor quality housing, and lack of social and leisure opportunities all complicate the social disablement that arises from severe mental disorders. The unmet needs of the mentally disabled have pointed the way toward long-term and comprehensive rehabilitation services.

IMPLEMENTATION OF PSYCHIATRIC REHABILITATION

Despite the proven efficacy of psychiatric rehabilitation techniques, the implementation of psychiatric rehabilitation in the public and private sector has been insufficient to meet the need for these services. For instance, Young and colleagues (1) studied 224 patients at two public mental health clinics and found that 52% received inadequate psychosocial care. Similarly, the PORT project examined conformance of patterns of usual care for persons with schizophrenia with its treatment recommendations by surveying a stratified random sample of 719 persons diagnosed with schizophrenia (2). Findings indicated that usual treatment practices fall substantially short of what would be recommended based on the best evidence on treatment efficacy, with only 7% having been offered family psychoeducation and 12% receiving social skills training. The private sector fared no better as illustrated in a survey of U.S. psychiatrists in which fewer than 10% of respondents reported using any of the evidence-based methods (3).

What is the effect of the limited availability of psychiatric rehabilitation techniques on ethnic minority populations? Unfortunately, research has not systematically studied patterns of use of psychiatric rehabilitation services among persons from ethnic minority groups who have severe mental illness. One exception is a study by Barrio and colleagues (4) that examined case management service use by ethnic group in a sample of 4249 Euro-American, Latino, and African-American patients with a diagnosis of schizophrenia or schizoaffective disorder who were receiving services in the public mental health sector of San Diego County during fiscal year 1998 to 1999. This report found that Latinos were less likely than Caucasians to receive services from specialized case management providers, a finding that persisted after adjustment for language indicating that the ethnic difference was not simply a function of language. Other psychiatric rehabilitation modalities, however, were not examined.

Despite the lack of specific information about the participation of ethnic minorities in psychiatric rehabilitation treatments, the importance of finding ways to increase the availability of these approaches is clear given the fact that the gap in mental healthcare utilization between whites and ethnic minorities is large and growing. Cook and colleagues reported recent evidence of this phenomenon. By applying Institute of Medicine definitions of mental healthcare disparities to data from the Medical Expenditure Panel Survey from 2001 to 2004, they found significantly increased disparities between Latinos and whites in mental healthcare expenditures between 2001 and 2002 and 2003 and 2004 and a trend for a larger gap between African Americans and whites (5). Such findings point to the need to understand the barriers to mental healthcare for ethnic minority patients as they pertain to psychiatric rehabilitation.

PSYCHIATRIC REHABILITATION FOR COMMUNITIES OF COLOR

The President's New Freedom Commission on Mental Health highlighted the fragmented state of mental healthcare and pointed out the need for an improved model of mental healthcare that would eliminate the many truncations of current service arrangements. This is particularly the case when considering the mental healthcare for members of ethnic minority groups. The Surgeon General's 2001 *Report on Mental Health: Culture, Race, and Ethnicity* provided ample evidence that minority groups as a whole underutilize mental health services and when they do avail themselves of such services, they often receive lower quality of care than Euro-Americans. The roots of the problem are multiple, but much of the explanation comes from the interaction among the patient, the clinician, the environment or system of care and the prevailing attitudes toward racial and ethnic minorities in society. At each step in the treatment process these interactions influence the patient's access and ability to enter mental healthcare, remain in care and adhere to treatment recommendations.

The many factors that contribute to the observed disparities in mental healthcare can be grouped into three general domains: individual, service, and community. To illustrate the type of research in this area we consider selected studies that primarily relate to service use or to quality of care.

Individual Factors

One research area within the individual factors domain is that of mental health literacy. The Institute of Medicine (6) defines literacy as the extent to which individuals are able to obtain, process, and understand health information and services to make health decisions. Although there are many components of health literacy, including print and oral literacy (e.g., reading prescriptions and communicating with health professionals), one area that has received recent attention concerns mental health knowledge. Lopez and colleagues (7) found that Spanish-speaking community residents living in the Los Angeles area have limited literacy with regard to psychosis. When presented with a hypothetical case in which a recently divorced woman was experiencing depressed mood, possible hallucinations, and possible delusions, most residents described the problem as depression/sadness (86%) and social disruptions (54%), whereas few residents referred to psychosis (2%) or to a more general reference to a mental health problem (7%). Although it is not clear if the residents viewed the depression/sadness as a treatable condition, it is clear that the residents have very low literacy with regard to psychosis. This is just one of many individual factors that contribute to the apparent delay in treatment seeking for Spanish-speaking adults with serious mental illness

Service Factors

A fundamental service consideration is the availability of health insurance. The Latino population is the least likely of U.S. ethnic groups to enjoy health insurance or a usual source of healthcare. Health insurance increases use of specialty mental health providers among Latinos. It is estimated that between 35% and 40% of the U.S. Latino population does not have health insurance (8). The tendency of low-income Latinos to be employed part-time and to have multiple employers, or employers how do not offer insurance benefits, produces a higher uninsured rate during the course of any 12-month interval (9). Furthermore, Latinos are more likely to have a limited scope of insurance benefits, and individual families may have different insurance programs, or no coverage, for different family members such as children. Because of the large influx of documented and undocumented people in the Latino population, many are not eligible for public insurance, and their access to safety net providers is also restricted (10). The result is a higher fraction of income dedicated to out-of-pocket expenses for medical care, or possibly delaying or foregoing medical care altogether. Regrettably, the economic behavior of Latinos related to receiving mental healthcare and related medications is inadequately documented. Having a usual source of care is least likely among the undocumented and newer immigrants, and this sector of the Latinos population is numerous, comprising possibly one-quarter of the U.S. Latino population, and they are the most impoverished, and have the lowest educational attainment.

Not only does the differential availability of health insurance affect the mental healthcare of ethnic minority communities, but the specific financial policies of insurers may also differentially affect their care. Snowden and colleagues' examination of the mental healthcare for youth in foster care is particularly relevant (11). First, mental health problems occur at a relatively high rate among those in the child welfare system. Second, African American and Latino youth are overrepresented in out-of-home placements. Third, mental healthcare provided to foster care is primarily carried out in the public sector and supported through Medicaid. As a result, these services and their financing can be studied using available databases. Snowden and colleagues examined whether the shift from fee-for-services to capitated managed care in the state of Colorado affected the use of inpatient and outpatient care among the over 60,000 youth from 1994 to 1997 (11). Some critics argue that relative to fee-for-services, capitation may lead to minorities receiving less mental healthcare because of the perception that they are hard to treat and require special services with additional costs (e.g., medical interpreters). The findings indicated that managed care had relatively no impact on the use of inpatient or outpatient care for African American and Latino youth. Under both the fee-for-service and managed care plans, African American and Latino youth received disproportionately less services than whites. There was an increase, however, in the use of Residential Treatment Centers for the minority youth that was caused by the implementation of managed care. Because it is not clear whether such services are effective, it is not known whether this is a positive or negative outcome. This study of financial policy and its impact on service use of youth in foster care represents one of the important directions of organizational and service characteristics as they relate to minority groups' service use (see Reference 25 for the study of quality improvements in the treatment of depression in primary care and their effect on the quality of care for ethnic minority adults).

Community Factors

Whereas it is important to consider individual factors and service or organizational factors, it is equally important to consider the social context in which services are embedded. One way to do so is to examine the geographical location of services. In a secondary analysis of the National Comorbidity Survey, Alegría and colleagues (12) found that minority adults' use of specialty mental health services differed by geographical region. Specifically, African Americans from the South or the West had a significantly lower probability of using specialty mental health services than non-Latino whites. Sturm, Ringer and Andreyeva (13) also observed geographic differences, specifically state differences in children's use of mental health related services. In a secondary analysis of the 1997 and 1999 waves of the National Survey of America's Families ($N = 45,247$ children aged 6 to 17) based primarily on 13 states, they found that differences in service use between states was greater than differences in service use because of race/ethnicity and other sociodemographic variables. They argued that disparities across states are more likely to be a consequence of state policies and healthcare market characteristics than the sociodemographic makeup of the states.

Aguilera and Lopez (14) also examined the use of services by geographic region, but in a local area, specifically two service or catchment areas within one county—Los Angeles County. They identified one service area that has had a longstanding presence of Latinos whereas the other was largely an African American community until a large influx of Latino immigrants recently moved in. As expected, Aguilera and Lopez found that Latinos' use of services was greater in the established immigrant community than in the recent immigrant community. In addition, they found that characteristics of the communities were differentially associated with service use. For example, for the recent immigrant community, Latinos' mental health service use was consistently low regardless of the density of foreign-born immigrants within that community's census tracts. In contrast, for the established immigrant community, service use and density of foreign immigrants in census tracts were related. With increasing density of foreign immigrants there was a corresponding decrease in Latinos' use of services. These findings indicate that public mental health services in both service areas do a poor job of reaching Latinos living in high-density immigrant neighborhoods, but that in the established immigrant community public mental health services do a better job in reaching Latinos from the lower density neighborhoods than do services in the recent immigrant community.

The important point of the findings regarding context is that race and ethnicity are limited predictors in advancing our understanding of service use. As we examine mental health service use by minority adults and children, it is important to consider the social and community context of the services and of the residents. Even within the same system of care, Latinos, for example, can differentially use mental health services. The observed contextual differences in service use likely represent variability in the available resources within given communities, states or regions, as well as the likely variability in the services' responsiveness across those contexts. The important point is that minority youth and adults are not monolithic groups that underutilize services regardless of the context. Community factors are important to consider as well as individual and service factors.

INTEGRATING CULTURAL CONSIDERATIONS WITH TREATMENT OF FAMILIES

The previous discussion of the barriers to mental healthcare points out the need for special initiatives to improve the treatment and rehabilitation of ethnic minorities. One approach, supported by both the *President's New Freedom Report on Mental Health* and the *Surgeon General's Report on Mental Health: Culture, Race, and Ethnicity*, is to provide culturally competent care. Such care requires culturally-informed communication between patient and clinician, including recognizing patients' expectations about treatment and resolving cultural-linguistic disconnects, developing treatment plans that are culturally appropriate, engaging families or social networks in support of treatment and successful patient management and relapse prevention, and developing culturally tailored models for psychiatric rehabilitation. Effective psychiatric rehabilitation of mental disabilities involves the implantation of cultural competence within phase-linked, consumer-oriented, and evidence-based practices. We now consider the methods used to ensure that cultural considerations are integrated into psychiatric rehabilitation techniques. Family psychoeducation will be used as an exemplar.

One strategy for ensuring that family psychoeducation is culturally congruent is by building on basic research of family processes and serious mental illness. Although the adaptive function of family life may be considered universal, family structure and organization vary across different societies and are subject to intracultural patterning. For instance, within Anglo-Saxon culture, it is assumed often that affective over-involvement and dependency among family members is dysfunctional. This contrasts with clinical observations of several minority ethnic groups that consider family cohesion, interdependence and a family-centered lifestyle healthy and normal. Examples abound of minority ethnic groups that value family closeness more than autonomy: Hispanic groups of Mexican Americans, Puerto Ricans, and Cuban Americans as well as Asian groups represented by Koreans and Chinese. One Puerto Rican mother of a patient with schizophrenia expressed the sentiment this way, "I don't want my son to be independent. To be a family, we need to be interdependent." A Korean father put it this way, "In my country, only homeless people are independent."

Current family interventions have been significantly influenced by basic family research. One line of research is the examination of families' expressed emotion and its relation to the course of schizophrenia. This work, carried out in predominantly Anglo-Saxon cultural groups, has found that posthospitalization patients returning to households marked by high criticism, hostility or emotional overinvolvement are more likely to relapse than those patients who return to households found to be low in these characteristics (15). Consequently, clinical investigators developed family interventions focused largely on reducing family conflict and tension through communication training, problem solving strategies and psychoeducation. Unfortunately, it is easily forgotten that teaching communication and problem solving skills must be orchestrated according to the specific values, expectancies and norms of the family's culture. When the goals of treatment are congruent with the family's cultural expectations, these evidence-based techniques of family psychoeducation can be directed in effective ways.

Investigators have identified ethnic differences in the relationship between family characteristics and course of schizophrenia. While in Euro-American families, criticism and emotional overprotectiveness proved to be key predictors of relapse, for Mexican Americans a lack of family warmth was the significant predictor of relapse (16). The fact that family warmth matters most for Mexican Americans suggests that family interventions targeted at reducing what might appear to be excessive face-to-face contact and compliance with family obligations, may not be appropriate for many Latino families harboring a severely mentally ill relative. For example, the first author of this chapter is conducting a research project that is studying culturally determined interventions for rehabilitation of Latinos with schizophrenia. Multifamily therapy groups, in which the focus is on the enhancement of family affective ties, are hypothesized to be more effective for Mexican Americans with schizophrenia than the standard family therapy approach with its emphasis on building communication and problem solving skills that promote individual expressiveness, assertiveness and autonomy.

Another approach used to incorporate culture into the family intervention enterprise examines a given family intervention from the perspective of what is culturally competent, and then assesses the potential fit of the intervention's domains for the group under study. Cultural competence is conceptualized as the congruence between the cultural perspectives of the clinician and the family (17). As such, cultural competence reflects an openness on the part of the clinician to adapt his or her intervention methods to the patient's or family's expectations. For example, the clinician can incorporate the family's folk conception of illness into the treatment process as in the following example.

Maria and Jorge Garcia moved from Zacatecas to Los Angeles in 1982, when their three children were less than 5 years old. Over the years, they adapted well to life in America, but Juan, the oldest child, developed schizophrenia at age 19. His siblings, Carmen and Jose, generally were very supportive and understanding of Juan's problems. However, they were very concerned about Juan's smoking in his room at night, fearing that he might fall asleep smoking in bed and start a fire. Their parents decided to raise the issue at the next multifamily group session.

The multifamily group therapist elicited each family member's point-of-view about the problem. Juan saw the problem as his siblings' nagging him about his smoking habits. Carmen and Jose expressed the belief that their parents coddled Juan when he acted loco (crazy) and felt that he needed limits on his behaviors. Maria and Jorge, however, felt that Juan suffered from nervios, an idiom of distress that emphasizes both the somatic and mental aspects of schizophrenia and tends to reduce blame directed at the ill relative. In fact, Maria and Jorge believed that Juan benefited from smoking cigarettes by decreasing the stress associated with his nervios.

Rather than dismiss the parents' folk concept of mental illness, the multifamily group therapist chose to incorporate their ideas by reframing the act of cigarette smoking as leading to the worsening of Juan's nervios. The therapist explained that smoking cigarettes increases the chemicals in the brain responsible for causing nervios. Consequently, not discouraging Juan from smoking was making his nervios worse. Buoyed with this new information, Maria and Jorge agreed to engage in problem-solving with the goal of putting reasonable conditions on Juan's smoking behavior. ■

This clinical example highlights another culturally relevant dimension; namely, in Latino and Asian cultures, the role of the therapist or psychiatrist is expected to be authoritative, albeit not authoritarian. The problem-solving that led to a satisfactory resolution of the intrafamily conflict was engineered by the therapist, rather than thrown open to the various family members to debate and try to reach some sort of compromise.

There is some evidence to suggest that by incorporating culture into psychiatric rehabilitation approaches, utilization of such services can be increased and better outcomes can be achieved. As an example of the former, Gilmer and colleagues probed the use of San Diego County Adult and Older Adult Mental Health Services between 2000 and 2005 by people with severe mental illness (18). The subjects were non-Latino whites, and Latinos and Asians with and without English proficiency. The investigators found that Hispanics and Asians with limited English proficiency were significantly less likely than those with English proficiency to use emergency services and more likely to use outpatient mental health services. Even more telling, the investigators found that Hispanics and Asians with limited English proficiency were much more likely to visit clinics with a primary focus on cultural competence, including bilingual staff. The findings suggest that ethnically focused programs may be an effective approach to engaging populations that are underrepresented in the mental health system.

In terms of outcomes, a study that investigated cross-ethnic variations in prospective treatment outcomes over a period of 12 months from community-based, psychosocial rehabilitation interventions for people with schizophrenia found that Euro-American, Hispanic and African-American patients each demonstrated statistically significant rehabilitative improvement with no ethnic-related differences in outcome. These findings suggest that community-based psychosocial rehabilitation interventions result in similar benefits across ethnic groups provided that cultural considerations are taking into account (19).

A specific example of how culture can be incorporated into the rehabilitation enterprise comes from a study of social skills training conducted by Kopelowicz and colleagues (20) in which 92 Latino outpatients with schizophrenia and their designated relatives were randomly assigned to three months of illness management skills training versus customary outpatient care in a typical community mental health center.

The skills training approach was culturally adapted in several ways. First, the participation of key relatives was encouraged to facilitate acquisition and generalization of disease management skills into the patients' natural environment. The importance of involving family members is highlighted by a recent study demonstrating that Latino patients with severe mental illness are considerably more likely than Euro-American patients to live with their family members and to receive active family support (21).

Family members of patients were included in weekly "generalization sessions" aimed at utilizing relatives as generalization agents. These group sessions used skills training "modules" from the UCLA Social and Independent Living Series (22) as focal points for educating relatives as coaches for their ill family member. The modules include a Training Manual that provides a step by step guide to teach the relevant skills; a Patient Workbook, which allows participants to take notes, review what they learned and practice the learned skills at home; and a Videotape that includes demonstrations of the skills to provide modeling of the relevant behaviors.

Relatives were thoroughly informed about the skills the subject had been taught in each module as well as the problem solving skills and homework exercises that were provided. The relative was then assisted in mapping these skills to the patient's environment by examining how the home environment could provide opportunities for skill use. For example, a place, such as a bulletin board or the refrigerator, was identified where a copy of the Side Effects Checklist could be displayed for convenient completion by the patient on a daily schedule as prescribed in the Medication Management Module. The prescribed steps to be followed by the relative on how to coach the patient in the use of the Checklist were also covered. In essence, relatives were trained to offer opportunities, encouragement and reinforcement to their mentally ill relatives for applying the skills in everyday life. Equally essential to this training was that relatives would never take over the patients' responsibilities; for instance, they were instructed to not complete the Side Effect Checklist for the patient.

Another important method for relatives' amplifying generalization, namely monitoring and reinforcing the use of the skills by the patient, was instituted. The relatives were instructed to set aside time each week to discuss adherence to the module's skills and learning activities with the patient and resolve obstacles that impeded performance. Most importantly, the relative was asked, for instance, to use a checklist to verbally reinforce the patient for successful performance. Pictorial representations were used with illiterate relatives. The use of praise was thoroughly explained, modeled, and practiced using role plays. In addition, two home visits were conducted during the follow-up period; the first one about 1 month after the skills training and the second four months later. The purpose of these visits was to review progress and help solve problems identified by the therapist, the family or the patient in the process of transferring the skills to the home environment. Specific problem-solving exercises were conducted to address the identified difficulties. The therapist offered support and encouragement for continued use of the skills.

The wording of items on the training materials, checklists and monitoring sheets and the training procedures were culturally adapted for use with the study population. To create a culturally relevant translation, a work group of six bilingual mental health professionals met weekly, with each member assigned a section of the English-language version of the module to translate. The Spanish-language version was reviewed and modifications were made. Adaptations that were made in translating the modules for the study population included using Spanish vocabulary at the elementary school level, careful consideration of he wide range of dialects and colloquialisms used by the variety of Latino subgroups, and the attempt to forge a "universal

Spanish" that would be comprehensible to all. A bilingual, bicultural psychologist who worked at the mental health center conducted a back-translation for the Spanish-language version to ensure the accuracy of translation for the study population. Finally, four Mexican American actors dubbed the translated video scripts over the audio portion of the videotapes.

Additional cultural adaptations included the use of indigenous, bilingual and bicultural staff of the community mental health center as skills trainers, the participation of family members (rather than clinicians) as "generalization aides" and the modification of the trainer's activities during the sessions. As an example of the latter, skills trainers used an informal personal style with patients and relatives that included the sharing of food and encouragement of "small talk" before and after training sessions. These adaptations were made to encourage warm interactions among skills trainers, patients and relatives, thereby increasing retention in the study as well as enhancing the overall effectiveness of the intervention (23).

After the 3-month intervention, there was a significant advantage for the skills training group over the treatment as usual group on medication adherence, several symptom measures, skill acquisition and generalization, level of functioning, and rates of rehospitalization. These results persisted 9 months after the intervention had concluded. Most relevant for the present discussion, the results of a path analysis demonstrated that the skills training had a direct effect on skill acquisition and generalization, but that the utilization of illness management skills was a direct result of the involvement of family members in the skills training enterprise. Thus, family members were critical to the clients applying their newly learned skills.

CASE MANAGEMENT AND ACCESS TO CARE

Along with its focus on cultural competence, the report of the President's New Freedom Commission on Mental Health also called for a well-coordinated system of care that integrates treatment across relevant domains (primary care and specialty mental healthcare) and brings together multiple resources to reduce disability and improve functioning. Of course, such a system of care benefits all patients who require mental health services, but the need is especially great for ethnic and racial minority groups given their high reliance on primary care providers. Supporting this view, recent research from the Commonwealth Fund 2006 Health Care Survey demonstrated that affording a few core service elements in primary care has a major impact on reducing disparities in healthcare for U.S. ethnic groups, with about 75% of all groups receiving the care they needed (24). These service elements included patient access to a regular source of care, reducing or eliminating difficulties in contacting providers by telephone, availability of care and medical advice after hours, and provision of well-organized and on-time office visits. The impact of these elements in behavioral healthcare for Latino and other ethnic group patients has not been evaluated but they could be important factors in effective long-term care for reducing family burden and improving access to psychiatric rehabilitation services for ethnic minority patients with severe and chronic psychiatric disorders. Most importantly, the mechanism for providing this continuity of care is well established in mental health organizations in the form of the clinical case manager.

The clinicians who provide or broker a wide array of mental health and psychiatric rehabilitation services are the key to the delivery of continuous, comprehensive and coordinated care. Case managers are the final common pathway for the seriously mentally ill whose manifold needs—from medication and psychosocial treatments to social and human services—depend on the cadre of local case managers for responsiveness, timeliness, access and accountability. At its best, a case manager is often a masters level social worker, psychologist or nurse who delivers direct treatment services as well as soliciting, obtaining, monitoring and coordinating other services and resources that are provided by a large assortment of geographically dispersed, community agencies. These disparate services include psychiatric rehabilitation modalities, housing, financial entitlements, family support and, when needed, inpatient care. The direct treatment service that the clinical case manager provides depends on his/her caseload, duties and discretionary time. With a caseload of one case manager to 10 to 15 clients, it is feasible for the clinical case manager to offer supportive therapy, crisis intervention and access to human service agencies.

Those service delivery models with an intensive case management framework are often able to reduce hospitalization, increase the utilization of relevant services and lengthen the community tenure of patients with serious mental illness. The effectiveness of intensive case management has been empirically validated and adapted or "reinvented" according to the resources and constraints for a variety of settings.

Effective case management can be the mechanism for integrating psychiatric treatment and rehabilitation by overcoming the manifold obstacles to connecting their clients with the appropriate services. A case manager in a psychiatric rehabilitation setting has multiple specific tasks and responsibilities. These include:

- assisting patients in building natural social networks
- facilitating the acquisition of housing and employment
- helping patients interact with the various social and human service agencies for financial support, Medicaid, or Medicare insurance and home care
- teaching patients the skills they require for illness self-management
- monitoring the clinical progress of the patients and, when necessary, undertaking timely clinical interventions

Ultimately, the success of any case management approach depends on whether or not patients receive the appropriate services to meet their needs. The problems encountered when attempting to draw conclusions from the current generation of case management studies include: a failure to assess the needs of the individuals receiving the services; inadequate definition of the activities that comprise a given model of case management; and, little consideration given to the relationship between process and outcome measures (i.e., how a particular type of case management leads to salutary results). Improvements in the yield from empirical evaluations of case management require better specification of case management methods and objectives, characterization of the symptomatic impairments, medication status and psychosocial deficits of the study population, use of multiple outcome measures, and studies of longer duration that follow the trajectory of clients over 3- and 5-year periods.

To date, the majority of studies of case management have been concerned with the comparison of intensive case management or one variant, Assertive Community Treatment (26), with more traditional models of service delivery. While helpful, this type of research generates unwieldy comparisons of different models of clinical case management in markedly different care systems, with poorly defined or heterogeneous patient populations. The next generation of case management research will seek to compare different models of case management or specific interventions within case management services to tease out which service elements are responsible for the various outcome domains including the increase in access to psychiatric rehabilitation services for ethnic minority patients.

CONCLUSION

Psychiatric rehabilitation contributes principles and practices that are relevant to a wide array of patient populations that are characterized by physical and behavioral disabilities. As interest rises in medicine and psychiatry for promoting wellness and recovery from disability, we can expect to see further expansion of rehabilitation in future years with an increased knowledge base of what works to improve long term outcome for persistent and disabling biobehavioral disorders. In the short term, increasing the utilization of psychiatric rehabilitation interventions by ethnic minority patients can be accomplished by making the treatments sensitive to cultural considerations and accessible through the auspices of well-informed clinical case managers. Ultimately, making health insurance widely available, combined with offering equitable mental health benefits, is the foundation for supporting the changes in the delivery system to assure improved patient management and treatment outcomes for ethnic minority populations in the United States.

References

1. Young AS, Sullivan G, Burnam MA, et al. Measuring the quality of outpatient treatment for schizophrenia. *Arch Gen Psychiatry* 1998;55:611–617.
2. Lehman AF, Steinwachs DM. Patterns of usual care for schizophrenia: Initial results from the Schizophrenia Patient Outcomes Research Team (PORT) client survey. *Schizophrenia Bull* 1998;24:11–20.
3. West JC, Wilk JE, Olfsom M. Patterns and quality of treatment for patients with schizophrenia in routine psychiatric practice. *Psychiatr Serv* 2005;56:283–291.
4. Barrio C, Yamada AM, Hough RL. Ethnic disparities in use of public mental health case management services among patients with schizophrenia. *Psychiatr Serv* 2003;54:1264–1270.
5. Cook BL, McGuire T, Miranda J. Measuring trends in mental health care disparities, 2000–2004. *Psychiatr Serv* 2007;58:1533–1540.
6. Institute of Medicine. *Health Literacy: A Prescription to End Confusion.* Washington, DC: National Academies Press, 2004.
7. Lopez SR, Lara MC, Kopelowicz A, et al. *La CLAve* to increase psychosis literacy of Spanish-speaking community residents and family caregivers. Manuscript submitted for publication.
8. Quinn K. *Working Without Benefits: The Health Insurance Crisis Confronting Hispanic Americans. The Commonwealth Fund Task Force on the Future of Health Insurance for Working Americans.* New York: Commonwealth Fund, 2000.
9. Brown ER, Lavarreda SA, Ponce N, et al. *The State of Health Insurance in California: Findings from the 2005 California Health Interview Survey.* Los Angeles, CA: UCLA Center for Health Policy Research, 2007.
10. Derose KP, Escarce JJ, Lurie N. Immigrants and health care: Sources of vulnerability. *Health Affairs* 2007;26:1258–1268.
11. Snowden LR, Cuellar AE, Libby AM. Minority youth in foster care: Managed care and access to mental health treatment. *Med Care* 2003;41:264–274.
12. Alegría M, Canino G, Rios R, et al. Inequalities in use of specialty mental health services among Latinos, African Americans, and non-Latino whites. *Psychiatr Serv* 2002;53:1547–1555.
13. Sturm R, Ringel JS, Andreyeva T. Geographic disparities in children's mental health care. *Pediatrics* 2003;112:308–315.
14. Aguilera A, Lopez SR. Community determinants of Latinos' use of mental health services. *Psychiatr Serv* 2008;59:408–413.

15. Butzlaff R, Hooley J. Expressed emotion and psychiatric relapse. *Arch Gen Psychiatry* 1998;55:547–552.
16. Lopez SR, Nelson KH, Polo AJ, et al. Ethnicity, expressed emotion attributions and course of schizophrenia: Family warmth matters. *J Nervous Ment Dis* 2004;113:428–439.
17. Lopez SR. Cultural competence in psychotherapy: A guide for clinicians and their supervisors. In: Watkins CE, ed. *Handbook of Psychotherapy Supervision*. New York: Wiley, 1997.
18. Gilmer TP, Ojeda VD, Folsom DP, et al. Initiation and use of public mental health services by persons with severe mental illness and limited English proficiency. *Psychiatr Serv* 2007;58:1555–1562.
19. Bae SW, Brekke JS, Bola JR. Ethnicity and treatment outcome variation in schizophrenia: A longitudinal study of community-based psychosocial rehabilitation interventions. *J Nerv Ment Dis* 2004;192:623–628.
20. Kopelowicz A, Zarate R, Gonzalez Smith V. Disease management in Latinos with schizophrenia: A family-assisted, skills training approach. *Schizophrenia Bull* 2003;29:211–228.
21. Snowden LR. Explaining mental health treatment disparities: Ethnic and cultural differences in family involvement. *Culture Med Psychiatry* 2007;31:389–402.
22. Liberman R, Wallace C, Blackwell G, et al. Innovations in skills training for the seriously mentally ill: the UCLA Social and Independent Living Skills Modules. Innovations and Research 1993;2:43–60.
23. Lopez SR, Kopelowicz A, Canive J. Strategies in developing culturally congruent family interventions for schizophrenia: The case for Hispanics. In: Lefley HP, Johnson DL, eds. *Family Interventions in Mental Illness: International Perspectives*. Westport, CT: Praeger, 2002:61–92.
24. Beal AC, Doty MM, Hernandez SE, et al. *Closing the Divide: How Medical Homes Promote Equity in Health Care*. New York: The Commonwealth Fund, 2007.
25. Miranda J, Schoenbaum M, Sherbourne C, et al. Effects of primary care depression treatment on minority patients' clinical status and employment. *Arch Gen Psychiatry* 2004;61:827–834.
26. Stein LI, Santos AB. *Assertive Community Treatment of Persons with Severe Mental Illness*. New York: W. W. Norton & Co., 1998.

21 Mentally Ill Populations

Suzanne Vogel-Scibilia

> *"May you live in interesting times. . ."—Unattributed, ancient Chinese curse*

Persons living with mental illness weather a "perfect storm" of adverse living conditions that create a pervasive range of disparities. It is common to experience a lack of access to both psychiatric and medical healthcare, a lack of a safe haven for recovery from serious relapses, increased fragmentation of both medical and psychiatric healthcare, limitations in the nature and scope of care by for-profit managed care entities, criminalization caused by psychiatric symptoms, lack of timely access when disabled to income and health insurance, cutbacks in the funding for affordable housing, and entitlement cutbacks that jeopardize even a marginal standard of living. Additionally there is no accountability from a single government agency to resolve problems with care for persons with serious and persistent mental illness (SPMI). Some duties fall to the states and others to the federal government. Even within the state and federal governments, multiple agencies also share portions of the responsibility. This diffusion of responsibility with no one agency or individual accountable for these systemic disparities impairs living well with mental illness. Each individual or agency will maintain that they have done all they can do or suggest that the most pressing problems are too complex for them to change or lie within another agency. Let us highlight this "perfect storm" of disparities by following a hypothetical consumer named Theo:

Hypothetical Case Vignette

Theo is a 29-year-old night custodian who worked for many years with low-level psychotic symptoms that he did not feel needed treatment. He has a 30-year mortgage on a one-bedroom bungalow in a rural area outside of town and has never had as much as a parking ticket. He develops pneumonia one winter and then experiences increased psychotic symptoms over a 3-month period.

Disability determinations are made either by for-profit companies or overburdened government agencies. This system presents a huge hurdle for clients with brain disorders to navigate.

When Theo begins baptizing coworkers with water, he is placed on medical leave. After more than 2 months with no income, Theo has exhausted his savings and finds out that the disability company has rejected his short-term disability claim because he has not adequately answered the disability company's phone calls. His meager savings make him ineligible for welfare, so Theo tries to pinch pennies anywhere he can. The lack of viable income for Theo becomes a nightmare. He falls behind on his mortgage; his utilities are turned off. He tries to go to the social security office to fill out a long-term disability application, but the crowds are overwhelming. The worker talks too rapidly to him while emphasizing that he needs to fill out a thick wad of complex forms by himself. Theo gives up. Even if he had filed out the application, many people like Theo who have no concrete, disabling medical illness and a past history of gainful employment are denied through two rounds of paper appeals and have to go to a hearing with a judge. The court docket is currently backed up over 14 months. If Theo had eventually received social security insurance payments, he still would have had to endure a 24-month waiting period to receive Medicare coverage. Because he also inherited a run-down, abandoned house across the street from the bungalow, he is not eligible for Medicaid. ▪

The lack of dependable income for persons with psychiatric illness is a major barrier against recovery. Many advocates describe adverse outcomes in individuals during the 24-month wait after disability determination before Medicare coverage is granted. Additionally, private disability company procedures are often not accommodating of clients with brain disorders. If they are perceived as not cooperating with the company and have no persons to advocate for them, their claims may be denied. This not only presents a tremendous financial hardship and hinders recovery but often pushes an individual into a cascade of further problems.

Managed care plans often control costs with short-sighted measures such as plan-specific restrictive drug formularies that present hurdles for both providers and consumers. This impairs clients from staying on a regimen that works. Intermittently, prescriptions will be denied because of technical difficulties in authorization or limits on approved dosages or pill counts. This is a huge obstruction to stable adherence with prescribed medication regimens in clients who have trouble problem-solving and may be only marginally motivated to stay on medication that gives side effects without immediate perceived benefits.

When Theo goes to the drugstore to fill the prescription, the pharmacist tells him the medication is not covered and it will cost him $329.47. Theo cannot afford that, but he is afraid to tell his doctor. He buys over-the-counter medicine that is supposed to help his memory and leaves the pharmacy. The clinic nurse calls 3 days later to see how Theo is doing after he misses an appointment and finds out from Theo that the prescription was denied. She instructs Theo to come to the clinic for free samples. Because samples are only dispensed in limited quantities from the pharmaceutical representatives, Theo has to come every week to pick them up. Sometimes he forgets or arrives too late. He often goes without medication for several days. The clinic obtains authorization about 3 weeks later for the medicine but that only lasts 8 months before Theo's managed care vendor changes. Despite Theo's good success on the "nonpreferred" medicine, his policy states that clients cannot be grandfathered in on another plan's authorization. The plan requires him to have failed two other similar medications first. Theo starts on one of the "preferred" managed care medications. Within a week, the voices of God increase. ▪

One of managed care's cost containment strategies is to disincentivize doctors from prescribing costly medication instead of less costly generics. This is accomplished using preauthorizations, time-consuming documentation, and complex, automated restrictions on which medications can be filled at the pharmacy without prior approval that produce constant office calls or require physician intervention to secure the "nonpreferred," more costly medication. Medicare Part D management has been found to increase the administrative work for psychiatrists by 45 minutes of paperwork time for every hour spent seeing clients (1). This affects clients' access to long-term medication regimens and timely treatment changes while impairing the quality of care. Many states have adopted these formulary strategies for Medicaid consumers including preferred drug lists, fail-first protocols, cumbersome prior approval procedures, and substantial copays for psychotropics, which are not interchangeable with preferred drugs within the same class. Clients who by definition have a brain disorder find the system frustrating and confusing. If the client lacks insight into the importance of care, these experiences may be used as a reason to discontinue treatment.

Clients with symptoms that impair their ability to adhere to treatment are likely to experience difficulty accessing services when they are in crisis or need medication changes because of the overloaded and understaffed outpatient care system.

> *Theo feels more "psychic interference" from the outside so he isolates more in the bungalow. He begins loosing track of time and forgetting his outpatient appointments. The clinic discharges him from care after three missed appointments. Months later, he presents to the emergency room with several infected lacerations on his back. When the nurse attempts to clean his wounds, he begins loudly proclaiming the coming of Jesus Christ. This convinces the crisis social worker to urge the clinic to take Theo back.*

In 1963, John F. Kennedy's administration envisioned a network of community mental health clinics, called CMHCs, to be created utilizing federal funds. Following a series of legislative, political, and financial decisions, only a proportion of these public mental health clinics were established. This lack of crucial psychiatric outpatient capacity has never been rectified. The parallel lack of psychiatric providers especially psychiatrists, both adult and pediatric, have become another hurdle to ramping up outpatient services.

Another pressing issue is financial. Over the years, declining reimbursement for outpatient services has caused community psychiatry programs to be unfunded. One research group found both private managed plans and Medicaid had serious access problems for psychiatric care (2). This jeopardizes the viability of the service delivery system and forces providers to focus on services that are more profitable. Programs that provide crisis services or intensive community care are money-makers that balance the deficit from traditional outpatient services. This shift of staff resources and priorities often produces fragility in the system as traditional public outpatient services contract.

Clients in need of increased care often are unable to receive more frequent traditional services but instead are routed to partial programs or crisis services that are more costly and therefore tightly managed. More intensive services have less capacity so a smaller number of consumers benefit. For-profit managed care companies then place limitations on access to these intensive, pricey services while simultaneously ratcheting down the reimbursement for traditional outpatient care appointments to the minimum the market will allow. Clinics may only maintain fiscal solvency by seeing patients for medication monitoring in high volume utilizing brief contacts. This structure does not lend itself to solving complex social or service access problems. Teaching long-term recovery strategies becomes impossible.

The current focus on fee for service reimbursement that has declining rates instead of fixed grants that support deficit-laden services causes missed appointments to be unreimbursed. Therefore, many clinics discharge clients who miss appointments. The financial impact of missed appointments is minimized by utilizing queuing strategies that are feasible with briefer medication monitoring appointments. One may schedule four clients to an hour and expect three to show up.

Outpatient psychotherapy sessions, because of their longer time length, are unable to be queued. Missed psychotherapy appointments are more likely to produce a monetary loss. Because therapy is often a money loser based on managed care reimbursement rules, mental health systems do not focus on providing therapy for all clients despite evidence that shows its benefits. Many managed care systems carve out behavioral health services to a financially at-risk administrative entity. One study in persons with schizophrenia showed that when these organizations were at-risk financially for individual therapy, group therapy and psychosocial rehabilitation, these services were sharply decreased by the providers based on the managed care's involvement (3). Interestingly, in this same study, costly newer generation antipsychotic medication were not limited by the presence of the carve-out entity. This incongruous finding is noteworthy because the entity was not at-risk for costs of medication!

Adverse financial conditions designed by for-profit care management not only affects consumer's care directly—fiscal underfunding also discourages practitioners from entering public psychiatry positions and causes clinician turnover to be high. Workforce shortages increase as new providers are discouraged from entering the outpatient system, while some remaining providers opt out of Medicaid or managed plans. The result is a further restriction of access to outpatient services.

Many costly, intensive services are in short supply and may not even be available to clients with private insurance. Often the "squeaky wheel" is the one that gets the intensive services but the necessary "squeaking" often occurs when consumers experience adverse outcomes such as costly inpatient admissions, criminalization, or decompensation that leads to dangerous behavior.

> *A clinician can see Theo no more frequently than every 2 months because of staffing shortages. A crisis worker informs Theo that there are no case managers available because state hospital dischargees use all the available openings. He joins a waiting list for a case manager, but Theo hears other community clients at the local drop-in center report that they were on the list after him and were recently assigned a case manager. They mentioned that the case managers always ask for their clients' welfare cards because they can bill welfare but not private insurance for intensive services. Theo confronts the program manager about his lack of progress on the waiting list and wonders whether or not his private health insurance is the reason he is not receiving more comprehensive services like a continuous treatment team or a case manager. The program manager states that welfare coverage is only one factor in who gets any intensive services but the big problem is their short supply. He urges Theo to be patient.* ■

When a service system is unable to appropriately see the large number of clients that require care, various strategies occur to care for the clients as best able. There is not much tolerance for late arrival appointments or transportation problems. Clients even in crisis may be told to wait for the next available appointment, possibly weeks away. Stating that one cannot wait or is in crisis may allow a referral to a "safety net" service.

Programs often develop a reliance on "safety net" services such as crisis teams, emergency rooms, partial hospital programs and assertive community treatment teams to manage clients with acute symptoms who need more care than the standard medication monitoring. Higher intensity support services such as case managers, rehabilitation day programs or supported housing is often limited in capacity and costly to finance. These slots are reserved from individuals who utilize costly services or who exhibit repetitive dangerous or decompensated symptomatology.

Physician extenders often care for a proportion of routine appointments previously handled by psychiatrists while time-consuming and underfunded outpatient care such as psychotherapy or partial hospital services are scaled back and develop limited access. Often there is only one public mental health clinic in an area with many potential customers and no competition. The motivation to change practice to solve problems, become more recovery oriented or empower consumers and families may be absent. These changes may be frightening because clinicians do not want to change prior clinical norms, fear litigation or feel threatened by the necessary surrender of some control or power. Public clinics that are being urged to change or are in financial crisis can threaten to close or limit practice in some way since they have a monopoly in many rural or underserved areas. These announcements cause much fear and turmoil among consumers who are engaged in care and cause many to be anxious or overwhelmed.

The lack of an easily accessed, universal healthcare payment plan for all persons in our society is a huge barrier for care with persons with SPMI.

> *Theo runs out of money to pay for his health insurance through Cobra and loses his prescription benefits. He is not able to afford his medication and the clinic is now sending Theo bills for his mental health appointments. They assist him in filling out his welfare application but case workers are scarce. No one goes down with him to the agency. Remembering his last experience at the welfare office, Theo takes the application and throws it away. He convinces himself that he is just fine on his own and stops his medication. One month later he drops out of care.*

While most modern societies provide universal access to healthcare, the United States lags behind its more progressive neighbors. As with many chronic diseases, mental healthcare suffers when the individual has no means of paying for preventive, acute and maintenance care. Uninsured consumers are not the only casualties. Reduced access to medication and treatment from cost containment by for-profit managed care providers while decreasing costs in one area may increase costs in another. These transferred costs offset any short-term savings while reeking increased pain and suffering. In one New Hampshire study of the effect of a three-prescription limit on psychotropic drugs for Medicaid clients, these limits produced increases in acute outpatient visits, emergency services and partial hospitalization which increased the average cost per person by $1530 (4). After the cap was discontinued, the use of medication and services returned to previous baseline levels. Grappling with ongoing frustrations, many consumers like Theo simply give up and try to manage their illness on their own.

Consumers who are savvy to the system will figure out how to get what they need and that often is by utilizing costly services such as emergency rooms and inpatient beds when less costly, but not readily accessible services would suffice. This drives up system-wide costs.

> *Theo talks to one of the long-time consumers at the drop-in center. This gentleman advises Theo to present repeatedly at the emergency room and threaten suicide. He should plan to have at least four short admissions over the next few months. The long-time consumer told Theo that the social worker at the hospital obtained Medicaid coverage, a*

case manager, and a bed in supported housing for him when he used this strategy. He warned Theo that it may take several admissions close together before people try to squeeze him into already overloaded, but more intensive benefits. Theo rejects this idea because he fears they will lock him up and send him to a state hospital. Little does he know that entry to state hospital beds is no longer readily available. ■

Inpatient psychiatric care is another vital "safety net." Cost control by managed care often restricts admission to individuals exhibiting acute dangerousness or marked inability to care for self. General hospital psychiatric units shoulder the revolving door of clients who are admitted over and over again because readily accessible long-term state-sponsored institutional care is no longer available. These clients are individuals who are not able to achieve long term stabilization in the community or need more help than is available from outpatient services. Before the whittling down of managed care reimbursement for inpatient care, hospitals had money to absorb occasional uncovered hospital stays, fund a more intensive rehabilitative group program, and invest in higher staff to patient ratios. Inpatient stays were longer and gave clients a greater chance to stabilize before return to the community.

Inpatient physicians were paid fee-for-service that increased in amount because of the length and complexity of the care contact. Managed care strategies included bundling the physician charge into a fixed amount per day paid to the hospital for all psychiatric and medical care. Now physicians receive a fixed amount for all care to the client so longer sessions and routine contacts or meetings with family by the psychiatrist decreased as hospitals increased volume to control costs.

Since medical care was also bundled into a per diem inpatient charge that managed care slowly ratcheted down to a bare minimum, clients who needed necessary but not emergent medical care were told to follow up after discharge when the cost would not be assumed by the hospital. Clients once released were often nonadherent with important, often life-saving tests or treatment at the cost of their physical health. These changes over the last 30 years have diminished inpatient acute care's therapeutic environment as well as some of its protective effect toward consumers.

Repeated inpatient treatment was once a common criterion for state hospital care. These state hospitals, another crucial "safety net," allowed longer term care that was vital to the recovery of many severely ill consumers and was completely financed by the individual states. These high costs have motivated many states to close state hospital beds further destabilizing community based services.

Because of these infrastructure deficits and service access issues, vital "safety net" services are becoming increasing overwhelmed. The result is inadequate emergency room crisis treatment and overcrowded inpatient units. The very public death of Esmin Elizabeth Green, unnoticed and unaided in a New York City emergency room during the summer of 2008 after she had waited more than 24 hours for an inpatient psychiatric bed, highlights the struggles that consumers face to get care within a dysfunctional service system (5).

It is no wonder that savvy consumers learn how to game the system to get what they need. Only the complicated nature of psychiatric systems and man's inherent impulse to be honest prevents many from being the squeaky wheel that gets the grease. If everyone did squeak, the system would be overwhelmed.

Clients who are not savvy to the system cannot understand how to get what they need and often fall through the cracks. Others who lack insight reject care and slip away unnoticed. Many need longer term care than the acute inpatient hospital and outpatient

system can provide. These individuals remain symptomatic and are at high risk for criminalization, becoming homeless, or dropping out of care.

> *One day when walking home from the drop-in center, Theo finds his bungalow padlocked by the bank. Now homeless and without treatment for 5 months, he walks to the local pharmacy and takes a bottle of over-the-counter sleeping pills in the parking lot. After the emergency response personnel take him to the hospital, he is admitted to the ICU under an involuntarily commitment based on his combativeness in the emergency room. Theo gets an 8-day inpatient psychiatric stay and a restart of antipsychotic medication. Unfortunately, he will assume a new series of burdens on discharge.*

Excluding people with mental illness in jails or locked facilities, one recent study found a 15% rate of homelessness in people with schizophrenia and bipolar disorder (6). This study highlighted two risk factors—a lack of Medicaid and substance use disorders—that hold promise for targeted corrective strategies. This is crucial given the lower documented rates of homelessness in prior decades. This recent data suggest that current levels of homelessness for persons with mental illness are increasing (7).

Discussion about how to prevent criminalization of consumers focuses on two strategies—expanding community services and increasing "leverage" in the forms of representative payees to manage consumer's finances and outpatient commitments to compel care. Despite these ideas, the lack of a broad continuum of nonforensic psychiatric hospital bed capacity extending from acute through intermediate to long-term treatment are needed for those individuals who do not respond to less restrictive strategies (8).

Homelessness is found to be a significant risk factor for subsequent criminalization. In our country, jails have replaced longer term state-funded mental hospitals as the place for persons with psychiatric symptoms who are disruptive in the community.

> *On his day of discharge from the psychiatric unit, Theo is informed that the police are charging him with fighting them in the pharmacy parking lot and for stealing the pills he used in the overdose. A hospital social worker applies for medical assistance which provides Theo's first steady income source in one year. Theo's case is plea bargained into probation for 3 years but he now has a parole officer who has little patience for Theo or his psychiatric symptoms. He often accuses Theo of "rambling" in their meetings and threatens to reincarcerate him for offenses such as being disorderly in the probation office or missing scheduled check-ins. One day when Theo is getting loud in the waiting area, the officers search him and find a concealed club in his army jacket that he carries "for protection." They charge him with a probation violation, disorderly conduct, terroristic threats, and carrying a concealed weapon. Theo does 3 years in a state prison with the maximum sentence because there are no easy options for his psychiatric care or acceptable housing to allow parole.*

There is an extensive body of evidence that shows clients with mental illness are also more likely to be homeless, unemployed, and incarcerated (9,10). Previously cited outpatient care deficits along with critical shortages of support services and housing create a process whereby deinstitutionalization leads to transinstitutionalization.

Transinstitutionalization is the process whereby clients with mental health needs are placed in one institution such as acute care hospitals and jails instead of another restrictive facility such as psychiatric state hospital beds. Fred Markowitz's (11) research shows eloquently that as one decreases state hospital beds in an area, an increasing number of people develop homelessness leading to arrest and incarceration. Many government administrators have focused on increasing extended acute care beds in general hospitals to address clients who need longer stays to achieve clinical stabilization, but Markowitz's paper highlights the inadequacy of this plan.

Lack of adherence to psychiatric medication is another significant risk factor for incarceration. One study of inmates in an urban county jail documented that 92% of the inmates with severe mental illness were nonadherent with their psychiatric medication before arrest (12). Because of acute service deficits and a reluctance of community providers of healthcare and housing to accept individuals with a criminal record, obtaining an early discharge from jail is extremely difficult.

Mental health consumers do not receive comprehensive treatment for their mental illnesses in the criminal justice system. The nature of the criminal justice system often leads to persons with mental illness having harsh treatment and an overall worsening of their mental health condition.

> *Since Theo was out of treatment prior to his prison stay, the clinicians in the prison list him as not being on any medication. Theo has minimal understanding about his illness, so he denies all symptoms on questioning. Theo's untreated psychotic symptoms lead to frequent disruptions in the jail and his disciplinary citations garner him long periods in isolation. The adversarial, rigid criminal justice system and the long periods of isolation worsen his illness.*
>
> *At one point when they are transferring him from one cell to another and he is handcuffed, he refuses to let the officer uncuff him. He is TASERed three times while still cuffed before he stops moving around. Eventually the mental health clinician talks to Theo about taking an older antipsychotic medication that is on the prison formulary managed by the for-profit behavior health provider because of its reduced cost. Theo refuses it because of past side effects. The more costly medication that Theo did well on is not offered.* ■

Jail nurses document every time Theo refuses the inexpensive medication they offer. The jail administration sets a greater priority on writing up his behavioral outbursts than on treating the cause of them. Theo remains off medication for the whole 3 years.

There is a much research devoted to the rising number of persons with mental illness in our jails and prisons (12). Many of the problems suffered by consumers of mental health services who become incarcerated stem from the criminal justices system's inherent inability to identify persons in need of mental healthcare as well as barriers to comprehensive and timely care. While experts acknowledge the growing number of persons with mental health issues in jails and prisons, a dangerous triad of outdated policies, limited finances, and a lack of education limit the system's ability to change in response to this reality.

Advocacy organizations such as the National Alliance on Mental Illness routinely document personal accounts of violent often punitive treatment of persons with psychiatric symptoms within U.S. jails and prisons. While most organizations focus on increasing collaboration between criminal justice and mental health providers, improving education of staff within the correction system and focusing on diversion away from incarceration, some organizations are finding that litigation may be the most expedient way to advance these goals.

Mental health consumers who attempt to reenter the community from jails, prisons, or after periods of homelessness face barriers including obtaining housing, seeking employment and re-establishing benefits.

After Theo is discharged from prison, he has no Medicaid coverage, which prevents him from securing an apartment in the community. Since he's been incarcerated and identified as being at-risk for rearrest, he is assigned a case manager who helps him restart his welfare benefits. No one will hire him because of his criminal record, but the lack of any daytime work allows Theo to start back at the outpatient clinic and receive medication again. Unfortunately, he is still denied supported housing. His 22 disciplinary citations for yelling or not following staff directions in prison were a factor in four separate housing agencies in the community rejecting him. Facing homelessness again, he is granted a 30-day respite bed at a personal care home. Theo states he will not stay at a personal care home for the long term because he is the only young person in the house, but in his heart he realizes he has no other options. He joins the old men sitting in rocking chairs on the porch.

The lack of viable housing options that are easily accessed by consumers who need support in the community or have a past history of being unable to maintain housing is as significant a barrier to recovery as a lack of access to psychiatric treatment. Many individuals with severe mental illness at risk for homelessness have comorbid substance abuse issues that further complicate this situation. Novel programs such as Housing First, which provides housing to consumers with substance abuse diagnoses that is not tied to treatment or sobriety, has shown that long-term housing stability and improved outcomes is possible for this population (13). Housing First models are also being implemented in consumers with chronic homelessness without substance use. Not tying housing to treatment, sobriety or nondisruptive behaviors will improve living opportunities for consumers and decrease the coercion that is implicit in the older strategies.

The medical needs of consumers are often not prioritized by mental health clinics. Clients may not be monitored for metabolic complications of their medication or their illnesses.

Theo agrees to stay on at the personal care home and he begins to attend the outpatient clinic regularly and take his prescribed medication. Three years later, he begins feeling thirsty all the time and his house supervisor takes him to the emergency room. They diagnose both elevated blood pressure and early diabetes of unknown duration. The psychiatric clinic has not been monitoring his blood work even though his medication regimen puts him at risk for metabolic complications.

Over the last decade, an increased understanding of the metabolic consequences of mood stabilizers, anticonvulsants, and antipsychotic medication has lead to much discussion but less practical follow-through on both monitoring and interventions for at-risk consumers—especially those with schizophrenia and bipolar disorder (14). The risk of cardiovascular disease can be influenced by physicians (improved healthcare and monitoring), lifestyle improvement (smoking cessation, exercise, dietary changes), and treatment changes (less poly-pharmacy and improved choices of medications with lower metabolic risks). Many providers make excuses about why they cannot assume more responsibility to monitor clients for adverse medical conditions or collaborate more closely with medical providers as other specialists do (15). Often clients have been symptomatic for some time before being referred back to their primary care physician for treatment.

Many medical doctors do not aggressively treat metabolic complications in patients with SPMI assuming they will not adhere with medication, appointments, or lab work.

> *The emergency room refers Theo to his family practice doctor, who tells him that the values are really not that elevated yet. He defers starting any medication and suggests diet and exercise. Despite Theo not improving his risk factors, the doctor waits until Theo's blood sugar and hypertension progress over the next 8 years before starting any medication. Theo continues to gain weight on his current regimen and increases his cigarette smoking to two packs a day. The staff at the personal care home discourage Theo from leaving for very long so he stops his long walks, which were his best form of exercise.* ■

Consumers as a group lack aggressive medical care for their medical conditions and find their psychiatric providers disinclined to practice primary medical prevention or monitor for medical comorbidities (16). Suboptimal medication treatment for consumers has continued despite greater publicity about cardiovascular disease being the leading cause of death in persons with mental illness and diabetes (17).

When problems occur, they are often misidentified. Coordination of care between medical doctor and mental health clinicians is frequently lacking.

> *Nineteen years later after gaining more than 75 pounds, Theo is diagnosed with sleep apnea. The pulmonologist has trouble getting a C-Pap machine authorized because Medicaid is claiming he has another insurance that no one else knows about. When Theo begins having persistent fatigue throughout the day and periods of shortness of breath, his family practice doctor does a cursory evaluation and tells the care home worker to urge the pulmonologist to prioritize getting Theo his C-Pap machine. His psychiatrist prescribes an antidepressant medication for presumed increasing depression. Three days later, Theo is found dead in his bed by his roommate of an apparent heart attack and congestive heart failure. Theo was 51 years old.* ■

Recent research has shown multiple factors that produce less help-seeking and a decreased quality of physical healthcare in persons with mental illnesses (18). Several provider issues are noteworthy including a lack of understanding about the nature of mental illness, poor prognostic beliefs about mental illness and negative views of persons with mental illness. In Theo's case, Thronicroft's (18) "diagnostic overshadowing" or misidentifying physical illness as psychiatric symptoms can impair treatment and be ultimately responsible for a reduced life span.

Public sector consumers with schizophrenia have a life expectancy more than 25 years less than members of the general population (19,20). Causes of the decreased life expectancy may be critical life style issues that are associated with severe mental illness such as obesity, alcohol and illicit substance abuse, accidents or suicide caused by symptoms, cigarette smoking, poor diet, a sedentary life style, as well as metabolic complications of some medications. Currently, the medical profession as a whole is struggling to decide how to better care for the bodies as well as the minds of consumers. As medical and psychiatric providers debate the alternatives of increased collaboration between internists and psychiatrists versus imbedding primary care providers within traditional mental health clinics, years pass and the message about the importance of monitoring and treatment only slowly trickle into the clinical community. The lack of aggressive attention and solution building to such an urgent public health priority validates the belief among some advocates that disparities for consumers even when life threatening fail to illicit the concern and outrage compared with other subgroups of American society.

STIGMA ABOUT MENTAL ILLNESSES

"A society expresses itself positively in the mental illness displayed by its members, whether it places them at the centre of its religious life, as is often the case amongst the primitive peoples, or whether it seeks to expatriate them by situating them outside social life, as does our culture" (21).

Many advocates believe the root cause of most of the disparities in care that individuals with serious mental illness experience is pervasive, egregious stigma within Western society. This is based on the reasonable assumption that stigma either creates, encourages, or allows all the other aspects of disparities in care and enriches barriers to societal opportunity.

A process first delineated by Link and Phelan (22) describes sequential acts that create stigma by defining the cognitive aspects of greater society's reaction to stigmatized individuals. Applying these principles, we will now discuss how this model creates stigma for persons with mental illness.

First, individuals with SMI are labeled on the basis of specific differences from the "chronically normal" community. Corrigan and Kleinlein (23) posit that persons with mental illness are distinguished from others on the basis of four features: overt psychiatric symptoms, social skill deficits, physical appearance, and labels. Second, the larger community affixes undesirable or negative stereotypes to this subgroup. One example of stereotyping that advocates have identified as extremely injurious is the perception that persons with mental illness are unpredictable and dangerous. Third, individuals are separated or avoided in some way to create a distance through isolation or social ostracism creating "us" versus "them" categories. Last, labeled, isolated individuals experience discrimination and social status decline that produces a disparity in outcomes.

Stigma has two main forms. First, there is external stigma that reflects the views and behaviors of greater society as well as specific individuals who interact with persons with mental illness. The second form is internal or self-generated stigma that impacts the individual and mirrors the external form but occurs from the individual's own beliefs and perceptions about mental illness.

Eternal stigma focuses on negative views about persons with mental illness which leads to fear, avoidance, and anger from other people. These emotions translate into the behavioral manifestations of discrimination. This discrimination comes in the many forms:

- restriction of work, housing, education, and rehabilitative opportunities
- increased risk of coercion as an accepted aspect of psychiatric care
- increased criminalization
- abusive methods of confinement
- increased judicial penalties such as capital sentences or barriers to parole and probation
- lack of adequate medical treatment

- acceptance of inadequate psychiatric or substance abuse services
- lack of parity for insurance coverage of psychiatric disorders
- diminished access to medical and psychiatric care
- withholding of appropriate personal or community-based assistance in emergencies.
- abusive treatment when seeking assistance for psychiatric crises
- social ostracism
- socially sanctioned or tolerated ridicule or abuse

In addition to persons with mental illness, external stigma impacts other members of society. People who have relationships with consumers such as family members and friends report perceived stigma, lowered self-esteem, and damaged family relationships (24,25). Family members with higher educational levels or who have had a relative experience a relapse within the last 6 months were more likely to report greater avoidance by others (26).

Psychiatrists and the psychiatric profession have been noted to experience stigma not only from the general public but also from other medical professionals (27).

Additionally, there is the impact to society as a whole in terms of the loss of personal potential and financial productivity from stigma and discrimination toward persons with mental illnesses.

Internal or self-directed stigma may well be more damaging to consumers of mental healthcare than external stigma since it robs individuals of hope, stifles initiative, and squashes resiliency. One survey of 1031 consumers who belonged to the National Alliance on Mental Illness was followed up with 100 personal interviews. Respondents described their attempts to conceal their disorders and to worry that others would become aware of their mental illness (28). They described discouragement, hurt, anger, and decreased self-esteem from the stigmatization.

In 2003 the National Alliance on Mental Illness (NAMI) launched an ambitious antistigma campaign, In Our Own Voice (IOOV), throughout the grassroots of the United States. IOOV is a single presentation utilizing a short video sectioned into six parts: Introduction, Dark Days, Acceptance, Treatment, Coping Skills, and Successes, Hopes and Dreams. Two nationally trained consumer presenters play each section of the video and intersperse personal comments about their illnesses using first person, "I statements."

Using time-tested audience ice-breaker questions, the IOOV speakers stimulate group discussion within the standardized 60- to 90-minute format. Target audiences include consumers, family members, professionals, law enforcement, legislators, and/or the general public. A George Mason University study in 2006 indicated that this type of mental illness education program that portrays consumers as real people improves audience knowledge and attitudes about mental illnesses (29). To arrange an IOOV presentation in your area, please contact NAMI at 703-524-7600.

WHERE TO GO FROM HERE

Historically the general public, consumers, family members—even other medical practitioners—have had misconceptions about psychiatric treatment and care. The lack of a clear etiology for mental illness and the resultant subjectivity in diagnosis and treatment often leads to belief in the community that mental illnesses are less medically based and less treatable.

Unspoken within the current mental health parity debate on Capitol Hill in Washington, DC, is the viewpoint by some that economic equality in treatment for mental disorders will not lead to substantially improved outcomes but will increase healthcare costs. Since many other medical disciplines, for example cardiology, have made huge strides in disease management and improved outcomes in less than 40 years, knowledgeable experts believe similar expectations are possible in psychiatry. Despite the marked complexity of the organ in question and the current limitations in conceptualization of brain pathophysiology for mental disorders, genomic DNA research presents an option to improve the quality of recovery.

The long delays in new research gains filtering into the grassroots of the United States is another huge frustration for consumers and their family members. Barriers to clinical advances identified in this chapter should be addressed but the root causes remain alive and intact in our society—stigma and discrimination. These resultant disparities in care, research, and policy implementation hinder consumers from realizing their full potential.

References

1. Wilk JE, West JC, Rae DS, et al. Medicare Part D prescription benefits and administrative burden in the care of dually eligible psychiatric patients. *Psychiatr Serv* 2008;59(1):34–39.
2. Wilk JE, West JC, Narrow WE, et al. Economic grand rounds: Access to psychiatrists in the public sector and in managed health plans. *Psychiatr Serv* 2005;56:408–410.
3. Busch AB, Frank RG, Lehman AF. The effect of a managed behavioral health carve-out on quality of care for Medicaid patients diagnosed as having schizophrenia. *Arch Gen Psychiatry* 2004;61:442–448.
4. Soumerai SB, McLaughlin TJ, Ross-Degnan D, et al. Effects of limiting Medicaid drug-reimbursement benefits on the use of psychotropic agents and acute mental health services by patients with schizophrenia. *N Engl J Med* 1994;331(10):650–655.
5. *ChicagoTribune.com*. Available at http://newsblogs.chicagotrubune.com/triage/2008/07/a-psychiatrist.html. Accessed July 11, 2008.
6. Folson DP, Hawthorne W, Lindamer L, et al. Prevalence and risk factors for homelessness and utilization of mental health services among 10,340 patients with serious mental illness in a large public mental health system. *Am J Psychiatry* 2005;162:370–376.
7. Culhane DP, Averyt JM, Hadley TR. The rate of public shelter admission among Medicaid-reimbursed users of behavioral health services. *Psychiatr Serv* 1997;48:390–392.
8. Lamb RL, Weinberger LE. The shift of psychiatric inpatient care from hospitals to jails and prisons. *J Am Acad Psychiatry Law* 2005;33:4:529–534.
9. Greenberg GA, Rosenheck RA. Homelessness and mental health: A national study. *Psychiatr Serv* 2008;59:170–177.
10. Mc Neil DE, Binder RL, Robinson JC. Incarceration associated with homelessness, mental disorder and co-occurring substance abuse. *Psychiatr Serv* 2005;56:840–846.
11. Markowitz FE. Psychiatric hospital capacity, homelessness and crime and arrest rates. *Criminology* 2006;441:45–47.
12. Lamb RL, Weinberger LE, Marsh JS, et al. treatment prospects for persons with severe mental illness in an Urban County jail. *Psychiatr Serv* 2007;58:782–786.
13. Stefancic A, Tsemberis S. Housing first for long term shelter dwellers with psychiatric disabilities in a suburban county. *J Primary Prev* 2007;28(3–4):265–279. Epub 2007 Jun 26.
14. Newcomer JW. Medical risk in patients with bipolar disorder and schizophrenia. *J Clin Psychiatry* 2006;67(Suppl 9):25–30; discussion 36–42.
15. Newcomer JW, Nasrallah HA, Mc Intyre RS, et al. Elevating the standard of care in the management of cardiometabolic risk factors in patients with mental illness. *CNS Spectrums* 2008;13(6 Suppl 10):1–14.
16. Vogel-Scibilia S. Addressing inadequacies in the care of patients with schizophrenia and bipolar disorder. *CNS Spectrums* 2008;13(6 Suppl 10):11–12.

17. Kreyenbuhl J, Medoff DR, Seliger SL, et al. Use of medications to reduce cardiovascular risk among individuals with psychotic disorders and type 2 diabetes. *Schizophrenia Res* 2008;101(1–3):256–265. Epub 2008 March 19.
18. Thornicroft G, Rose D, Kassam A. Discrimination in health care against people with mental illness. *Int Rev Psychiatry* 2007;19(2):113–122.
19. Colton CW, Manderscheid RW. Congruencies in increased mortality rates, years of potential life lost and causes of death among public mental health clients in eight states. *Prev Chron Dis* 2006;3(2):A42.
20. Miller BJ, Paschall CB, Svendsen DP. Mortality and medical co-morbidity among patients with severe mental illness. *Psychiatr Serv* 2006;57(10):1482–1487.
21. Foucault Michel (1966). Maladie Mentale et psychologie. 3rd edition Paris: Presses Universitaires de France, p. 75 (1st ed 1954. This passage trans. Claire O'Farrell). Available at http://www.michel-foucault.com/quote/2008q.html (accessed on 6/28/08).
22. Link BG, Phelan JC. Conceptualizing stigma. *Ann Rev Sociology* 2001;27:363–385.
23. Corrigan PW, Kleinlein P. The Impact of Mental Illness: Stigma. In: Corrigan P, ed. *On the Stigma of Mental Illness*. Washington, DC: American Psychological Association, 2005:13.
24. Wahl OF, Harman CR. Family views of stigma. *Schizophrenia Bull* 1989;15(1):131–139.
25. Larson JE, Corrigan P. The stigma of families with mental illness. *Academic Psychiatry* 2008;32:87–91.
26. Phelan JC, Bromet EJ, Link BG. Psychiatric illness and family stigma. *Schizophrenia Bull* 1998;24(1):115–126.
27. Fink PJ. Dealing with psychiatry's stigma. *Hosp Community Psychiatry* 1986;37(8):814–818.
28. Wahl OF. Mental health consumers' experience of stigma. *Schizophrenia Bull* 1999;25(3):467–478.
29. Wood AL, Wahl OF. Evaluating the effectiveness of a consumer-provided mental health recovery education presentation. *Psychiatr Rehabil J* 2006;30(1):46–53.

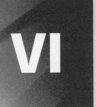
Addressing Disparities

22 The Culturally Sensitive Evaluation

Ora Nakash, Daniel Rosen, and Margarita Alegría

INTRODUCTION

Mental healthcare systems that were originally designed to serve predominantly native-born, English-speaking patients must now meet the needs of patients from many different cultural, linguistic, and socioeconomic backgrounds. The increasing interactions between health providers and ethnically and socially discordant care recipients bring unexpected challenges, with clinicians unprepared to deal with such encounters. With a growing number of mental health intakes being cross-cultural, clinicians vary tremendously in the extent to which they address ethnic and racial differences in clinical practice. Yet mental health providers rarely get trained in communicating essential concepts and information for effective mental healthcare in different languages; working effectively with patients who have limited health literacy; or effectively adapting services for diverse populations. These clinicians face new demands connecting diverse patients with healthcare personnel who may not be accustomed to working with non–English-speaking populations with different customs, values, and experiences. Addressing these challenges may prove critical to determine whether minority patients will enter mental healthcare and remain in care, which is central in addressing disparities. This chapter describes the challenges of conducting the initial mental health interview with multicultural populations and presents recommendations to improve the clinical assessment during the intake process.

CHALLENGES IN CONDUCTING MENTAL HEALTH INTAKES WITH MULTICULTURAL POPULATIONS

The mental health intake is often the first point of contact for patients seeking mental health services. It poses significant challenges to clinicians as they are faced with the need to accomplish multiple goals, including, but not limited to, establishing diagnosis, facilitating rapport, providing psycho-educational tools, and planning treatment. The observations providers make during the intake directly affect patients' retention in care and guide providers' decisions regarding treatment planning. These decisions are exceptionally taxing as they are often made under conditions of time pressure and uncertainty. Such conditions are even more pronounced in service delivery for multicultural populations, which are typically in safety net health settings.

Despite growing awareness of the importance of addressing the needs of diverse populations, these patients continue to face barriers even before reaching mental health intakes. Among these barriers are structural factors (e.g., transportation; availability of specialty services); language and literacy (e.g., providers who speak their native language, access to interpreter services); and financial (e.g., insurance, reimbursement) and cultural barriers relating to acceptable norms and perception of mental illness and treatment.

Patients also bring their cultural backgrounds, beliefs, practices, and languages into the mental health intake; these require attention to provide quality care that reduces disparities. Patients and providers may have a different understanding of the etiology of an illness and the acceptable forms of treatment as a result of their cultural background. What patients want from their providers in the mental health intake may vary as a result of their ethnic/racial background.

Communication styles may also differ as a result of the patient's background. A person's ethnic and racial background may impact what s/he reports, what the clinician asks him/her to report, and how the clinician interprets the information provided. For example, forms of communicating, such as asking questions, may not be considered appropriate behavior in some cultures. Alegría and colleagues (1) also found that the symptoms patients discussed with their providers during the mental health intake varied as a function of their ethnic and racial background. Exposure to traumatic events was more likely to be discussed with Latino patients, while substance abuse–related symptoms were more likely to be discussed with non-Latino white patients. These differences in assessment appear to be mechanisms leading to diagnostic bias in the clinical encounter.

Language challenges are also detrimental factors in non–English-speaking patients trying to explain their mental health problems. When patients and providers speak the same language, patients have reported better physical and mental health outcomes. Alternately, when patients are not able to communicate in their native language with their providers, they are less likely to adhere to treatment and more likely to dropout of care. Stigmatization of mental healthcare, which is common in many minority populations, can also impede the willingness of these patients to come to care (2). Having "depression" or "mental illness" may be perceived by the patient in a deficit model rather than as a curable and manageable medical condition.

In addition, multicultural patients' expectation of being stereotyped may lead to mistrust in mental health services (3). For ethnic and racial minority patients, there appears to be a strong distinction between being looked *at* or looked *over* as a patient, in a way that hinders the clinician's ability to "see" them as a person. Themes of respect and healthy cultural paranoia have been acknowledged as being culturally relevant in the clinical intake and crucial for clinicians to appreciate when working with black patients (4). This requires clinicians to embark on strategies to uncover the uniqueness of a distinct individual and avoid stereotyping these patients. Multicultural patients may feel prejudice or perceive a negative attitude from their provider, reducing the likelihood that these patients will remain in care.

These barriers, in addition to others, will make multicultural patients delay entry into treatment, presenting for care usually in a crisis or emergency state (5). Furthermore, members of minority groups are more likely to dropout after the intake session as compared with their non-Latino white counterparts. For these reasons, the intake session is critical as the entry point to engage these patients in mental healthcare.

BARRIERS CONFRONTED BY CLINICIANS IN THE CLINICAL INTAKE WITH MULTICULTURAL POPULATIONS

Providers face many institutional and clinical challenges in conducting the mental health intake with diverse minority populations. Time pressure, which has significantly increased in the past two decades under managed care, is one of the most significant institutional barriers providers face. Further, existing research leaves no doubt that providers' decision-making is complicated by cultural and sociocontextual differences between patients and clinicians (6). Providers are often socialized and trained in making clinical decisions (e.g., the patient's diagnosis) in a universalistic way, without a clear understanding of the cultural and socio-contextual factors that influence the endorsement of psychiatric symptoms and the diagnosis of illness. Where practice guidelines exist, they often do not include common manifestations of symptoms among ethno-cultural populations. To make diagnostic decisions, providers must collect relevant information related to the particular problem at hand, while organizing this information within a classification system such as that of the *Diagnostic and Statistical Manual* (DSM-IV) (7). However, providers vary widely in the way in which they utilize the DSM-IV to evaluate each of nearly 80 criteria used to establish the presence or absence of psychiatric disorders. In this role, providers are expected to use decisions to estimate the probability of the disorder, while statistically quantifying uncertainties as subjective probabilities in the process of arriving at the correct diagnosis. Additionally, reduced reliability of diagnoses is related to poor knowledge of the criteria by providers, which is often connected with the failure to obtain key information.

Another source of reduced reliability relates to the interpretation of the diagnostic criteria, particularly when clinicians need to decide on the clinically significant characteristics. Given the complexity of such predictions, it is not surprising that to date there are no well-validated algorithms for decisions regarding diagnosis and treatment plans. Under such conditions, clinicians may inadvertently incorporate a prior diagnosis when the decisions are more discretionary than evident. This may lead clinicians to disregard individual data, using what they expect will be the typical symptom presentation and consequently mismatch services to needs.

The quality of the information gathered during the mental health intake is particularly demanding when working with multicultural patients and may vary as a result of the patient's ethnicity/race. The general literature on disparities shows that symptom presentation varies across racial and ethnic groups and can differ from what most clinicians are trained to expect. For example, recent epidemiological research has raised questions about the relationship between the endorsement of psychotic symptoms and the diagnosis of psychotic disorders among culturally diverse groups (8). In addition, another study showed that African Americans with posttraumatic stress disorder endorsed more items suggesting psychosis than non-Latino whites, which has led to misdiagnosis (9).

Misdiagnosis can also occur in the form of underdiagnosing when clinicians ignore genuine manifestations of mental illness, misguided by a misinterpretation of cultural sensitivity. Also, clients likely respond to the therapeutic situation in ways that are consistent with their cultural socialization regarding care, but which may be atypical to the expectations of the clinician.

It remains unclear how clinicians organize and weigh the complex information presented to them during the clinical interview to make decisions regarding diagnosis. Recent research suggests that unconscious processes or "deliberation without attention" provide an advantage for making decisions in complex matters (10). Dijksterhuis and colleagues (10) distinguish between conscious thought, which is rule-based and precise, and unconscious thought, in which large amounts of information can be integrated into an evaluative summary judgment in decision-making. In this regard, intuition plays an important role in many clinical decisions. Intuition is characterized as an implicit cognitive process where a decision is made without the explicit knowledge of how it was made. Also, intuition is more likely to play a significant role in decisions that involve uncertainty, such as those faced in clinical practice with multicultural populations. Yet, implicit cognitive processes could have detrimental effects on the care multicultural patients receive, as they are less subject to analysis or supervision and less amenable to change when compared with explicit processes. Providers may not be aware of diagnostic bias or stereotyping, which can guide their implicit clinical decisions with minority patients, thus making it even more difficult to address service disparities in caring for these patients.

The structure of the clinical interview, which is often at the core of the mental health intake, can also directly affect the implicit processes linked to providers' clinical decisions. Most notable is the tension between structured and unstructured clinical interview models. Structured clinical interviews employ systematic ways of collecting critical information about patients such as evaluation of the specific symptoms and behaviors in a standardized manner. Such systematic ways of collecting information have often been recommended to improve clinical utility by increasing the reliability of the diagnosis and the predictive validity of the assessment. Increasing the reliability of the information gathered by using structured interviews is particularly important when working with minority/multicultural patients, as they can reduce bias and prejudice that have been noted to affect decisions regarding diagnosis and care. However, structured interviews may challenge the existence of open communication between patients and providers, and therefore may hinder the development of a therapeutic alliance. Alternatively, unstructured models of conducting the mental health intake view it as an opportunity to "tell a story" and emphasize the role of good listening and responsiveness on the part of the provider in facilitating good rapport. Open interviews which employ effective listening can allow for contextualizing the patient's presentation and facilitate "knowing" the patient as an individual person. Such contextualization is pertinent to the initial encounter in which patients often present an intimately complex and unique story (11). Although unstructured interviews can facilitate the development of rapport during the intake, they may challenge the attainment of information required for assessment and decisions regarding diagnosis given the time pressure to which most intakes are subject. Furthermore, unstructured interviews may lead to greater reliance on stereotypes and bias in these decisions.

THE ROLE OF STEREOTYPING AND BIAS WHEN PROCESSING MINORITY PATIENT'S CLINICAL INFORMATION

The Institute of Medicine's (12) analysis highlights the role of stereotyping and biases as contributors to service disparities. In our recent study (1), we observe that during the intake interview providers consistently gathered scarce diagnostic information about the patient's symptom presentation and tended to base their decisions about mental health diagnosis on generalized statements of illness, patients' treatment history, and family history of mental health. Moreover, discussion of mental health symptoms varied as a result of the patient's ethnicity and race. Differential discussion of symptom areas appeared to lead to differential diagnosis and increased likelihood of diagnostic bias. Even with similar information collected during the intake, such as history of abuse, clinicians sometimes weighed the information differently to assign a diagnosis depending on the race/ethnicity of the patient. For example, information about trauma was more likely used to assign a depression diagnoses for Latinos in contrast to non-Latino whites or blacks. However, clinicians appeared to use these shortcuts to maximize the time they could devote to getting to know the patient and engaging her/him in treatment.

Patient's initiation of information affected providers' evaluation of the credence and valence of this information (13), as well as their assessment of the rapport during the initial interview. Providers perceived information that was volunteered by patients as more trustworthy and valuable as compared with information they elicited themselves. However, patients' initiation of information varied depending on whether patients had previous experience in mental health treatment. Novice patients, such as many of the minority populations who are unfamiliar with the expectations of the intake, limited their initiation of diagnostic information. Providers tended to perceive these patients as less engaged and attribute less value to the information that was exchanged during these intake sessions.

Furthermore, unconscious bias on the part of providers has been shown to have significant impact on treatment recommendations for minority patients. For example, Green and his colleagues (14) documented that although clinicians expressed no explicit preference for white versus Black patients, an investigation of their unconscious bias revealed an implicit preference for white patients and an implicit stereotype of Black patients as less cooperative. This unconscious bias directly impacted decisions regarding patient medical care. The likelihood of treating the white patient and not treating the black patients increased as their implicit pro-white bias increased. Bias may also disrupt the formation of the therapeutic alliance, which is fundamental for successful engagement in treatment (15). When significant bias is present in treatment, the result may be alienation and lack of trust compounded by cultural misunderstanding.

Clinicians have frequently described the challenge of collecting, interpreting, and integrating sociocultural information in making decisions about the diagnosis and care of minority patients (16). Most notably, providers have struggled with questions related to the attribution of symptomatology. Deciding what of their patient's presentation can be attributed to psychopathology, and what can be attributed to sociocultural stressors, such as belonging to a minority status, has been found to be particularly challenging. For example, for some clinicians, certain types of trauma are "in the eye of the beholder"; if it is culturally acceptable for a man to hit his wife, then that may not be considered as traumatizing (17). However, these assumptions clinicians may make about the greater acceptance of domestic violence as making certain events less traumatizing for certain immigrant groups may be incorrect.

RECOMMENDATIONS TO IMPROVE THE INTAKE PROCESS WITH CULTURALLY DIVERSE GROUPS

Despite the numerous challenges clinicians face during the initial intake session, best practices do exist for providing effective services to culturally diverse populations. The Cultural Formulation of Diagnosis (CFD), found in the Appendix IX of the DSM-IV (7), was developed to make the manual more culturally sensitive. The CFD model expands on the guidelines and diagnostic criteria published in DSM-IV to better incorporate cultural contexts and meanings in establishing psychiatric diagnoses for ethnic minorities and diverse populations (18). It assesses five components for formulating diagnosis and treatment needs that include (i) cultural identity (e.g., group affiliation, acculturation); (ii) cultural explanations of the illness; (iii) cultural factors related to the psychosocial environment and levels of functioning (e.g., family and social support); (iv) cultural elements of the clinician-patient relationship; and (v) the overall impact of culture on diagnosis and care.

Kleinman and Benson (19) emphasized that providing care to minority patients is a complex and nuanced process that requires an inquisitive and curious stance, without easily identified parameters to establish when cultural elements explain psychopathology. A balance between an anthropological approach (which emphasizes an effective and attuned listening that views the patient as an individual), and an epidemiological approach (which emphasizes the ability to generalize without stereotyping) may aid in providing quality care to minority patients. Drawing from both theory and empirical research, additional recommendations will be made related to provider awareness of cultural issues and dynamics, contextual and systemic issues and strategies for enhancing the therapeutic alliance.

PROVIDER AWARENESS OF CULTURAL ISSUES AND DYNAMICS

When meeting a patient during the intake visit, previous professional and personal encounters help shape the clinician's initial understanding and assessment of the patient, including his or her cultural, linguistic, and socioeconomic background. Whether this is conceptualized as related to cognitive schemas and scripts, counter transference, or otherwise, such information exists prior to the first meeting and manifests itself during the initial session of treatment. Prior experiences inevitably influence the way each person makes sense of him or herself and how s/he experiences others.

Among the factors impacting the worldview of the clinician (and patient) are the values of the dominant culture. In the United States, beliefs in the importance of individualism and independence, logic and rationality, and success through the achievement of personal goals are embedded in U.S. mainstream culture. The degree to which any clinician may subscribe to these and other ideas informing his or her worldview obviously varies. Such variation appears to be based on racial and ethnic identity, socioeconomic status, gender identity and socialization, religious and spiritual beliefs, and multiple other factors (20). Reliance on such beliefs without reflection increases dependence on unchallenged personal biases, assuming that one's own version of "normal" has broader application to the lives of others. Challenging these culturally encapsulated views is often the first step toward providing more effective patient care. Additionally, recognizing how racist attitudes and stereotypes impact one's thought processes is essential when serving ethnic and racial minority patients. Both race and the racial identity status of the patient have been shown to be significant factors in research investigating therapy process and outcome (21).

Clinicians from dominant social groups (e.g., white, Christian, male) are particularly susceptible to assuming their experiences are generalizable to others based on higher levels of reinforcement received from the larger society. To ensure accurate diagnosis and appropriate treatment, patient behavior needs to be understood within the patients' cultural context. While interpreting reality through one's own cultural lens is unavoidable, the mental health profession requires a higher standard. Among the competency areas suggested for practitioners to increase awareness of values and biases are: understanding how one's cultural background influences attitudes related to psychological processes such as problem-solving, decision-making, and information processing; recognizing the limitations of one's cultural competency to make appropriate referrals or seek cultural consultation; being cognizant of sources of discomfort related to differences with others; and understanding areas in which one holds privilege and power relative to marginalized groups (22).

In addition to understanding the relevance of cultural variables in one's own life, it is essential that clinicians are aware of these factors in the lives of the patients they serve. Expanding one's awareness from the intrapersonal world of the patient to his or her broader context may prove instrumental to arriving at an accurate diagnosis and avoiding either over or underpathologizing diverse patient populations. Recognizing the intergenerational impact of past events, such as slavery, the *Shoah* (Holocaust), and the destruction of American Indian culture may provide a context for the beliefs, values, and current presentation of patient issues for individuals from communities that have experienced past traumatic events.

Understanding the extent to which racism has been directed toward a patient has been given recent attention in the context of mental health. Carter (23) highlighted the importance of assessing experiences of racism without pathologizing the patient, proposing that such encounters may result in race-based traumatic stress injury. Sue and colleagues (24) have called attention to the shift from direct and explicit acts of racism to subtler, sometimes invisible occurrences. They have proposed that daily indignities experienced by people of color, even if unintentional, may have detrimental consequences to one's psychological functioning and to the therapeutic alliance in mental health treatment. While individuals vary in the way such acts impact their psychological well-being and functioning, these implications must be considered in the assessment and treatment process. To connect with and accurately conceptualize a patient's condition, it is necessary to understand current manifestations of racism as well as other forms of oppression that have previously shaped such interactions in clinical encounters.

CONTEXTUAL CONSIDERATIONS AND SYSTEMIC RECOMMENDATIONS

Mental health services in the United States are delivered within a specific cultural context. The values, practices, and beliefs held by society are inevitably present in the clinical intake. As evidenced by the disparities presented earlier in this chapter, racism and discrimination permeate the field of healthcare. Therefore, the intake session represents a critical opportunity for patients to assess their clinicians and the overall mental health treatment process. Recent contributions to the literature (25) have highlighted the importance of systemic factors that enhance effective treatment for culturally diverse communities. Each of the following recommendations holds in common a need for institutional support through clinician advocacy and effective organizational leadership.

A patient's experience with any mental health system begins by interacting with the lager clinical environment of the organization. For many, a few key factors are worth serious attention: (i) ensuring that signs throughout the building are written in the primary language(s) of patients served; (ii) providing easy access to the facility regardless of physical ability; (iii) hiring receptionists with the language skills and attitude necessary to serve a diverse patient population; (iv) constructing treatment rooms large enough to hold multiple family members whom the patient may wish to include in her or his care; and (v) attending to the cultural relevance of the magazines/literature and artwork in the building. Attention to these issues can be the first steps in building confidence and trust in the treatment process.

Clinic policies related to treatment delivery represent another systemic factor critical to ensuring success in the intake session. Ineffective policies may prove detrimental to even the most well-intentioned practitioner; particularly policies dictating the structure of the intake interview, such as a standardized protocol, that can largely determine the flow of the session. While the advantages to the structured interview have already been discussed, it is important to emphasize that culturally relevant areas of inquiry be included. Time constraints for "completing" the intake are another area often determined by clinic policy. The notion that a patient's entire clinically relevant history may be gathered in a single session is unworkable in many instances, and flexibility must be offered for extended evaluations in complex cases. At an administrative level, this includes offering clinicians the opportunity to schedule follow-up appointments with such patients in a timely way, as well as making provisions for documenting the extended evaluation. Other policies central to providing competent care during the intake session include requiring collaboration with professional interpreter services for individuals who prefer to conduct the interview in a language not spoken by their provider, ongoing mandatory training in cultural issues for clinic staff, and an organizational commitment to creating a diverse workforce reflective of the patient community.

A final area in which systemic practices have proven important concerns the materials and resources available for patients' care. In addition to hiring reception personnel with appropriate language proficiency to answer phone calls and providing access to interpreter services based on patient needs and preferences, it is vital that clinically relevant documents be available in multiple languages. The process of obtaining informed consent to treatment is among the key tasks of the intake session, and such consent is most often acquired through written documentation. The need for accurate forms in the patient's primary language is obvious. Attention must also be placed to providing accessible educational handouts and resources. The use of culturally appropriate assessment instruments is also pertinent to patient services, as many diagnostic tools have not been normed across diverse populations and may prove invalid and unethical for use with certain cultural groups. Further, practitioners must ensure that translated instruments are valid in terms of their linguistic translation as well as being conceptually and functionally equivalent.

STRATEGIES FOR PROMOTING THERAPEUTIC ALLIANCE

Fostering a therapeutic alliance with the multicultural patient is central to the mental health intake. A clinician's ability to establish an effective rapport has the potential to set the tone for future work and contribute to positive treatment outcomes. For those who enter treatment with uncertainty or skepticism, patient's expectations are particularly important to address as early as possible. This will be relevant for those patients who had past negative experiences in the mental health system. Spending sufficient time guiding the patient through some of the potentially difficult and/or uncomfortable procedures, such as administering a standardized battery to better assess the diagnostic information, will prove critical. Cultural mistrust related to a specific clinician or the mental health system in general may be accompanied by doubts that a provider can offer effective help or understand their specific situation. Addressing such concerns with openness and cultural humility and showing an interest in learning from and listening to the patient may help establish the necessary affective bonds. Concerns about being stigmatized as a "mental health patient" and fears of breaking cultural norms by talking with others about personal matters may present additional challenges to creating a therapeutic alliance during the intake session. Further, ensuring confidentiality and guaranteeing a nonjudgmental approach is crucial when working with multicultural patients.

Patient-provider communication holds a central role in developing a collaborative therapeutic relationship. Alegría and colleagues (26) have called attention to the necessity of patient activation in the treatment process. To this end, they developed an intervention focused on preparing patients to gather information from providers and formulate questions during appointments. Results showed intervention participants were more likely to attend sessions and follow-up with practitioners than a comparison group. Consistent with these findings, a clinician's ability to elicit patient questions and concerns, provide information about the treatment process and options available, and facilitate the patient's participation in actively making decisions in support of her or his goals may prove instrumental to both treatment process and outcome.

Creating a truly collaborative relationship during the intake process requires openness to hearing questions (including those to which answers may be unknown) and a commitment to transparency and authenticity in communication. In addition to spending time obtaining informed consent for treatment, the therapeutic alliance can be enhanced by discussing: (i) the purpose of the intake session; (ii) the process and format of the intake session; (iii) the likelihood that treatment will be of benefit to the patient based on the intake session, (iv) an initial treatment plan; and (v) what patients can expect during the next session if they return to treatment. This information can empower individuals to becoming active participants in their care, particularly for patients who may be unfamiliar with the mental health system.

Through continually enhancing and refining one's knowledge of various cultural groups is of great importance, this chapter's emphasis on humility reflects a willingness to listen to and learn from the patient. Setting aside one's assumptions about the patient and one's role as "expert" opens the space for an inquiry of cultural variables relevant to the patient's psychological functioning and well-being. Among those areas to be considered in the assessment process are the patient's multiple cultural identities, including race and ethnicity, religion and spirituality, socioeconomic status, and relationship status/sexual orientation. Questions related to language and literacy may also prove relevant, including the preferred language spoken during the interview, at home, in dreams and prayers, and to best communicate emotions. Additional attention must be placed on significant family and/or kinship networks (including extended family, community involvement, and religious community), immigration history and acculturative stress (including pre-migration history, events precipitating immigration, the migration experience, and experience following immigration), definitions of health and illness and sources of strength and resilience. These and other culturally relevant questions have the potential to enhance both the therapeutic alliance and the effectiveness of care provided (27).

ACKNOWLEDGMENTS

This chapter references data from the Patient-Provider Encounter Study (PPES), provided by the Advanced Center for Latino and Mental Health Systems Research of the Center for Multicultural Mental Health Research at the Cambridge Health Alliance. This study was supported by NIH Research grant No. 1P50 MHO 73469 funded by the National Institute of Mental Health. We acknowledge Sheri Lapatin and Anna Nillni at the Center for Multicultural Mental Health Research for their contributions.

References

1. Alegría M, Nakash O, Lapatin S, et al. How missing information in diagnosis can lead to disparities in the clinical encounter. *J Public Health Manage Pract* 2008;14 suppl:S26–35.
2. Hinshaw SP, Stier A. Stigma as related to mental disorders. *Ann Rev Clin Psychol* 2008;4: 367–393.
3. Burgess D, Fu S, van Ryan M. Why do providers contribute to disparities and what can be done about it? *J Gen Intern Med* 2004;19:1154–1159.
4. Whaley AL. Paranoia in African American men receiving inpatient psychiatric treatment. *J Am Acad Psychiatry Law Online* 2004;32(3):282.
5. Snowden LR, Masland MC, Libby AM, et al. Racial/ethnic minority children's use of psychiatric emergency care in California's public mental health system. *Am J Public Health* 2008;98(1):118–124.
6. Malgady RG, Zayas LH. Cultural and linguistic considerations in psychodiagnosis with Hispanics: The need for an empirically informed process model. *Social Work* 2001;46(1): 39–49.
7. American Psychiatric Association. *Diagnostic and Statistical Manual of Mental Disorders-4th edition*. Washington, DC: American Psychiatric Association, 1994.
8. Vega W, Lewis-Fernandez R. Ethnicity and variability of psychotic symptoms. *Curr Psychiatry Rep* 2008;10:223–228.
9. Alim TN, Graves E, Mellman TA, et al. Trauma exposure, posttraumatic stress disorder and depression in an African American primary care population. *J Natl Med Assoc* 2006; 98(10):1630–1636.
10. Dijksterhuis A, Bos M, Nordgren L, et al. On making the right choice: The deliberation-without-attention effect. *Science* 2006;311:1005–1007.
11. Weiner S. Contextualizing medical decisions to individualize care. *J Gen Intern Med* 2004; 19:281–285.
12. Institute of Medicine. *Unequal Treatment: Confronting Racial and Ethnic Disparities in Health Care*. Washington, DC: The National Academies Press, 2002.
13. Nakash O, Darghouth S, Oddo V, et al. Patient initiation of information: Exploring its role during the mental health intake visit. *Patient Educ Couns* 2005; Dec 3 [epub ahead of print].
14. Green AR, Carney DR, Pallin DJ, et al. Implicit bias among physicians and its prediction of thrombolysis decisions for black and white patients. *J Gen Intern Med* 2007;22(9): 1231–1238.

15. Hovarth A. Reliance on the alliance. In: Hovarth A, Greenberg L, eds. *The Working Alliance: Theory Research and Practice*. New York: John Wiley & Sons, 1994:121–155.

16. Snowden L. Bias in mental health assessment and intervention: Theory and evidence. *Am J Public Health* 2003;93(2):239–243.

17. Fortuna L, Porche M, Alegría MA. A Qualitative Study of Clinicians' Use of the Cultural Formulation Model in Assessing Posttraumatic Stress Disorder. *Transcult Psychiatry* (in press).

18. Lewis-Fernandez R, Diaz N. The cultural formulation: A method for assessing cultural factors affecting the clinical encounter. *Psychiatr Q* 2002;73(4):271–295.

19. Kleinman A, Benson P. Anthropology in the clinic: The problem of cultural competency and how to fix it. *PLoS Med* 2006;3(10):e294.

20. Alarcón DR, Bell CC, Kirmayer JL, et al. Beyond the funhouse mirrors. In: Kupfer JD, First BM, Regier A, eds. *A Research Agenda for DSM-V*. Washington, DC: American Psychiatric Association, 2002:219–281.

21. Carter RT, Williams B, Juby HL, et al. Racial identity as mediator of the relationship between gender role conflict and severity of psychological symptoms in black, Latino, and Asian men. *Sex Roles* 2005;53(7):473–486.

22. Arredondo P. Operationalization of the multicultural counseling competencies. *J Multicultur Counsel Dev* 1996;24(1):42–78.

23. Carter RT. Racism and psychological and emotional injury: Recognizing and assessing race-based traumatic stress. *Counsel Psychologist* 2007;35(1):13.

24. Sue DW, Capodilupo CM, Torino GC, et al. Racial microaggressions in everyday life: Implications for clinical practice. *Am Psychologist* 2007;62(4):271–286.

25. Powe NR, Cooper LA. Diversifying the racial and ethnic composition of the physician workforce. *Ann Intern Med* 2004;141(3):223.

26. Alegría M, Canino G, Shrout PE, et al. Prevalence of mental illness in immigrant and non-immigrant U.S. Latino groups. *Am J Psychiatry* 2008;165:359–369.

27. Caraballo A, Hamin H, Lee JR, et al. Appendix A: A Resident's Guide to the Cultural Formation. In: Lim R, ed. *Clinical Manual of Cultural Psychiatry*. Washington, DC: American Psychiatric Publishing, Inc, 2006:243–267.

The Role of Cultural Competence

Russell F. Lim

This chapter will discuss the various policy issues involving cultural competence and psychiatric disparities and suggest ways that mental health professionals can be advocates for the training and application of cultural competence as a way to reduce mental health disparities in ethnic minority populations. Policy can be influenced by many federal agencies, state legislatures, national accreditation boards, professional societies, foundations, and academic literature, and all of these influences will be discussed in turn. The most logical place to start is the federal level, as the U.S. Congress determines spending priorities of the country, which then influences the delivery of services to minority patients with mental disorders.

FEDERAL POLICIES

Nationally, policy follows governmental oversight by the federal government, which will determine funding priorities. In 1998, the U.S. Department of Health and Human Services (USDHHS) Office of Minority Health (OMH) conducted a review and comparison of existing cultural and linguistic competence standards and measures on a national level, to propose a draft of national standards (1). The standards were informed by an analytical review of key legislation, regulations, contracts, and standards currently in use by federal and state agencies and other national organizations. Proposed standards were then developed with input from a national advisory committee of policy administrators, healthcare providers, and health services researchers. Fourteen standards were created, defining culturally competent care; i.e., care that is compatible with cultural health beliefs, and in the preferred language, how to provide services in the appropriate languages for the client, such as providing signage, literature, and interpretation in their preferred language so that family members would not be used as interpreters, and supporting cultural competence in the organization, such as having a strategic plan that includes instituting hiring and retention practices that encourage a diversity in the staff that matches the patient population, and that they be trained in cultural competence principles, such as working with the community, as well as an ongoing assessment of cultural competence practices, and the demographics of the patient population, and a review process that is available to the public (Table 23.1).

TABLE 23.1	National Standards for Culturally and Linguistically Appropriate Services

Culturally Competent Care

1. Healthcare organizations should ensure that patients/consumers receive from all staff members effective, understandable, and respectful care that is provided in a manner compatible with their cultural health beliefs and practices and preferred language.

2. Healthcare organizations should implement strategies to recruit, retain, and promote at all levels of the organization a diverse staff and leadership that are representative of the demographic characteristics of the service area.

3. Healthcare organizations should ensure that staff at all levels and across all disciplines receive ongoing education and training in culturally and linguistically appropriate service delivery.

Language Access Services

4. Healthcare organizations must offer and provide language assistance services, including bilingual staff and interpreter services, at no cost to each patient/consumer with limited English proficiency at all points of contact, in a timely manner during all hours of operation.

5. Healthcare organizations must provide to patients/consumers in their preferred language both verbal offers and written notices informing them of their right to receive language assistance services.

6. Healthcare organizations must assure the competence of language assistance provided to limited English proficient patients/consumers by interpreters and bilingual staff. Family and friends should not be used to provide interpretation services (except on request by the patient/consumer).

7. Healthcare organizations must make available easily understood patient-related materials and post signage in the languages of the commonly encountered groups and/or groups represented in the service area.

Organizational Supports for Cultural Competence

8. Healthcare organizations should develop, implement, and promote a written strategic plan that outlines clear goals, policies, operational plans, and management accountability/oversight mechanisms to provide culturally and linguistically appropriate services.

9. Healthcare organizations should conduct initial and ongoing organizational self-assessments of CLAS-related activities and are encouraged to integrate cultural and linguistic competence-related measures into their internal audits, performance improvement programs, patient satisfaction assessments, and outcomes-based evaluations.

10. Healthcare organizations should ensure that data on the individual patient's/consumer's race, ethnicity, and spoken and written language are collected in health records, integrated into the organization's management information systems, and periodically updated.

11. Healthcare organizations should maintain a current demographic, cultural, and epidemiological profile of the community as well as a needs assessment to accurately plan for and implement services that respond to the cultural and linguistic characteristics of the service area.

12. Healthcare organizations should develop participatory, collaborative partnerships with communities and utilize a variety of formal and informal mechanisms to facilitate community and patient/consumer involvement in designing and implementing CLAS-related activities.

13. Healthcare organizations should ensure that conflict and grievance resolution processes are culturally and linguistically sensitive and capable of identifying, preventing, and resolving cross-cultural conflicts or complaints by patients/consumers.

14. Healthcare organizations are encouraged to regularly make available to the public information about their progress and successful innovations in implementing the CLAS standards and to provide public notice in their communities about the availability of this information.

From USDHHS, OMH, CLAS Standards, 2000, Available at http://www.omhrc.gov/clas/.

The first report created by a government agency was "Cultural Competence Standards in Managed Care Mental Health Services: Four Underserved/ Underrepresented Racial/Ethnic Groups," in 1998 (2), which detailed overall system standards and implementation guidelines, such as cultural competence planning, community outreach and education, and quality monitoring and improvement, as well as human resource development. The standards also included clinical standards, such as access, triage, assessment, treatment, and discharge planning, as well as case management. Finally, it delineated guidelines for communication and patient self-help, as well as carefully outlined provider competencies, such as knowledge, attitudes, and skills.

In the year 2000, the Office of Civil Rights (OCR), empowered by Executive Order 13166: Improving Access to Services for Persons with Limited English Proficiency, from the White House, required that all federal agencies formally address how they would provide access to their services to those clients with Limited English Proficiency (LEP). The USDHHS issued a guidance that includes an "Effective Plan on Language Assistance for LEP Persons," which states that programs receiving federal funds must (i) identify individuals who need language services, (ii) have language assistance services, (iii) train staff to appropriately work with clients who need language assistance, (iv) provide notice for clients that services are available, such as signs in their language, and (v) that such programs must be monitored and updated (3).

Also in 2001, the Supplement to the Surgeon General's Report on Mental Health, *Mental Health: Culture, Race, and Ethnicity* (4), was released by the Surgeon General, which established that ethnic minorities do not utilize services as much as the majority population and that "culture counts." The supplement documented striking disparities in mental healthcare for racial and ethnic minorities involving access to care, appropriateness of treatment, overall quality of care, and treatment outcomes. Minorities were also noted to be poorly represented in most research studies. Taken as a whole, these mental health disparities impose a greater disability burden on racial and ethnic minorities. Some examples from each of the four chapters on the major racial and ethnic groups follow:

- Disproportionate numbers of African Americans are represented in the most vulnerable segments of the population—people who are homeless, incarcerated, in the child welfare system, victims of trauma—all populations with increased risks for mental disorders.
- As many as 40% of Hispanic Americans report limited English-language proficiency. Because few mental healthcare providers identify themselves as Spanish-speaking, most Hispanic Americans have limited access to ethnically or linguistically similar providers.
- The suicide rate among American Indians/Alaska Natives is 50% higher than the national rate; rates of co-occurring mental illness and substance abuse (especially alcohol) are also higher among Native youth and adults. Because few data have been collected, the full nature, extent, and sources of these disparities remain a matter of conjecture.
- Asian Americans/Pacific Islanders who seek care for a mental illness often present with more severe illnesses than do other racial or ethnic groups. This, in part, suggests that stigma and shame are critical deterrents to service utilization. It is also possible that mental illnesses may be undiagnosed or treated later in their course because they are expressed in symptoms of a physical nature (4).

The report concluded with "A Vision for the Future," in which recommendations were grouped in six areas: (i) continue to expand the science base, (ii) improve access to treatment, (iii) reduce barriers to treatment, (iv) improve quality of care, (v) support capacity development, and (vi) promote mental health.

Finally, in July 2003, the President's New Freedom Commission on Mental Health issued its report entitled "Achieving the Promise: Transforming Mental Health Care in America (5)." Of the six overall goals that were discussed as strategies to transform the mental health system, two are most relevant to minority mental health disparities: (i) mental healthcare is consumer and family driven and (ii) disparities in mental health services are (to be) eliminated. Some of the specific recommendations concerning racial and ethnic disparities that affect healthcare delivery included the following:

Recommendation 3.1: Improve access to quality care that is culturally competent. "The Commission recommends making strong efforts to recruit, retain, and enhance an ethnically, culturally, and linguistically competent mental health workforce...These efforts could include (i) recruiting and retaining racial and ethnic minority and bilingual professionals, (ii) developing and including curricula that address the impact of culture, race, and ethnicity on mental health...(iii) training and research programs targeting services to multicultural populations, (iv) engaging minority consumers and families in workforce development, training, and advocacy....All Federally funded health and mental health training programs should explicitly include cultural competence in their curricula and training experiences.

Recommendation 3.2: Improve access to quality care in rural and geographically remote areas.

Recommendation 4.4: Screen for mental disorders in primary healthcare [settings], across the life span, and connect treatment and supports (sic) [systems].

Recommendation 5.3: Improve and expand the workforce providing evidence-based mental health services and supports. "Every mental health education and training program in the Nation should voluntarily assess the extent to which it....emphasizes developing cultural competence in clinical practice and ensures that the diversity of the community is reflected among trainees and in the training experience."

Recommendation 5.4: Develop the knowledge base in four understudied areas: mental health disparities, long-term effects of medications, trauma, and acute care (5).

Thus, the Bush Administration has produced a policy document guiding how mental health services should be delivered, where research should be done, and how future health professionals should be recruited and trained.

Finally, in 2005, the National Institute of Health (NIH) and the National Institute of Mental Health (NIMH) have instituted a policy that all investigators must describe how they will recruit underrepresented groups, such as ethnic minorities, women, and other nonmajority groups in their experimental protocols. According to the guidance, "NIH also requires a description of the proposed outreach programs for recruiting sex/gender and racial/ethnic group members as subjects (6)." Thus, investigators are required to describe how they will recruit subjects that represent all of the major underrepresented groups, and not just the mainstream and majority group, or they risk not being approved for funding.

STATE LEGISLATION

States are free to develop their own policies and these can in turn be adopted by the federal government, as seen in the creation of the CLAS Standards earlier. California was one of the first states to institute cultural competence standards. In 1993, California began the process that became known as the California Cultural Competence Plan (7).

TABLE 23.2	Massachusetts Department of Mental Health Cultural Competence Action Plan Goals for FY 2005 to 2007

1. Partner with multicultural communities in the planning, development, and implementation of culturally and linguistically effective mental health services within a unified public behavioral health system.

2. Promote leadership in cultural competence/diversity to reduce mental health disparities.

3. Integrate cultural competence and diversity into staff training, staff development, and educational activities.

4. Recruit and retain a culturally diverse workforce at all levels of the organization that reflects the cultural communities in the Commonwealth.

5. Ensure strengthened access and availability of culturally and linguistically competent services throughout the entire DMH service delivery system.

6. Promote communication and information dissemination on issues related to cultural competence and diversity.

7. Use demographic information about DMH clients and applicants to inform decisions about policy development, clinical practice, research, program development, service delivery, and workforce development.

From MDMH Cultural Competence Action Plan FY 2005–07, 2005. Available at http://www.mass.gov/Eeohhs2/docs/dmh/p_cultural_action_plan.pdf

Each of the 58 California counties has to assess the percentages of the languages spoken by their patients and providers and requires that they provide services and brochures in any language spoken by 3000 Medi-Cal (California's version of Medicaid) members or 5% of the Medi-Cal population in that county. The State of California also requires that all Continuing Medical Education (CME) courses include material on cultural competence by the passage of AB 1195, Chapter 514 (8). Massachusetts was one of the first states to implement mandated program and professional experience requirements related to racial/ethnic basis of behavior, as cultural competence became a proficiency necessary for the licensure of professional psychologists in 1993 (9). The Massachusetts Department of Mental Health has had a Cultural Competence Action Plan since 2002, and its latest version, spanning 13 pages, was released in 2005 (10). The plan outlines major goals, such as developing community partnerships, encouraging leadership in cultural competence, promote cultural competence training and education, ensure culturally competent hiring practices, provide culturally appropriate services, support research efforts to document successes in implementing programs, and disseminate information about culturally competent practices that are effective (Table 23.2).

NATIONAL ACCREDITING AGENCIES

National accreditation boards, such as the Liaison Council of Medical Education (LCME), and the Residency Review Committee (RRC) of the Accreditation Council of Graduate Medical Education (ACGME) also have an influence on how students and trainees are taught. The LCME requires that the medical school curriculum include instruction on cultural competence, as seen in this excerpt from the accreditation standards: ED-22. Medical students must learn to recognize and appropriately address gender and cultural biases in themselves and others, and in the process of healthcare delivery.

The objectives for clinical instruction should include student understanding of demographic influences on healthcare quality and effectiveness, such as racial and ethnic disparities in the diagnosis and treatment of diseases. The objectives should also address the need for self-awareness among students regarding any personal biases in their approach to healthcare delivery (11).

According to the LCME, medical student must know more than just that the ethnicity of the patient may influence the diagnosis and treatment of disease, but that they must also develop the ability to self assess their levels of bias and stereotyping that may lead to health and mental health disparities. The RRC for residencies in psychiatry has similar requirements, that residents must see a sufficient variety of patients to allow the resident to be trained on how to deal with different ethnic minority groups (12).

PROFESSIONAL ORGANIZATIONS

Professional organizations, such as the American Psychiatric Association (APA), the American Psychological Association, the National Association of Social Workers, and the International Society of Psychiatric-Mental Health Nurses have all issued policy statements on how their members should utilize principles of cultural competence. In 1994, the APA published its ground-breaking *Outline for Cultural Formulation in the Diagnostic and Statistical Manual, Fourth Edition* (DSM-IV), as well as a glossary of culture bound syndromes, and new culturally related diagnoses, such as an Acculturation Problem and Spiritual Crisis, and in the updated DSM-IV-TR (Text Revision) (13). In the *Practice Guidelines for the Assessment of Patients*, the APA included being aware of cultural issues (14). Finally, in 2006, the APA initiated a plan to implement the recommendations of the Supplement to the Surgeon General's Report on Mental Health (15), which recommended to: (i) continue efforts to increase cultural awareness and competence at all levels of APA organization, including Board [of Trustees], Assembly, District Branches (DBs), components, and staff, (ii) strengthen efforts to recruit members of underrepresented minority groups into psychiatry, including efforts to increase interest in psychiatry as early as high school, (iii) strengthen efforts to recruit members of underrepresented minorities to become psychiatric researchers, reviewing the outcomes of the 15-year-old PMRTP (Program for Minority Research Training In Psychiatry) and developing a new strategic plan for additional development of minority research programs, (iv) strengthen efforts to recruit and develop racial and ethnic psychiatrists to serve as administrators and policymakers, both within and outside APA, such as post residency fellowships, (v) strengthen efforts to support faculty development in cultural competence, cultural diversity, and reduction of mental health disparities, (vi) strengthen efforts to include cultural competence in the residency curriculum, (vii) strengthen efforts to mentor underrepresented minority medical students, residents, and early career psychiatrists, and (viii) strengthen efforts to provide CME on cultural competence and diversity, with specific focus on reducing mental health disparities.

The American Psychological Association published its "Guidelines on Multicultural Education, Training, Research, Practice, and Organizational Change for Psychologists (16)," which contains six guidelines, including (i) psychologists should recognize that they are cultural beings and may hold attitudes and beliefs that can negatively influence their perceptions of and interactions with individuals who are ethnically and racially different from themselves, (ii) psychologists are encouraged to recognize the importance of cultural sensitivity/responsiveness, knowledge, and understanding the varied values and beliefs of ethnically and racially different individuals, (iii) psychologists are encouraged to use the constructs of multiculturalism and diversity in undergraduate and post graduate education, (iv) culturally sensitive psychological researchers are encouraged to recognize the importance of conducting culturally centered and ethical psychological research that includes persons from ethnic, linguistic, and racial minority backgrounds, (v) psychologists should strive to apply culturally appropriate skills in clinical and other applied psychological practice such as psychological testing, and (vi) psychologists are encouraged to use organizational change processes and participate in the organization to support culturally informed policy development and practices (16).

The National Association of Social Workers (NASW) published their "NASW Standards for Cultural Competence in Social Work Practice" in 2001, and they included 10 standards of practice for social workers, including [culturally competent] ethics and values, [cultural] self-awareness, cross-cultural knowledge, cross-cultural skills, [culturally competent] service delivery, [encouraging] empowerment and advocacy [for social workers and clients], [developing a] diverse workforce, [cultural competent] professional education, language diversity, and cross-cultural leadership (17).

Finally, the International Society for Psychiatric and Mental Health Nursing (ISPN) issued its "ISPN Position Statement on Diversity, Cultural Competence, and Access to Mental Health Care (18)," which notes that the World Health Organization in its Global Burden of Disease identifies depression, substance abuse, suicide, and violence as major problems affecting the world's population, and stated that the ISPN would like to reduce health disparities. Therefore, their goals and objectives are to advocate for better access for diverse individuals, provide direct services in a culturally competent manner, advocate for more research with diverse groups, support policy initiatives for culturally competent care, recruit mental health practitioners who possess diverse backgrounds, advocating for the prevention of mental illness, and for research in providing mental healthcare within primary care services. Their immediate action plan includes (i) having at least one presentation on cultural competence at its national meeting, (ii) giving an award to an individual, program, or organization that has been exemplary in its practice of cultural competent care or advocacy for policy in cultural competence, (iii) having members participate in outreach to high schools with predominately minority populations to encourage them to consider a career in mental health nursing, and (iv) developing a minority mentor network for interested students.

ACADEMIC LITERATURE AND FOUNDATIONS

The academic literature and the foundations have many examples of policy articles, but I will discuss only two examples, an academic article by Brach and Fraser, entitled, "Can Cultural Competency Reduce Racial and Ethnic Health Disparities? A Review and Conceptual Model" (19), a white paper for the Commonwealth Fund, and Betancourt's "Improving Quality and Achieving Equity: The Role of Cultural Competence in Reducing Racial and Ethnic Disparities in Health Care" (20). Both articles are excellent reviews of the literature in showing that applying cultural competence principles can reduce health disparities. Brach and Fraser suggest that providing nine cultural competency techniques, such as interpreter services, recruitment and retention policies, training, coordinating with traditional healers, use of community health workers, culturally competent health promotion, including family/community members, immersion into another culture, and administrative and organizational accommodations, would reduce health disparities. Interpreter services would improve communication; improve access, diagnosis, and treatment (Fig. 23.1).

Recruitment and retention is important, as minority staff improve communication and understanding and create a more welcoming environment. Training staff in cultural competence principles would add knowledge and skills and change attitudes that may interfere with the proper delivery of healthcare. Using traditional healers improves the relationship of the treating agency with the patient and the community, as it shows that they accept the patient's health beliefs. The use of community health workers decreases mistrust and misunderstandings that can interfere with the culturally appropriate treatment being accepted by the patient. Health promotion can modify behaviors that increase risk for illnesses, and identify diseases at earlier stages of development, when treatment may be more effective, as well as decrease the stigma of illness. Including family and/or community members is critical to engaging the minority patient and his or her support system, and failing to engage them usually results in non-adherence to recommendations. Immersion is the best way of learning about another culture and would be a helpful training modality if available. Finally, administrative structures can be detrimental to engaging ethnic minority groups whose concepts of time are non-Western. A common practice it to reschedule a patient when they are fifteen minutes late, but the patient may not feel that they were late, because it was "close enough." Lack of appropriate signage or operating hours that exclude working parents can convey a message that the patient or his or her family is not welcome, and geographic concerns may make it impossible for patients to make their appointments. The more that we can see the healthcare encounter from the patient's perspective, and adjust accordingly, the more likely that a client will make their appointments and engage in treatment with the physician (Fig. 23.2). Thus, a diverse population plus cultural competence techniques equals improved therapeutic alliance, culturally appropriate services that lead to improved outcome and a reduction of health disparities.

Finally, Betancourt states how cultural competence can reduce racial and ethnic disparities in healthcare by applying the six principles outlined in the Institute of Medicine's (IOM) 2001 report, *Crossing the Quality Chasm* to cultural competence, which include (i) safety, or making the appropriate culturally sensitive diagnosis, (ii) effectiveness, or providing proper interpretation, (iii) patient centeredness, or respect for the patient's values, preferences, and needs, such as family support, (iv) timeliness (v) and efficiency, or care that is not delayed because of a lack of interpreters, and (vi) equity, or eliminating clinical decisions made based on ethnic stereotypes.

According to Betancourt, the IOM's 2002 report, *Unequal Treatment*, identifies a set of root causes for racial and ethnic health disparities, including (i) health system factors such as its complexity, (ii) care-process variables, such as stereotyping, impact of ethnicity on clinical decision-making, and poor communication, and (iii) patient level variables, such as refusal of services, poor adherence to treatment recommendations, and delays in seeking care. Cultural competence can reduce disparities at three levels. First, at the organizational level, the members of the administration and staff should be from diverse backgrounds, and have strategies for increasing diversity in all hiring practices and recruitment. Second, at the systemic level, community assessments

Interpreter services can improve the following:

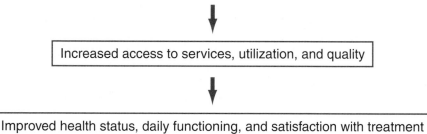

1. Improved patient education reduces risk producing behavior and risk exposure.

Lower incidence of disease

2. Patients, knowing that they will be understood, increase use of clinics.
3. Formation of trusting relationships based on a healthy therapeutic alliance increases likelihood that patient preferences coincide with best medical practices.
4. Increased knowledge (through training) of genetic background, risk behavior, and risk exposure leads to appropriate screening.
5. Increased information on medical history and symptoms leads to improved accuracy of diagnosis.
6. Increased knowledge (through training) of home/folk remedies prevent complications due to drug interactions and can reduce harmful culturally appropriate practices.
7. Greater understanding of treatment requirements and benefits by the patient and more culturally appropriate treatment regimens implemented by providers will improve adherence.
8. Ability of patients to communicate with English-only speakers increases patient choices of high-quality providers.

Increased access to services, utilization, and quality

Improved health status, daily functioning, and satisfaction with treatment

Figure 23-1. How interpreter services could reduce health disparities. (Adapted from Brach C, Fraser I. Can cultural competency reduce racial and ethnic health disparities? A review and conceptual model. *Med Care Res Rev* 2000;57(Suppl 1):181–217.)

can be done, as well as data collection on ethnicity and language, and providing literature and signage in appropriate languages, as well as supporting health promotion. Finally, at the clinical level, clinicians can be trained to increase their awareness of how sociocultural factors affect the health encounter in the health beliefs of the patients, and being aware of how ethnicity affects clinical decision-making.

Betancourt also describes quality improvement approaches, such as (i) identifying patients who need care by ethnicity and illness data; (ii) providing care by tailoring the methods used to the patient's needs, such as using translated materials that are at the appropriate level for the patient's literacy; (iii) supporting physicians and

Nine cultural competency techniques

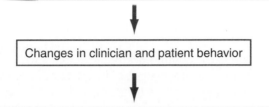

1. Interpreter services
2. Use of community health workers
3. Recruitment and retention policies
4. Culturally competent health promotion
5. Including family/community members
6. Training
7. Immersion into another culture
8. Coordinating with traditional healers
9. Administrative and organizational accommodations

Changes in clinician and patient behavior

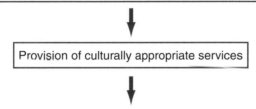

ı Improved communication between patient and physician and improved trust.
ı Greater knowledge of differential epidemiology and treatment efficacy.
ı Expanded understanding of patients' cultural behaviors and environment.

Provision of culturally appropriate services

1. Patient education, other prevention activities, and screenings, targeting conditions either prevalent in population or indicated by risk behaviors or risk exposures.
2. Culturally appropriate and accurate diagnosis of conditions, and education of patients on relative merits of treatment options, recognizing cultural beliefs and other cultural factors and incorporating them into the treatment regimen.
3. Education of patients on how to follow chosen treatment regimens in their cultural environment. Adaptation of treatment to be culturally appropriate.

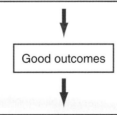

Good outcomes

ı Higher level of health status
ı Increased social and occupational functioning
ı Improved satisfaction with treatment

Figure 23-2. How nine cultural competency techniques could reduce health disparities. (Adapted from Brach C, Fraser I. Can cultural competency reduce racial and ethnic health disparities? A re-view and conceptual model. *Med Care Res Rev* 2000;57(Suppl 1):181–217.)

multidisciplinary teams in their initial decision-making, such as encouraging physicians to elicit their patient's explanatory model for their illness; (iv) supporting patients in their ability to help manage their own illnesses, such as providing support or educational groups in their own language; and (v) providing physicians, teams, and physician organizations with feedback on their performance, by tracking outcomes based on ethnicity to discover any issues caused by ethnic stereotypes.

CONCLUSION

We have discussed many guidelines and policy statements in this chapter, but many common threads run through all of them. All of them agree that cultural competence is an important goal to strive for, as many clinicians are Caucasian, and increasing numbers of patients are of ethnic minority backgrounds. Therefore, clinicians need to be able to communicate accurately with the patient, using interpreters, and having some knowledge about the culture of the patient, and their health beliefs. Clearly, training will be helpful in this regard, as well as the recruitment and retention of diverse staff to create an environment welcoming of diversity, as well as providing cultural brokers. Administrators need to understand cultural values such as time orientation and family structure when creating the policies and procedures of treatment centers, as well as provide appropriate signage, literature, access to properly trained interpreters, and allowing for community and family involvement will allow stigmatized ethnic minority patients to get treatment for their mental illness.

Finally, any mental health practitioner who wishes to utilize the principles of cultural competence has many levels of policy that he or she can quote or implement, either from federal guidelines, or professional standards and academic literature to support their use of these principles. For those practitioners not in a state that has cultural competence guidelines, there are many examples of states that have implemented their own, such as California, Massachusetts, New Jersey, and New York, that can be used to encourage their own legislatures to follow. Mental health practitioners need to be familiar with the mental health disparities academic literature and policy statements from foundations and professional organizations to empower them to act on behalf of their patients who belong to underrepresented and are subject to mental health disparities because of their racial or ethnic backgrounds and provide better access and quality of care to these vulnerable populations.

References

1. Western Interstate Commission for Higher Education (WICHE), Center for Mental Health Services/Substance Abuse and Mental Health Services Administration (CMHS/SAMHSA). *Cultural Competence Standards in Managed Care Mental Health Services: Four Underserved/ Underrepresented Racial/Ethnic Groups* (Publication No. SMA00-3457). Washington, DC: SAMHSA, 1998. Available at http://www.wiche.edu/mentalhealth/cultural_comp/ ccstoc.htm. Accessed January 28, 2008.
2. Office of Minority Health. *Assuring Cultural Competence in Health Care: Recommendations for National Standards and an Outcomes-Focused Research Agenda, 2000.* Available at http://www.omhrc.gov/clas/. Accessed January 28, 2008.
3. USDHHS. *Guidance to Federal Financial Assistance Recipients Regarding Title VI Prohibition Against National Origin Discrimination Affecting Limited English Proficient Persons, 2000.* Available at http://www.hhs.gov/ocr/lep/revisedlep.html. Accessed August 27, 2005.

4. USDHHS. *Mental Health: Culture, Race, and Ethnicity: A Supplement to Mental Health: A Report of the Surgeon General*. Rockville, MD: U.S. Department of Health and Human Services, Public Health Service, Office of the Surgeon General, 2001.

5. New Freedom Commission on Mental Health. *Achieving the Promise: Transforming Mental Health Care in America. Final Report*. USDHHS Pub. No. SMA-03-3832. Rockville, MD: United States Department of Health and Human Services, 2003.

6. NIMH. *Terms and Conditions for Recruitment of Participants in Clinical Research, 2005*. Available at http://www.nimh.nih.gov/research-funding/grants/terms-and-conditions-for-recruitment-of-participants-in-research.shtml. Accessed June 28, 2008.

7. [California] DMH (Department of Mental Health) Information Notice No: 02-03. *Addendum for Implementation Plan for Phase II Consolidation of Medi-Cal Specialty Mental Health Services—Cultural Competence Plan Requirements; 2003, superseding [California] DMH Information Notice No: 97–14. Addendum for Implementation Plan for Phase II Consolidation of Medi-Cal Specialty Mental Health Services–Cultural Competence Plan Requirements, 1997*. Available at http://www.dmh.cahwnet.gov/DMHDocs/docs/notices02/02-03_Enclosure.pdf. Accessed February 16, 2008.

8. California State Assembly. Assembly Bill No. 1195, Chapter 514: An act to amend Section 2190.1 of the Business and Professions Code, relating to physicians and surgeons. Available at http://www.healthlaw.org/library/attachment.78947. Accessed June 28, 2008.

9. Chin JL. *Cultural Competence and Health Care in Massachusetts: Where are we? Where Should We Be?* Boston: The Massachusetts Health Policy Forum, 1999. Available at http://www.forumsinstitute.org/publs/mass/issue_brief_5a.pdf. Accessed June 28, 2008.

10. Massachusetts Department of Mental Health (MDMH). *MDMH Cultural Competence Action Plan FY 2005–7, 2005*. Available at http://www.mass.gov/Eeohhs2/docs/dmh/p_cultural_action_plan.pdf. Accessed June 28, 2008.

11. LCME. *Standards for Accreditation of Medical Education Programs Leading to the M.D. Degree*. Chicago, 2007. Available at http://www.lcme.org/functions2007jun.pdf. Accessed January 28, 2008.

12. ACGME. *Program Requirements for Residency Training in Psychiatry*. Chicago, 2008. Available at http://www.acgme.org/acWebsite/downloads/RRC_progReq/400_psychiatry_07012007_u_04122008.pdf. Accessed May 30, 2008.

13. APA. *Diagnostic and Statistical Manual, Fourth Edition, Text Revision (DSM-IV-TR)*. Washington, DC: American Psychiatric Publishing, 2000.

14. APA. *Practice Guidelines for the Psychiatric Evaluation of Adults, 2nd edition* Arlington, VA: APPI, 2006.

15. Lu FG, Primm A. Mental health disparities, diversity, and cultural competence in medical student education: How psychiatry can play a role. *Acad Psychiatry* 2006;30:9–15.

16. American Psychological Association. Guidelines on multicultural education, training, research, practice, and organizational change for psychologists. *Am Psychologist* 2003;58:377–402. Available at http://www.apa.org/pi/multiculturalguidelines.pdf. Accessed February 15, 2007.

17. National Association of Social Workers (NASW) Standards for Cultural Competence in Social Work Practice, 2001. Available at http://www.socialworkers.org/sections/credentials/cultural_comp.asp. Accessed February 3, 2008.

18. ISPN. *ISPN Position Statement on Diversity, Cultural Competence, and Access to Mental Health Care, 2003*. Available at http://www.ispn-psych.org/docs/diversity-st-final.pdf. Accessed June 28, 2008.

19. Brach C, Fraser I. Can cultural competency reduce racial and ethnic health disparities? A review and conceptual model. *Med Care Res Rev* 2000;57(Suppl 1):181–217.

20. Betancourt JR. *Improving Quality and Achieving Equity: The Role of Cultural Competence in Reducing Racial and Ethnic Disparities in Health Care*. New York: The Commonwealth Fund, 2006. Available at http://www.commonwealthfund.org/publications/publications_show.htm?doc_id=413825#areaCitation. Accessed January 28, 2008.

24 The Role of Emergency Care

Benedicto Borja and Steven S. Sharfstein

There is a crisis in mental healthcare in America today. Millions of Americans lack health insurance, or, if they have health insurance, it is not adequate to meet the needs of individuals or families who experience a serious illness and its costly treatment. This is particularly true for the mentally ill and the addicted. Whether covered by private insurance or the public sector, those with insurance must confront a dysfunctional system of care that relies heavily on the emergency room, the acute inpatient bed, and community-based alternatives.

This chapter will describe the state of affairs in America today where many, if not most, Americans with an acute psychiatric illness must rely on the emergency department and the struggle to find an available acute inpatient bed. Various models of care have emerged to link the emergency department to other community-based resources, and this will be reviewed as well. Disparities in access to care will be highlighted, and one model (the Psychiatric Emergency Service) will be described as an example of how to decrease the workload on emergency departments and inpatient services, which will be of great value in the design of accessible acute care throughout the United States.

Rene Muller in his book, "Psych ER," describes an interesting case: "Kim was brought to the ER late one evening by the police on emergency petition. Kim, 38, was first hospitalized at age 26 and diagnosed with a psychotic mood disorder. It is not clear when the schizophrenia diagnosis was made. Kim told me she had stopped taking her medication because she had died in the recent fire that damaged her house, had been reborn with a new body and a new head, and so no longer needed to take the medication that her former body required (she was not injured in the fire). Kim told me that God spoke to her directly, but she did not offer any further details. I can see Europe, she said. I have very different eyes. Her answers to even the simplest questions revealed strong underlying psychotic processes. A man claiming to be Kim's boyfriend came to the ER and volunteered to escort her home. He told us he was negotiating with the insurance company on Kim's behalf for a settlement on the fire damage to her house and was making arrangements with contractors to have the repairs made. Three weeks after I discharged Kim from the ER, she was admitted to the inpatient psychiatric unit. She was admitted again 5 weeks later and 8 weeks after that, and 12 weeks after that. Clearly, she was noncompliant with treatment. During her last admission to our hospital, Kim was restarted on Clozaril. She remained grossly psychotic, delusional, and thought-disordered. The staff thought that she needed intensive, long-term inpatient treatment, and she was transferred to a state mental hospital" (1).

THE DECLINE IN STATE HOSPITAL BEDS

There has been a great deal of national discussion about the decrease in availability of inpatient beds for psychiatric patients. In Maryland, there has been the closure of several hospitals (including Crownsville State Hospital, Liberty Medical Center, and Gundry Glass) and the downsizing of beds in two other state facilities (Spring Grove Hospital and Springfield Hospital). Many patients, perhaps a million, have been discharged into communities that are ill-prepared to provide the therapeutic and rehabilitative services they need, such as halfway houses, aftercare programs, sheltered workshops, and psychosocial rehabilitation (2). With the availability of mental health services declining nationwide, psychiatric patients have become a growing presence in hospital Emergency Departments (EDs). To accommodate the influx—which may exacerbate capacity problems and distract providers from other cases—facilities are assembling psychiatric rapid response teams, designating ED space specifically, and forging community partnerships.

Although emergency rooms have existed for at least 100 years, the concept of publicly-funded psychiatric emergency services was introduced on a national level in 1963 with the Community Mental Health Act, which mandated emergency services as part of a comprehensive system of community mental healthcare. Ten years later, the Emergency Medical Systems Act provided that the ability to provide services for psychiatric emergencies was a critical component of emergency room care. The mid-1970s saw the beginning of the impact of deinstitutionalization, with EDs bearing the brunt of insufficient community services (3). The plan was that the funding for the clients would follow them into the community, but state hospitals often stayed open, consuming capital costs, and state funds remained institutionalized, locked in the hospital long after the patients had left the wards. There are today many deinstitutionalized patients who have nowhere to go to receive services that were once available in institutionalized settings. Disproportionately, these patients are African American and other minorities, poor, and disenfranchised. Maryland is an example of what is happening nationwide.

MENTAL HEALTH UTILIZATION

In the past decade, following national trends, mental health service need in the Baltimore area has increased, despite the shortage of available inpatient beds and community health programs (3). The shortage of mental health services is felt most acutely in emergency departments, which act as a barometer for community health shortages (4).

Homeless patients with mental illness are also utilizing emergency services. Bipolar disorder and schizophrenia are independently associated with an increased risk of being homeless (5). The reduced number of homeless shelters in our country, combined with the deinstitutionalization of the mentally ill who are unable to provide for themselves, means that we have an increasing number of mentally ill who are homeless (6).

Having a better therapeutic relationship with a primary care physician who collaborates with mental health professionals is associated with decreased utilization of community mental health services, including psychiatric ED visits (7). In our current healthcare environment, we have a shortage of primary care physicians and a shortage of psychiatric professionals with whom the primary care physician can collaborate. There are also other barriers that make it difficult for psychiatric patients to access services through their primary care physician.

PRIMARY CARE PSYCHIATRIC SERVICES

Many primary care physicians are deterred from treating patients with psychiatric health needs because of poor reimbursements, and they are less likely to conduct a thorough psychiatric screening because of the time constraints placed on them by payers. Many pediatricians will not provide treatment for depression because of recent warnings released by the FDA regarding the use of antidepressive medications in children. Although it is difficult to generalize, many, if not most, primary care physicians prefer not to evaluate and treat mental illness and/or addiction.

In Baltimore, whites are significantly less likely than African Americans of similar socioeconomic standing to discuss mental health concerns with a primary care physician, and both groups reported feeling uncomfortable seeking psychiatric care from a primary care provider (8).

The combination of patients' unwillingness to seek psychiatric care from primary care providers, the lack of reimbursement for providers, and decreased treatment of depression in pediatric populations means that many patients do not receive as much preventive mental health services. The lack of preventive mental health services increases the risk of emergency room visits for all patients, particularly for those suffering from schizophrenia who might have been permanently institutionalized in earlier eras (7). This adds to the burden on already-overcrowded EDs and creates an even greater need for a dedicated psychiatric space in EDs.

PROFILE

The Maryland Health Care Commission (MHCC) report on ED has found the following relative to the insurance profile of 96,413 individuals using the ED for mental health reasons (9): "When compared with overall emergency department use, a higher proportion of mental health–related visits are covered by public sector programs or have no reported insurance coverage. Of all visits with mental health related primary diagnosis in 2005, 26% had coverage under the Medicaid program and 15% were enrolled in the Medicare program; 28% reported no insurance (i.e., self-pay or no charge). For all ED visits, about 36% were covered by public sector programs (Medicaid, 18%; Medicare, 17.8%); 19% report no insurance. Although private insurance programs (including Blue Cross and commercial plans) accounted for 41% of all emergency department visits, they covered only 29% of visits for patients with diagnoses of mental health conditions in 2005." However, there has been a decrease in the number of Medicaid recipients covered by the Public Mental Health System using EDs for psychiatric reasons. Care for the uninsured population appears to be a major issue for EDs. In Maryland, with a population of 5.3 million in the year 2000, approximately 10% were uninsured individuals. In 2005, with a population of

5.6 million, approximately 14.5% were uninsured individuals. Thus, the uninsured population grew from approximately 530,000 to 810,000. As indicated previously, 28% of ED visits for mental health reason are by uninsured individuals. (The MHCC data indicate this percentage increased 3% from 2002 to 2005.) In addition, as of January 1997, individuals with drug and alcohol disabilities were no longer covered under Supplemental Security Income (SSI) or Social Security Disability Insurance (SSDI). As a result, these individuals are now uninsured and frequently utilize EDs for their healthcare.

PSYCHIATRIC READMISSION

Diagnosis of schizophrenia or schizoaffective disorder is independently associated with a greater chance of readmission after a psychiatric hospitalization. These patients are most frequently readmitted through an ED (10).

Patients suffering from schizophrenia and schizoaffective disorder were frequently confined in long-term treatment facilities prior to the closure of many state-run long-term care facilities and the reduction of state psychiatric hospital beds (11).

Patients with a previous psychiatric admission are much more likely to have a future psychiatric admission through an ED (12). There is an emergence of alternative scheduled drop-in clinics such as the Scheduled Crisis Intervention Program (SCIP) at Sheppard Pratt Hospital in Baltimore, and research is needed to show whether having scheduled community interventions can reduce the demand on psychiatric emergency departments.

EMERGENCY DEPARTMENTS EMERGE AS A DYSFUNCTIONAL MODEL OF HEALTHCARE

During the last decade, hospital EDs have emerged as de facto mental health providers as state cutbacks and declining reimbursements have forced inpatient psychiatric units to close; subsequent outpatient gridlock has rendered EDs as one of few remaining options. A study published in the February 2005 *Academic Emergency Medicine* (Hazlett et al.) provided statistical evidence of this dynamic, showing that psychiatric-related ED visits (those reflecting any of three common psychiatric ICD-9 codes) increased 15% nationwide from 3.7 million in 1992 to 4.3 million in 2002, representing 5.4% of all ED volumes. Moreover, in a national survey of 340 ED physicians, conducted by the American College of Emergency Physicians (ACEP), 67% of respondents said mental health services had declined in their community during the previous year, and 60% reported increased pressure on the frontline particularly because psychiatric patients consume provider attention, increase patient boarding, and force ambulance diversions (ACEP release, 4/27/04). Similarly, a recent analysis of 12 nationally representative communities published by the Center for Studying Health System Change cites psychiatric patient volumes as part of a "convergence. . .of pressures" currently taxing hospital EDs, restricting access to care, and increasing healthcare costs ("Rising Pressure: Hospital EDs as Barometers of the Health Care System," November 2005).

While roughly 12% of people who visit the ED for medical treatment are admitted to inpatient beds, the inpatient admission figure for people seen in the ED for psychiatric reasons is more than twice as high, and in some places exceeds 50% of people brought in for psychiatric emergency services (13). In one study that appears to be an outlier, more than 90% of the people who came to the ED for psychiatric reasons were hospitalized (14). This creates serious problems because of the scarcity of psychiatric inpatient beds, causing delay in disposition and resulting in overnight and multiple day "boarding" of patients, which is expensive and occupies emergency beds needed by other patients (15). The provision of adequate continuity of care to these patients is fundamental but usually is driven by the availability of community resources. Social services should assist in making these plans, and, at a minimum, the ED should have lists of community-based programs and, at best, linkages with several programs to ensure closer and tighter aftercare planning.

Most commentators agree that at least some people who present to EDs could be served in the community if appropriate community crisis services (including crisis housing and respite care) were more readily available. In some cases, the "fix" would be even simpler. Budget cuts in community mental health treatment have not only resulted in the loss of crisis services (16) but also in curtailment of particular medications and limitations on therapy. These, in turn, have resulted in an upsurge of visits by people in psychiatric crisis (17). Thus, EDs have become an expensive and inappropriate way of providing necessary mental health services, and the cost has been passed on to the hospital, which then passes it along to the state and insurance companies in the form of higher and unrecoverable costs.

SECONDARY UTILIZERS OF THE EMERGENCY DEPARTMENT

EDs are utilized by police, group home operators, and family members as a way to resolve conflicts perceived by these "secondary utilizers" as caused by an individual's psychiatric condition. Bringing the individual to the ED, in effect, solves the conflict for the family member, group home operator, or officer. The term "secondary utilizer" was coined in the book, *Emergency Department Treatment of Psychiatric Patients: Policy Issues and Legal Requirements*, to describe people and agencies that bring individuals to the ED because those individuals are creating problems for the persons or agencies who take the individual to the ED as a solution to their problem (for example, police remove a person from a neighborhood who is disruptive but has not actually broken any laws; group home operators resolve escalating personality conflicts between residents; or residents, staff, and exhausted family members get respite when mental health services are unavailable). Family caretakers of patients with severe and persistent mental illness have special needs as well—burnout and stress and their impact on the patient's well-being are all very important in many of these cases. Interventions with these caretakers should be attempted, and support resources in their community sought.

Secondary utilizers also include agencies such as mental health departments and state Medicaid agencies that rely on the fact that EDs are open around the clock; provide medication, testing, and disposition services; and cannot turn anyone away, unlike most providers of mental health services. As Factor and Diamond explain (18), "Often family, friends, housemates, emergency department staff, landlords, employers and police have their own views of the problems and their own needs that must be met. . .A decision to support a patient in the community may be an appropriate way to deal with the patient's crisis, but it may do little to help the family with their sense of responsibility, the landlord with his or her disturbing tenant, or the police...If the clinician understands the needs of all the people connected with the crisis, it will be easier to come up with a solution that all parties can accept. . ." A retrospective study of the use of EDs in Maine revealed that more than half of accompanied ED visits by people with psychiatric disabilities were the result of a conflict between the individual and those who accompanied him/her, and that taking the individual to the ED, in effect, "resolved" the conflict with the individual with a psychiatric disability (19).

One reason that mental health agencies and providers resort to the ED is that they know about its operations and location. On the other hand, ED staff are often unaware of mental health resources such as crisis beds, family foster care, and respite care. Hospital social workers consider "admit to inpatient bed" and "discharge to home" as the only options available to them. Oftentimes, they are not sufficiently informed about programs for clients of the mental health, substance abuse, and social service systems. The ED has become the gatekeeper in the public model of mental healthcare, the arbiter of inpatient services, and (all too often) the final drop-off point for the problem client or family member.

CREATING EMERGENCY DEPARTMENT PSYCHIATRIC SPACE

In light of a 25% increase in psychiatric ED visits since 2001, North Carolina–based Wake Forest University Baptist Medical Center is planning to construct a new, larger ED with a separate area for psychiatric patient care that includes six private, secure rooms.

Similarly, Forsyth Medical Center in North Carolina relied on a newly opened $18 million ED (featuring a designated area for mental health cases, staffed by specialized providers, and equipped with locking rooms) to absorb 4088 psychiatric ED patients during the first ten months of 2005—a 9% increase over the same period in 2004. The care of patients presenting to the University of Maryland Medical Center underwent a dramatic change with the opening of Psychiatric Emergency Services (PES) in November 2006. Prior to the implementation of PES, patients with psychiatric complaints were registered by the Emergency Department registration staff, triaged by an ED triage nurse, and then were sent to an area in the emergency department that was dedicated to the care of psychiatric patients. These patients were then evaluated by an ED resident and attending physician, and a medical screening examination was performed. Subsequently, the patient was evaluated by a psychiatry resident under the supervision of a psychiatry attending physician. The implementation of PES was geared toward decreasing the volume of the ED and providing more expedient care for psychiatric patients. The new procedure was to have the patients registered and triaged in the same way, but then the patient would be sent to the PES. There is currently a study at UMMC designed to examine several variables of patient care both before and after the implementation of PES, with the goal of determining if there are significant differences or improvements in the way that psychiatric care is now being provided.

OTHER MODELS OF CARE

Public mobile teams, traditionally operated by community mental health centers, serve the entire community and are more likely to go wherever the referral leads them without regard for ability to pay. While types of mobile crisis overlap to some extent, they also differ in terms of readiness, tactical training, equipment, and cross-training of police in mental health techniques and vice versa. Mobile teams can cover wide areas and may be particularly useful in rural communities where mental health services are distant and public transportation is lacking. What distinguishes mobile crisis from other kinds of mobile outreach is the perception of urgency surrounding the referral and the capability of the agency providing the service to respond in consistently rapid fashion.

Although it is also a form of 24-hour care, the crisis residency, in contrast to the hospital, attempts to create a normalized environment. Apartments, group and foster homes, even the client's own home have been used for this purpose. Fields and Weisman describe the acute diversion program as equivalent to voluntary hospitalization in terms of their capability (20). They have referrals from hospital emergency services on a "no refusal" basis, including suicidal, potentially violent, or psychotic clients as long as they are cooperative. Such programs operate outside hospitals but with significant numbers of full-time professional and paraprofessional staff and a part-time psychiatrist.

Assertive Community Treatment (ACT) is a service-delivery model that provides comprehensive, locally-based treatment to people with serious and persistent mental illnesses. Unlike other community-based programs, ACT is not a linkage or brokerage case-management program that connects individuals to mental health, housing, or rehabilitation agencies or services. Rather, it provides highly individualized services directly to consumers. ACT recipients receive the multidisciplinary, round-the-clock staffing of a psychiatric unit but within the comfort of their own home and community.

ACT strives to lessen or eliminate the debilitating symptoms of mental illness each individual client experiences and to minimize or prevent acute episode of the illness.

THE FUTURE

Today, 47 million Americans have no health insurance. Just who are these people? Most are not poor, for the poor have access to Medicaid—a government assistance program (21). Surprisingly, nearly one in three live in households that earn more than $50,000 a year. Most are self-employed or work for a small business. Most of them are young (41% are under the age of 25). And most do not go without insurance as a lifestyle choice—they simply cannot afford the monthly insurance premiums.

The number of inpatient psychiatric beds is not sufficient to meet the needs of our mentally ill. Primary care is not able to meet the demands of the psychiatric patient population. The lack of available community resources and the trend to reduce the number of available inpatient psychiatric beds mean that psychiatric emergency service demands will continue to grow. The crowding in today's emergency rooms means longer wait times than ever, and policy makers are trying to find ways to reduce the amount of time Americans spend waiting in EDs (22).

As Stephen Bezruchka (23), Barbara Starfield (24), and others have pointed out, the United States does very poorly when it comes to the standard measurements of health status. In fact, when compared with other developed nations, we rank about 20th or lower in such measures as life expectancy, infant mortality, and immunizations. Much of his disparity comes from the ever-widening gap in America between the rich and the poor. Bezruchka even theorizes that the wide gap itself is the reason for the differences. America has a higher percentage of people living in poverty than other developed countries. Unfortunately, too many Americans are forced to use EDs to obtain their healthcare. Many people, particularly the uninsured, lack a regular healthcare provider and have nowhere else to go. However, the EDs are the most expensive and inefficient way to deliver primary care. The ED physician usually does not know the patient, has no previous medical interaction with the patient, and is much more obliged to practice defensive medicine (i.e., more expensive, with more tests). Follow-up is incomplete and uncertain. The patient is often given a few sample pills and a prescription to take to a pharmacy only to discover that they can't afford to buy the medicine.

Emergency Departments are being stressed to the maximum. *USA Today* published a front-page story (25) about how the EDs in the United States were falling apart under the strain of too many patients. EDs are being inappropriately used for primary care in America because our system to deliver primary care is inadequate. Only in recent years has there been an increase in outpatient "urgent care" or "doc-in-the-box" clinics offering extended hours of service. But these clinics lack continuity of care. They deal only with the immediate problem.

The pressing need for an expansion of programs and services was made clear by a study showing that the mental healthcare gap between whites and minorities is growing rather than shrinking (26). Investigators (led by Benjamin Le Cook, Ph.D., M.P.H., and including Jeanne Miranda, M.D.) applied new Institute of Medicine definitions of mental healthcare disparities to data from the Medical Expenditure Panel Survey from 2001 to 2004 (27). These definitions adjust for variables that affect healthcare, such as age, gender, and health status. The team found significantly increased disparities between Hispanics and whites in mental healthcare expenditures in 2001 to 2002 and 2003 to 2004. Further analysis confirmed a trend toward a larger gap in any mental healthcare expenditures over time among both blacks and Hispanics compared with whites.

As more and more healthcare systems open PES clinics to help decrease the workload on overburdened EDs, Psychiatric Emergency Services are likely to emerge as the model for modern mental healthcare.

References

1. Muller R. *Psych ER*. London: The Analytic Press, Inc., 2003:59–62.
2. Borus JF. Deinstitutionalization of the chronically mentally ill. *N Engl J Med* 1981;305:339.
3. Bassuk EL, Apsler R. Managing the chronic patient in an acute care setting. *Psychosoc Rehabil J* 1982;6:20–21.
4. Bassuk EL, Birk AW. *Emergency Psychiatry: Concepts, Methods and Practices*. New York: Plenum Press, 1986.
5. Cooper-Patrick L, Gallo JJ, Powe NR, et al. Mental health service utilization by African Americans and Whites: the Baltimore epidemiologic catchment area follow-up. *Med Care* 1999;37(10):1034–1045.
6. O'Malley AS, Gerland AM, Pham HH, et al. Rising pressure: Hospital emergency departments as barometers of the health care system (Issue Brief). *Center Study Health System Change* 2005;101:1–4.
7. Clarke GN, Herinckx HA, Kinney RF, et al. Psychiatric hospitalizations, arrests, emergency room visits, and homelessness of clients with serious and persistent mental illness: findings from a randomized trial of two ACT programs vs. usual care. *Ment Health Serv Res* 2000;2(3):155–164.
8. Folsom DP, Hawthorne W, Lindamer L, et al. Prevalence and risk factors for homelessness and utilization of mental health services among 10,340 patients with serious mental illness in a large public mental health system. *Am J Psychiatry* 2005;162(2):370–376.

9. Craven MA, Bland R. Better practices in collaborative mental health care: An analysis of the evidence base. *Can J Psychiatry* 2006;51(6 Suppl 1):7S–72S.
10. Nutting PA, Gallagher K, Riley K, et al. Care management for depression in primary care practice: Findings from the RESPECT-depression trial. *Ann Fam Med* 2008;6(1):30–37.
11. Libby AM, Brent DA, Morrato EH, et al. Decline in treatment of pediatric depression after FDA advisory on risk of suicidality with SSRIs. *Am J Psychiatry* 2007;164(6):884–891.
12. Mackell JA, Harrison DJ, McDonnell DD. Relationship between preventative physical health care and mental health in individuals with schizophrenia: A survey of caregivers. *Ment Health Serv Res* 2005;7(4):225–228.
13. Bruffaerts R, Sabbe M, Demyttenaere K. Effects of patient and health-system characteristics on community tenure of discharged psychiatric inpatients. *Psychiatr Serv* 2004;55(6): 685–690.
14. President's New Freedom Commission on Mental Health. *Achieving the Promise: Transforming Mental Health Care in America. Final Report, July 2003.* Available at http://www.mentalhealtchcommission.gov. Accessed February 6, 2008.
15. Gustafson DH, Sainfort F, Johnson SW, et al. Measuring quality of care in psychiatric: Construction and evaluation of a Bayesian index (Abstract). *Health Serv Res* 1993;28: 131–158.
16. Stefan S. *Emergency Department Treatment of the Psychiatric Patient: Policy Issues and Legal Requirements.* London: Oxford University Press, 2006:30.
17. Maryland State Hospital Association. The Emergency Room Crunch. *Health Matters* 2006:1.
18. American College of Emergency Physicians. Emergency Departments. *See Dramatic Increase in People with Mental Illness—Emergency Physicians Cite State Health Care Budget Cuts as Root of Problem.* April 27, 2004. Available at http:www.acep.org/webportal/Newsroom/NR/general/2004/Emergency Departments. Accessed February 8, 2008.
19. Factor RM, Diamond RJ. Emergency psychiatry and crisis resolution. In: Vaccarro JV, Clark GH Jr, eds. *Practicing Psychiatry in the Community: A Manual.* Washington, D.C.: American Psychiatric Press, 1996.
20. Gustafson DH, Sainfort F, Johnson SW, et al. Measuring quality of care in psychiatric emergencies: Construction and evaluation of a Bayesian index (Abstract). *Health Svc Res* 1993;28:131–158.
21. Weisman G. Crisis-oriented residential treatment as an alternative to hospitalization. *Hosp Comm Psychiatry* 1985;36(12):1302–1305.
22. Cato Institute. *What Bush's Healthcare Plan Will Do.* Available at http://www.cato.org/pub.
23. Wilper AP, Woolhandler S, Lasser KE, et al. Waits to see an emergency department physician: U.S. trends and predictors, 1997–2004. *Health Affairs (Millwood)* 2008;27(2): w84–w95.
24. Bezruchka S. Is our society making you sick? *Newsweek,* February 26, 2001:14.
25. Starfield B. Is U.S. health care really the best in the world? *JAMA* 2000;284(4)483–485.
26. Emergency Care Safety Net Unraveling. *U.S.A. Today,* February 4–6, 2000.
27. Frei R. Studies elucidate complexity of delivering mental health care to minorities. *American Psychiatric News.* 2008:1(6).
28. LeCook BL, Miranda J. Medical expenditure panel survey. *Psychiatr Serv* 2007;58: 1533–1540.

25 The Role of Providers

Rodrigo A. Muñoz and Harold Eist

THERE ARE DISPARITIES IN HEALTH

Peter and Joe were classmates in Primary School. In the second grade classroom picture, they could have been taken for each other. Their homes were not far from each other, but far enough to establish a difference in health. Peter's family received medical care close to University Hospital, given by certified doctors affiliated with the largest medical group in town. Peter got all his vaccines, had regular follow-up visits with his pediatrician, saw him for most of his medical care, and knew that he would have medical attention when needed. Joe's mother would take him to the distant emergency department when there was no alternative, which was often, never thought of paying attention to vaccines or follow-up visits, and never knew who would see Joe if they ventured into the hospital. Quite often the treatments they got were long conversations with other people waiting without hope for long hours in the emergency department.

Peter and his family belonged to a working health system. Joe and his family belonged to no system. Peter and his family were conversant with doctors, medical insurance, hospitals, and help. Joe and his family had no organized medical care, and no hope of obtaining it. For that matter, Joe's family had never had a serious conversation about medical needs and the expenses associated with them. Even if they had, spending money in healthcare we definitely not a priority for Joe's family.

The differences between Peter and Joe are magnified in the country, so that the best medicine tends to go to Peter and others like him, and the worst or no medicine tends to go to Joe. On Peter's company, one easily finds the more affluent, the better educated, those with health insurance, and those who live in the better section of town. Joe is accompanied by those without resources, the less educated, the uninsured, the denizens of the less prosperous areas of town, and most of the minorities.

For all we know, when it comes to healthcare, Peter and Joe might as well live in very different countries. Joe's country belongs to the nonwhite country where care is difficult to obtain.

Blustein (1) presents very telling findings. Because healthcare delivery is substantially segregated by race/ethnicity, evidence from hospitals, nursing homes, and physicians' offices suggests that minority patients do not fair as well as others. For example, a study of Medicare beneficiaries hospitalized with myocardial infarction in 1994 and 1995 showed that the majority of facilities in the United States admitted no black patients during that period; 85% of all black acute myocardial infarction patients were admitted to only 1000 of 4690 acute care hospitals nationwide. Two-thirds of black residents in nursing homes are in 10% of the homes in the nation. 80% of all primary care visits by black Medicare beneficiaries are made to only 22% of physicians.

Hospitals and other centers of care are not easily accessible to minorities; their doctors may not have privileges in the key hospitals, and many minorities do not have easy access even to the emergency department.

Minority patients often rely on government insurance for their care. This means they are often not welcome in the hospitals, or their stay is reduced. Their care may be limited to the services allowed by Medicaid or Medicare, which often prevents proper treatment and follow-up. Because of growing budgetary restrictions, facilities that rely on government insurance end up curtailing care to the minorities. National Association of Public Hospital and Health Systems (NAPH) member institutions had an average operating margin of 1.2% in 2004 compared with an average operating margin of 5.2% for hospitals nationwide.

DISPARITIES LEAD TO DIFFERENT SYSTEMS OF CARE

Peter's mother had access to the medical diaries of her family, kept one for each of her children, and encouraged them to maintain them current. She knew that obesity, high blood pressure, and arthritis were common in relatives older than 50 years. There had been cases of diabetes and at least one of Alzheimer's disease.

In cooperation with his pediatrician and later with his family physician, Peter watched his diet, his weight, his blood sugar and cholesterol, and early in life decided to exercise regularly, not to smoke, drink only occasionally, and maintain a methodic life style. At 60 years of age, he was free of symptoms, had a Medical Savings Account, substantial savings in case of a medical emergency, and a life ahead of him.

Joe's contacts with healthcare during his early life were exclusively through the emergency rooms, for repair of broken bones in motorcycle accidents. John grew up smoking and drinking often. He did not have any worry about health until he was 42 years of age and underwent a medical examination for a new job. Much to his surprise, he was told he was grossly overweight, and had high blood pressure, high cholesterol and elevated sugar. Though initially impressed with these findings, Joe promised to check them up again, and progressively forgot them.

Joe was 48 years old and was at his usual work as a tool maker when he suddenly experienced severe pain chest and collapsed. He was taken to the Emergency Department of City Hospital. The doctors there told him he had had a myocardial infarction, and admitted him for 3 days. The cardiac catheterization showed coronary artery disease. Joe left the hospital with numerous prescriptions, an appointment with the heart surgeon and the cardiologist, and an enormous desire never to see a hospital again. As his life resumed its usual pace, Joe gradually forgot about the medications and the appointments.

By age 60 years, Peter had excellent health and had periodic check-ups by his family physician. By age 60 years, Joe had very poor health and numerous appointments for treatment of his obesity, high blood pressure, high cholesterol, and complications of diabetes. He was almost blind, was facing the amputation of one leg, and had lived on disability for several years.

Other than for annual office visits for checkups, Pete's relationships with physicians were social. His knowledge about medicine came from radio, television, newspapers, and magazines. His opinion was that the country had the best system of care, the most advances and the best attention for all.

Joe had tried to pay his medical bills, and developed an enormous debt before he qualified for Medicare because of his disabilities. To save money, he joined a Medicare HMO, and soon found himself going from office to office, often having to see a different physician, often misunderstanding prescriptions and recommendations for care, and often feeling as if his wellbeing did not count to anyone. He felt depressed, pessimistic, morose, and regularly expecting the worst from any of the professionals who saw him. He did not believe that any of them even remembered his name.

JOE'S DISTRESSES

Joe and many others, frequently those receiving care through government programs, have minimal say on their care, but face the following problems (2):

In more than 1000 audiotaped visits with 124 physicians, patients participated in medical decisions only 9% of the time.

When asked to repeat the physician's instructions, the patients responded incorrectly 47% of the time.

In a 2004 survey, 41% of the patients receiving regular prescriptions reported that their physicians had not reviewed their medications and had not explained side effects.

One study found that fewer than half of primary care physicians were provided information about the discharge plans and medications of their recently hospitalized patients.

In almost 33% of emergency department visits studied, information that included medical history and laboratory tests was absent.

A study by 122 pediatricians found that no information was sent to the specialist in 49% of referrals. The referring physicians received information from the specialist 55% of the time.

Adults with chronic illness who had seen a physician in the previous 2 years reported that test results or medical records were not available at the time of a scheduled visit or the physician ordered duplicate tests 22% of the time when seeing one physician and 43% of the time when seeing four or more physicians.

These problems are not equally distributed among patients. Pete, as an educated social leader, belongs to several organizations that are actively supporting community programs for well-being and sees several physicians at neighborhood gatherings and at meetings for the different causes he sponsors. The local none for profit hospital has included Pete in the Committee for Development of New Programs. He is not using services at this moment, but Pete is quite well informed about his medical system.

Though a frequent user of medical services, Joe is the opposite: nothing is stable or certain in his relationships with professionals and hospitals. His history, divided into too many pieces, rests in the care of too many facilities. His contacts with physicians, usually through Emergency Departments, are limited and transient. At a time when the experts talk of giving every patient a "medical home," Joe is a partial tenant at several medical shelters chosen by chance. Even if Pete and Joe had the same illnesses and the same diagnoses, one could predict that Joe would have more of the problems mentioned above than Pete. We could predict that Joe will die younger than Pete, from more illnesses, after more treatments and more use of facilities at a higher cost.

THE MEDICAL WORLD THAT WAS

Toward the mid-20th century there was the beginning of a profound transformation in the medical world. Before then, physicians saw their patients at their offices, usually consisting of one physician, a nurse or medical assistant, and a receptionist. Payment for the visit was usually in cash, and the cost of the prescription was usually within the finances of the patient. In this arrangement, Pete and Joe would perhaps have had an equal chance of receiving equal treatment, and the doctor would become aware very early of the difficulty he would have in obtaining Joe's compliance.

Insurance for medical expenses, intervention by employers, and the growth of medical facilities changed it all.

The original insurance companies offered to indemnify the patient for medical expenses. Insurance for medical bills was easily available and inexpensive. In 1942, during a period of price and wage control, the federal government started offering tax incentives to employers who offered health insurance. This arrangement grew immensely, to the point that employers eventually became the "providers" of healthcare to employees through the health insurances. In one of his last acts as President, Richard Nixon signed the papers creating the Health Maintenance Organizations, and the demise of patient centered medicine in many places.

While the insurance strategies for health and the employer interventions were growing, the small family practices and the small community hospital began to disappear, replaced by large medical groups and huge medical complexes. As time went by, the patient got excluded from the large money transactions among the newly appointed "providers" of health services: insurance companies, employers, and large medical centers. A wealthier and very powerful "provider" joined them very rapidly: the so called "Pharma," the pharmaceutical companies. These "providers" started to negotiate among themselves, and the medical field acquired a recognizable commercial atmosphere. Medical care became a commodity.

CONFUSION, MISDIRECTION, AND FAILURE

Emmanuel and Fuchs (3) write "Employers do not bear the cost of employment-based insurance; workers and households pay for health insurance through lower wages and higher prices." Employers also get tax benefits worth hundreds of millions of dollars as compensation for offering insurance to the employees. Their negotiations with insurance companies, and directly or indirectly with hospitals and pharmaceutical companies give them major advantages usually not available to the patient trying to pay directly for his health benefits. Employees surrender any pretension of freedom of choice when they accept that their health insurance be controlled by their employers. The employers define the benefits, choose the plan to manage the benefits, and collect the funds to pay the health plan. If one adds the progressively increasing deductibles and co-payments, the restrictions in drug formularies, and the persistent efforts by insurance companies to deny benefits, it becomes progressively clear that employers offer only partial help, and this help decreases constantly. The enormous discrepancies between corporate profits and average hourly earnings for workers are related to the bizarre arrangement by which the employer benefits from providing health insurances to his employees. In the last 30 years premiums have increased by about 300% after adjustment for inflation, corporate profits have had increases of 200% after taxes; and wages in private, non-agricultural industries have been stagnant.

It has become customary to announce on TV and in the press the availability of services often included in Medicare. That's the case with scooters for patients who have lost the use of their lower extremities. The message is clear "You won't have to pay a cent." Government has no source of funds other than taxes or borrowing to pay for healthcare. A more factual announcement would indicate that the federal government is willing to use tax money to buy the scooter.

Medicare and Medical cover a large number or patients who are not employed and generally have no other sources of healthcare funds. These programs are persistently under pressure. One strategy to try to do more with less money is by curtailing payments to the gradually smaller number of professionals that accept their reimbursement. The result is that the programs are meaningless for many who qualify for them, because the patient cannot find a professional who is willing to accept deeply discounted fees.

"PROVIDERS" AND THE DENIAL OF PAYMENT FOR HEALTHCARE SERVICES

Imagine for a moment that the absurd employer participation in healthcare payments existed in other aspects of the employee's life:

What if the employees had to consult with the employer to choose their children's schools?

What if the employees had to choose their house and their neighborhood from a list provided by the employer?

What if the employees had to buy their transportation from a catalogue created by the employer?

What if the employees had to get their clothes from a selection determined by the employer?

If employees would not tolerate these invasions of their privacy, what is different about healthcare financing?

Most employees first enter agreements about healthcare financing with their employers when they are young, do not expect to be sick, do not want to spend money or time in healthcare, and have less knowledge about the key issues. Most people do not have a budget for healthcare. When they get sick, they often find that the word "insurance" has no meaning, and they are at the mercy of the employers and the insurance companies.

PETER AND JOE AS NONCOMBATANTS IN THE HEALTH FINANCING WARS

Peter and his friends have often talked about the huge number, 47 million of Americans, who lack health insurance. His information from attending meetings at the community hospital, suggests that these people get care in the emergency department. He knows this is not optional, not even always effective or helpful, but Pete is proud that the hospital, representing the community, tries to help those who otherwise would die. Personally, he and his friends have no complaints, mostly because they are generally healthy.

Joe's personal experience has been the opposite. By now he has almost forgotten the days when he could make his own appointments with physicians, get attention, buy medications, and feel some relief.

Joe, as a young person, never cared to ask about the health history of his family. If he had, he would have learned that diabetes was common; most relatives gained much weight early in life, and most died young, often from heat conditions. When he first heard about his having high blood sugar, high blood pressure and excessive weight, it didn't occur to him that he was suffering several severe and chronic illnesses that would mar and shorten his life.

His first emergency visit to a hospital scared Joe, but not enough to change his life style, or even lead him to visit a physician regularly, take medication, or at least consider the implications regarding his future life.

Changes in jobs, changes in insurance coverage, illness and disability, progressively led Joe to being uninsured and uninsurable.

In his early fifties, Joe started to receive Medicare benefits, which he thought would provide adequate support for his medical needs. A casual patient who would miss appointments often, who never really paid attention to his medications schedule, who was drinking much and smoking constantly while gaining excessive way, Joe never lasted long in any Medicare program. His treatment continued to be mostly on an emergency basis, and primarily to procure treatment for the problem of the day. Mostly for the entertainment of his few friends, Joe was very vocal in his criticism of doctors, medications, hospitals, and treatments.

WHERE ARE WE NOW?

For about 4 decades there has been a building consensus that there is a crisis in healthcare financing in the United States.

The supporting evidence is quite clear:

The number of the uninsured has been increasing to 47 million people (4).

Since the year 2000 healthcare costs have increased from $1.4 million to $2.1 million.

Employer-sponsored insurance covers fewer employees for fewer services, with increasing copayments and deductibles. The expenses associated with employer-provided insurance lead to lower levels of coverage and higher levels of uninsurance: "1% (health insurance) premium increase results in a net increase in uninsured of 164,000 people" (4).

Government-provided insurance covers almost half the population, but this coverage is increasingly partial and undependable. Government policies regarding federal taxes, State guarantee issues, mandates for specific services, income eligibility, and care for children make government insurance unpredictable and unreliable.

The picture presented by the current combination of employer sponsored insurance and government financed programs is not encouraging: We have the most expensive health financing nonsystem in the world, providing incomplete services to large sectors of the population and leaving behind as many as 47 million people.

We may ask: How these very weak arrangements are kept alive?

1. They are supported in part by "a shifting patchwork of funds from Medicaid, the State Children's Health Insurance Program (SCHIP), the federal disproportionate share program, tax levies, foundation grants, state appropriations, commercial payers, and other sources" (5).

2. They are organized so that people like Joe, with many medical needs, can be kept out of the system. Joe may go many times to different emergency departments; receive appointments he will not keep, and prescriptions he won't fill. He will go home to complain again until a new emergency starts the same sequence again. If he ever made an effort to fill the prescriptions or to see the specialists, he would find it close to impossible to pay for all his medications or to set regular appointments for follow-up.

FORCES AGAINST CHANGE

For many years many voices, sometimes very loudly, have demanded that the current ineffective and very expensive accommodations for healthcare finance be changed. There are reasons for the current inertia:

1. The people who believe health problems are not their concern. They are healthy at the moment, are not paying attention to their ailments, or may be suffering serious and even lethal diseases that may not manifest themselves in many months or years.
2. The businesses that complain about the effects of employer-sponsored insurance but move toward new accommodations within the same plans instead of drastic changes. General Motors claims that it spends more in health than in metal, but has not come up with a plan that would permit it to compete more effectively in the area of health with manufacturers from Japan.
3. The large number of intermediaries that today is part of every transaction in healthcare. They are likely to see a threat in the simplification of the convoluted web of "providers" they have created, nourished, and enhanced.
4. The disillusionment of people like Joe who have the most need but are the least likely to obtain adequate services.
5. The incredible growth of administration webs that nourish the growth of the health enterprises but not necessarily the attempts to provide services to patients.
6. The powerful for profit corporations that have emerged to siphon resources from the care of patients in the name of centralization and coordination.

An examination of these factors would suggest that reform is thwarted by commercial and financial considerations that militate against the care of patients.

TAKING CHARGE

Will the American public challenge and change the current deplorable situation in healthcare finance? The challenge is not likely to come from employers, insurance companies, and the many intermediaries and administrators that are profiting from current arrangements. The challenge has to come from an educated public prepared to give credence to the following fact:

1. Perhaps only 20% of the people incur significant medical expenses at any given time. The other 80% cannot neglect themselves thinking that they will not have to face medical expenses. Health is everyone's business, and proper medical care starts with good prevention, healthy habits, and proper knowledge of the health

system. While still healthy, everyone should be aware of medical care and medical expenses. This is a personal responsibility, not likely to be successfully delegated to employers or insurance companies.
2. Though large medical expenses are not every day's experience, everyone has to be prepared for them. This requires **catastrophic insurance**, which is not expensive and offers protection when the worst strikes.
3. Most noncatastrophic medical expenses should be individually covered. Health Savings Accounts permit to save tax free moneys for these expenses. As in any other field of investments, savings in good times give the best chances when facing bad times.
4. Special consideration has to be given to the indigent, the chronically ill, and others whose condition or situations prevent them from participating in the health financing programs with their own funds.
5. Employers and insurance companies, including "healthcare plans," should no longer control medical services.

GETTING RID OF MULTIPLE "PROVIDERS"

Change in healthcare financing cannot be avoided, among other reasons, because there are so many people who can not pay for medical services, because many who get services are dissatisfied by the illogical limitations imposed by insurance companies, because the exorbitant budgets for health finances are misspent in administration, marketing, and other unnecessary expenses, and because the American public is finally coming to realize that medical services are controlled by a voracious and empty monster.

Change will not come from the health plans, the insurance companies, or the employers. They are not feeling enough pain, and still expect excessive financial benefits, power, and continued control on the employees.

Change will come when the grievances of mistreated patients, physicians, and other affected by the multiple health intermediaries will convince an indifferent public that the whole community faces a growing and lethal danger.

LET'S TALK FIRST ABOUT INSURANCE

This word is increasingly a misnomer when applied to health finance. Insurance companies are increasing their costs beyond the reach of many; offer fewer services; and often deny precisely the services that the patient needs.

Under current conditions, the insurance companies apply arbitrary rules directed at denying services, more often for those who need them the most.

A prescription for change includes at least the following:

1. **Reduce or eliminate capitation** as a former of reimbursement. Capitation, a flawed idea has never got any wide acceptance and is the mother of many injustices.
2. Reconnect consumers to **the cost of their day to day healthcare**. Insurance companies, by offering first dollar insurance coverage, have distorted the supply of services, so that many people ended up covered mostly for services they do not use, and not for those they badly need.

3. **Empower consumers** to discover the cost of healthcare services in advance of consumption.
4. Provide **full tax deductibility** for healthcare expenses. This is a point of fairness: give everybody the same advantages that employers have and employees **should** have.
5. Encourage **employer-defined contributions** as opposed to employer-defined benefits. The employees should know what money they get and should participate in deciding how to use it.
6. Promote **private ownership** of all health insurance policies.
7. Support mandatory, community-rated, **catastrophic health insurance**.
8. Require **adequate funding** mechanisms for the provision of government-provided health services.

EMPLOYERS: AMA

Since the early 1990s, the American Medical Association's (AMA) Council on Medical Services started to work on proposals that would change AMA policies and stop any support of employer-provided insurance. The reasons are clear: every individual should choose, buy, and independently use his health insurance; there is no clear fit between the employer's goals and the employee's needs; employer-sponsored insurance is subsidized by the employer but owned by the employer; employer's sponsored insurance promotes conditions of servitude, because aggrieved employee may not change jobs out of fear of losing their health insurance; finally, employer-sponsored insurance is a historical aberration that must be eliminated in the name of fairness.

The proposals of the Council on Medical Services against employer sponsored insurance have become policies of the AMA (6) and have given much support to the movement for alternative medical coverage plans, one of them, the Health Savings Account.

HEALTH SAVINGS ACCOUNTS

This form of protection became available in California at a time when health insurance was skyrocketing. Many physicians and others bought catastrophic insurance and started a savings account. Most of them were like Peter: they knew and tried to prevent their health risk. They also knew that money that would have gone before to an insurance company was now theirs. As time has gone by, some have started to see the savings account also as a source of protection in their retirement.

We have to assume that as young people, Pete and Joe would not have heard of Health Savings Accounts (HSAs) even if they had existed then, which they did not. Nevertheless, let's imagine that they did, and an expert in HSAs talked them into entering the HAS program.

Pete would probably have in the bank in excess of $100,000 in the HSA. Now that he is older than 65 years, he can spend the money as he wishes, without tax penalty. He has protected his health and profited from his planning.

Joe would have been much more difficult to predict. We assume that he obtained the HSA when he was in his late 20s and kept the savings account while he was working, for more than 20 years. We had to assume that he had much to think when he started getting money from the bank in his forties, and his illnesses gave every sign of becoming chronic. We believe he had more of a chance to keep appointments, listen to the physicians and take the medications, if he was clearly aware that his illnesses where increasingly expenses and draining his funds. Much research has found that even in the presence of chronic illness, very high expenses only occur for short periods. With good cooperation and good care, Joe might still have a savings account. Even better, he would have been likely to earn more and have less disability.

CONCLUSION

"Providers" are a word used by the health industry to deceive physicians and patients. The APA has wisely proposed the elimination of this word in its publications. This article gives reasons to eliminate it from any planning health services.

References
1. Blustein J. Who is accountable for racial equity in health care? *JAMA* 2008;299:814–816.
2. Bodenheimer T. Coordinating care: A perilous journey through the health system. *N Engl J Med* 2008;358:1064–1071.
3. Emmanuel EJ, FuchsVR. Who really pays for health care? *JAMA* 2008;299:1057–1059.
4. Emmanuel EJ: The cost-coverage trade-off. *JAMA* 2008;299:947–949.
5. Brown LD. The amazing noncollapsing US health care system: Is reform finally at hand? *N Engl J Med* 2008;358:325–327.
6. Palmisano DJ, Emmons DW, Wozniak GD: Expanding insurance coverage through tax credits, consumer choice, and market enhancements. *JAMA* 2004;291:2237–2256.

26 The Role of Quality Care

John M. Oldham and John S. McIntyre

Quality of care was described by Donabedian (1) more than a quarter century ago as being determined by the structure of care, clinical processes of care, and the outcome of care. Initial efforts at examining quality focused on the structure of care which is the easiest to measure. In 1917, the recently formed American College of Surgeons (ACS) published a document called Minimum Standards for Hospitals (2). This effort expanded over the next several decades and in 1951 the ACS, joined by the American Medical Association (AMA), the American College of Physicians (ACP), and other entities, formed the Joint Commission on Accreditation of Hospitals (currently designated as the Joint Commission [JC]). Over the past several decades, this process has expanded to include outpatient facilities and entities providing treatment of persons with mental illnesses, substance abuse, developmental disabilities, and long-term care. Gradually, the focus for the Joint Commission and quality improvement efforts in general has shifted from the structure of care to clinical process and outcomes. Current programs of JC focusing on behavioral health are described below.

Another private sector review and accrediting organization is the National Committee for Quality Assurance (NCQA), founded in 1990. The major focuses of NCQA's reviews are managed care organizations although more recently physician recognition programs have been developed. Using Health Care Effectiveness Data and Information Sets (HEDIS) and other tools NCQA reviews and provides a seal of approval to those entities that meet the identified criteria. Six basic features of a valid review process have been defined: (i) evidence-based criteria, (ii) current evidence, (iii) flexible criteria, (iv) shared criteria, (v) valid monitors, and (vi) professional reviewers (3).

The Institute of Medicine (IOM), in its seminal report "To Err is Human: Building a Safer Health System," precipitated many efforts, public and private, to improve the safety of healthcare and in general to improve the quality of care (4). A second IOM report in 2001, "Crossing the Quality Chasm: A New Health System for the 21st Century," identified issues and processes that impeded high-quality healthcare, enumerated six aims of high-quality care and described recommendations to guide the redesign of healthcare (5). The six aims of high-quality healthcare identified in this IOM report are that it be safe, effective, patient-centered, timely, efficient, and equitable. This report also describes "Ten Rules to Guide the Redesign of Health Care":

1. Care based on continuous healing relationships
2. Customization based on patient needs and values
3. The patient as the source of control

4. Shared knowledge and the free flow of information
5. Evidence-based decision-making
6. Safety as a system property
7. The need for transparency
8. Anticipation of needs
9. Continuous decrease in waste
10. Cooperation among clinicians.

A subsequent IOM report in 2004, "Improving the Quality of Health Care for Mental and Substance Use Conditions," considers the special features of the efforts to improve the quality of healthcare for patients who have mental illnesses and/or substance use disorders (6).

The IOM defines high-quality healthcare as "the degree to which healthcare services for individuals and populations increase the likelihood of desired health outcomes and are consistent with current professional knowledge" (7). Increasingly, evidence-based practices are identified as a core component of high-quality care. In the 2001 IOM report identified above, evidence-based practices are defined as combining the best research evidence, clinical judgment, and patient values. Evidence-based clinical practice guidelines have been widely adopted by most medical specialty organizations, as standards to guide such high-quality healthcare. Many systems of care and governmental entities have also promulgated guidelines. In the early 1990s, the federal government's Agency for Health Care Policy and Research (AHCPR) launched an ambitious guideline development project. Several guidelines were developed including a guideline for the Treatment of Major Depression in Primary Care (8). The AHCPR project was later modified and under its successor, the Agency for Healthcare Research and Quality (AHRQ), grants are provided to institutions that develop the evidence base to be used in guideline development. AHRQ has maintained on its website a Guideline Clearinghouse, which is a helpful reference source.

Several initiatives have developed to facilitate the use of screening instruments in both specialty care and primary care. For example, the National Quality Forum (NQF), in a report entitled "Integrating Behavioral Healthcare Performance Measures throughout Healthcare," identified screening for depression in general acute care and in primary care as one of several "priorities for immediate action" (9). One method to screen for depression that has been widely implemented is the Patient Health Questionnaire–9 Item (PHQ-9), along with a briefer two-question screen (PHQ-2) (10).

In psychiatry, the stage had been set for the creation of practice guidelines by the development of a criteria-based nomenclature, the *Diagnostic and Statistical Manual of Mental Disorders* (DSM). This diagnostic system brought clarity and increased reliability to psychiatric diagnoses and greatly aided psychiatric research. In the early 1990s, the American Psychiatric Association (APA) recognized the imperative to develop evidence-based practice guidelines (11). A transparent process of guideline development was developed and is available for review (12). A Steering Committee, which oversees the project, chooses topics for guidelines based on the degree of public importance, relevance to psychiatric practice, and the availability of data to drive the guideline recommendations. After a topic is chosen, a work group of recognized research and clinical experts is appointed. The work group conducts a search and evidence tables are created. An iterative process of drafts ensues (a total of some 800 individuals and organizations review a draft) and finally the guideline is considered and approved by the APA Assembly and Board of Trustees. A timetable for review and revision is established.

Using this process, APA has published seventeen guidelines since 1993 and six of these guidelines have been revised.

National surveys, however, indicate the need for substantial improvement in the quality of care including the increased use of evidence-based practices (7). In the 2004 IOM report described above, the IOM reviewed 21 studies of the use of clinical practice guidelines in treatment of patients with psychiatric or substance use disorders, finding that only 24% of these studies documented adequate adherence to specific guideline recommendations (6). To increase the use of practice guidelines by clinicians, a parallel initiative was also implemented by the APA, to develop a framework for clinically derived quality indicators, also referred to as performance measures, in psychiatry (13). As these projects moved forward, it became clear that specific quality indicators should be developed to be used to measure adherence to evidence-based practice guidelines. An example of this partnership is the development of quality indicators to measure the degree to which practitioners adhere to the recommendations of the APA practice guideline for the treatment of patients with bipolar disorder. Duffy and colleagues (14) described the development of a set of guideline-derived quality indicators to assess the quality of treatment of patients with bipolar disorder. Embedded within such efforts are concerns about whether indicators should be applied retrospectively to existing medical records or prospectively in the ongoing care of patients, and the cost, burden, and estimated validity of each approach.

A national momentum has been steadily building, emphasizing the use of performance measurement systems to assess the quality of healthcare. One example of this trend is the remarkable growth of the Physicians Consortium for Performance Improvement (PCPI), an AMA-sponsored organization with a broad multispecialty membership (15); the APA has participated in the PCPI since its inception and has a permanent seat on its Executive Committee. The PCPI was established to develop performance measures "by physicians for physicians" and its performance measure sets have been increasingly recognized as the "gold standard." Other organizations have developed performance measurement systems that have been widely implemented (e.g., the Veterans Administration [VA]) or are in pilot phases of development (e.g., Centers for Medicaid and Medicare Services [CMS], JC). A new "buzz word" has become popular, i.e., the importance of "harmonization" of the various measure sets with each other so that they use similar methodology and technical standards. In the context of this groundswell of attention to performance measurement, the National Quality Forum (NQF) has assumed a central and prominent role, as a national organization "vetting" performance measures to assure that they meet consistent standards and are derived from a scientifically sound evidence base. NQF is a voluntary standards-setting organization defined in the National Technology Transfer and Advancement Act of 1995 and in the Office of Management and Budget Circular A-119, where the formal process by which NQF achieves consensus on standards that it endorses is outlined (16). Performance measures can be submitted to NQF, in accordance with its published application timetable; measures approved by NQF are generally considered validated for widespread testing, a step facilitated by the Ambulatory Quality Alliance (AQA) and by other organizations (17).

The AQA was established in 2004 by the American Academy of Family Physicians, ACP, American Health Insurance Plans and AHRQ. The AQA has expanded and currently is a very active alliance of physician organizations, consumers, insurance plans, payers, and government agencies. Membership in the AQA is free, and the goal of the AQA is to facilitate physician-level performance measurement, data aggregation, and data reporting. The APA is a member of the AQA; collaborative pilot projects are underway, involving AHRQ, CMS, and other organizations.

In the hospital world, the Joint Commission has spearheaded a project referred to as the Hospital Based Inpatient Psychiatric Services (HBIPS) Core Measure Set, which has developed an initial set of performance measures now in pilot implementation:

1. Assessment of risk, substance abuse, trauma, and patient strengths;
2. Hours of restraint use;
3. Hours of seclusion use;
4. Documentation of adequate clinical rationale for maintaining patients on two or more antipsychotic medications after hospital discharge; and
5. Provision of discharge and aftercare recommendations to community providers after hospital discharge.

The Joint Commission has recently published a white paper entitled "Health Care at the Crossroads: Development of a National Performance Measurement Data Strategy," which calls for three major initiatives (18):

1. Create the framework for a national performance measurement system
2. Build a data highway to support the exchange of health information, and
3. Engage stakeholders and engender trust

A key element in any performance measurement system is the increased use of the Electronic Health Record (EHR). EHRs can facilitate quality improvement efforts as well as promote standardization of care, reduce errors, increase efficiency, and reduce costs. The VA has a single electronic health record system called VistA, which is achieving several of these goals. A major issue in the increased use of EHRs, especially in the area of behavioral health, is privacy concerns. The 1996 Health Insurance Portability and Accountability Act (HIPAA) has several mandates concerning access, storage, and transmittal of EHRs. Another key issue in the use of EHRs is the compatibility of multiple systems that now exist — "interoperability." There are several public and private entities that are addressing these issues (19).

As organizational participation in performance measurement activities proliferates, it is enormously challenging to coordinate efforts, minimize physician and provider burden, and safeguard against redundancy and unintended consequences. Two particular dimensions of the performance measurement movement will be highlighted here, which have the potential to affect practicing physicians: pay-for-performance (P4P) and maintenance of certification (MOC).

PAY-FOR-PERFORMANCE

In pay-for-performance programs providers are incentivized for meeting preestablished targets in the delivery of healthcare services. Over the past decade there has been a rapid growth in the development of such programs, public and private. A concern of practitioners is that such programs will focus on reducing costs and not on improving quality. The AMA has developed a set of principles and guidelines that should be met by such programs. The five AMA overarching principles are that P4P programs should be based on voluntary participation, data accuracy must be achieved, the incentives should be positive, the program should foster the patient-physician relationship and the guidelines for the program must be sufficiently detailed. An example of a successful P4P program for behavioral healthcare practitioners is one implemented by Anthem Blue Cross and Blue Shield of Virginia. In a review of this program, Pelonero and Johnson noted that important issues in the development of measures for the project included "application of the measures to all disciplines, feasible data collection processes for providers, creation of clinically meaningful and fair measures, and selection of measures with large baseline variability" (20). P4P programs have also been developed in other countries. In the United Kingdom, as part of the National Health Service, there is a Quality and Outcomes Financial program (QOF).

MAINTENANCE OF CERTIFICATION

Board certification in psychiatry, as in most medical specialties, has been restructured from its original practice of issuing lifelong specialty certification, to issuing limited certification for a specified period (usually 10 years), with a series of required steps to become re-certified. This ongoing process is generally referred to as Maintenance of Certification. The American Board of Psychiatry and Neurology has implemented a set of requirements that are being phased in, which include a "performance in practice" (PIP) component. Candidates for recertification will eventually be required to complete three PIP units, which include a requirement to demonstrate documented use of evidence-based best practices or practice guidelines in their patient care. Sample tools that could be used by psychiatrists to document the use of the American Psychiatric Association's Practice Guideline for the Treatment of Patients with Major Depressive Disorder, to meet the PIP requirement for MOC, have been described in a recent report by Fochtmann et al (21).

As noted in the IOM report referenced above, an essential aspect of quality programs is that they be patient centered. Although this appears to be self-evident, closer examination of many existing programs suggests that this is often not the case. Several studies have noted that patients and staff frequently have different priorities in issues that are to be the focus of treatment (22). Treatment plans that are actually developed by patients and staff working collaboratively, and whose language reflects collaboration, are central to these efforts. Being patient centered necessitates that issues driven by race and culture be addressed. In the report *Mental Health: Culture, Race and Ethnicity, A Supplement to Mental Health: A Report of the Surgeon General*, striking disparities are identified in mental health services for racial and ethnic minority populations (23). The report notes that these populations.

Are less likely to have access to available mental health services;
Are less likely to receive needed mental healthcare;
Often receive poorer quality care; and
Are significantly under-represented in mental health research.

The fundamental issue emphasized in this report of the Surgeon General is that "culture counts." Clearly, any comprehensive quality improvement program must address issues of culture and ethnicity for patients, family, and staff.

Another important issue related to person-centered care is that the physical health of persons being treated for mental health and/or substance use disorders must also be addressed. Comorbidity of physical illness and mental illness is frequent and complicates the treatment of either. Several models of integrated care have been developed and some have demonstrated improved outcomes across several measures.

CONCLUSION

Though still in evolution and development, the use of performance measures and quality indicators to demonstrate adherence to evidence-based practice guidelines is being broadly endorsed in all medical specialties. Accrediting and certifying organizations are increasingly recognizing the importance of collaborative efforts to standardize effective methods to demonstrate provision of quality care. Among the many challenges as we move forward is the need to demonstrate that such performance measurement systems do indeed lead to improvement in care. At the individual provider level, such programs can provide a mechanism to meet the performance-in-practice component of the emerging requirements for maintenance of board certification.

At the core of this chapter's message is the need to give priority and attention to "quality care" in the efforts to address and correct disparities in psychiatric care. It is of utmost importance that this principle and basic concept be an integral part in the resolution of psychiatric and mental health disparities; otherwise, disparities in the field of psychiatry will continue to exist because of the lack of appropriate understanding that disparities will always be present if quality care is not provided. This concept is of major importance in the context of this chapter.

References

1. Donabedian A. Evaluating the Quality of Medical Care. *Milbank Mem Fund Q* 1966; 44(3):166–203.
2. American College of Surgeons. *Minimum Standard for Hospitals.* Chicago, IL: American College of Surgeons, 1917.
3. National Committee for Quality Assurance. *Standards and Guidelines for the Accreditation of Health Plans.* Washington, DC: National Committee for Quality Assurance. Available at http://www.ncqa.org/tabid/499/Default.aspx.
4. Institute of Medicine. *To Err Is Human: Building a Safer Health System.* Washington, D.C.: Institute of Medicine, 1999.
5. Institute of Medicine. *Crossing the Quality Chasm: A New Health System for the 21st Century.* Washington, DC: Institute of Medicine, 2001.
6. Institute of Medicine. *Improving the Quality of Health Care for Mental and Substance-Use Conditions: Quality Chasm Series.* Washington, DC: Institute of Medicine, 2005.
7. Oldham JM, Golden WE, Rosof BM. Quality improvement in psychiatry: Why measures matter. *J Psychiatr Pract* 2007;14(2):8–17.
8. Agency for Health Care Policy and Research. *Depression in Primary Care: Treatment of Major Depression.* Rockville, MD: Agency for Health Care Policy and Research, 1993.
9. National Quality Forum. *Workshop Proceedings: Integrating Behavioral Healthcare Performance Measures Throughout Healthcare.* Washington, DC: National Quality Forum, 2005.
10. Kroenke K, Spitzer RL, Williams JB. The PHQ-9: Validity of a brief depression severity measure. *J Gen Intern Med* 2001;16:606–613.
11. Zarin DA, Pincus HA, McIntyre JS. Practice Guidelines. *Am J Psychiatry* 1993;150(2): 175–177.
12. American Psychiatric Association. *Practice Guideline Development Process.* Arlington, VA: American Psychiatric Association. Available at http://www.psychiatryonline.com/content.aspx?aID=58560.

13. American Psychiatric Association. *Quality Indicators: Defining and Measuring Quality in Psychiatric Care for Adults and Children.* Washington, D.C.: American Psychiatric Association, 2002.
14. Duffy FF, Narrow W, West JC, et al. Quality of care measures for the treatment of bipolar disorder. *Psychiatr Q* 2005;76:213–230.
15. American Medical Association Physician Consortium for Performance Improvement. Available at http://www.ama-assn.org/ama/pub/category/2946.html.
16. National Quality Forum. Available at http://www.qualityforum.org.
17. Ambulatory Quality Alliance. Available at http://www.aqaalliance.org.
18. The Joint Commission. *Health Care at the Crossroads: Development of a National Performance Measurement Data Strategy.* Oakbrook Terrace, IL: The Joint Commission, 2008.
19. Rosenthal MB, Landon BE, Normand SLT, et al. Pay for performance in commercial HMOs. *N Engl J Med* 2006;355:1895–1902.
20. Pelonero AL, Johnson RL. A pay-for-performance program for behavioral health care practitioners. *Psychiatr Serv* 2007;58:442–444.
21. Fochtmann LJ, Duffy FF, West JC, et al. Performance in practice: Sample tools for the care of patients with major depressive disorder. *FOCUS* 2008;6(1):22–35.
22. Krahn M, Naglie G. The next step in guideline development: Incorporating patient preferences. *JAMA* 2008;300:436–438.
23. U.S. Department of Health and Human Services. *Mental Health: Culture, Race, and Ethnicity — A Supplement to Mental Health: A Report of the Surgeon General.* Rockville, MD: U.S. Department of Health and Human Services, Substance Abuse and Mental Health Services Administration, Center for Mental Health, 2001.

27 The Role of Nonmedical Human Services and Alternative Medicine

William Sribney, Katherine Elliott, Sergio Aguilar-Gaxiola, and Hendry Ton

INTRODUCTION

In the United States, individuals with mental disorders who seek services are treated through various systems of care. Much of the extant mental health services research categorizes these systems of care in four broadly defined service sectors including the general medical sector (comprised of primary care physicians and other medical doctors), the specialty mental and addictive disorders sector (psychiatrists, psychologists, psychiatric social workers, and mental health counselors), the human services sector (counselors, social workers, nurses in a social service agency), and the informal sector (clergy, family, and friends) (1,2). Subsequent studies of mental health utilization on specific ethnic groups such as Mexican Americans have included in the informal sector providers such as folk healers (i.e., *curanderos*), natural healers, spiritualists, etc (3). As awareness of the diversity of service sectors choice among persons with mental illness has grown, there has been increasing research devoted to characterizing the variety of providers and provider preferences (1,3,4). There is evidence of disparities in access and utilization of healthcare for racial and ethnic minority clients when compared with non-Latino whites (5). In Health Care for Communities, a national telephone survey with nearly 15,000 adult participants, Wells and colleagues (6) documented that African American (25.0%) and Latinos (22.4%) experienced greater unmet need for mental healthcare and alcoholism and drug abuse treatment compared with whites (37.6%). In addition, African Americans and Latinos have been found to be less likely than whites to receive guideline-adherent treatment (7,8) and follow-up (9). This chapter presents service-use data from the Collaborative Psychiatric Epidemiological Surveys (CPES; see Chapter 7 by Alegría et al. for a detailed description of the CPES) for the purpose of examining disparities in mental healthcare across three sectors of care: medical (care provided by psychiatrists, family physicians, or other medical doctors, or mental health hospitalizations), non-MD clinicians and other human services (psychologists, social workers, counselors, other non-MD health professionals, self-help groups, or religious or spiritual advisors), and Complementary and Alternative Medicine (CAM). Based on the data presented, we address issues of recruitment, education, and training, focusing on nonmedical providers such as psychologists, social workers, counselors, and other nonmedical health professionals.

MEDICAL INTERVENTIONS FOR MENTAL HEALTH

Previous literature suggests that the general medical sector is the main point of entry for mental healthcare for many persons with mental health problems. In fact, 85% of all mental healthcare is currently delivered in the primary care setting by primary care practitioners (10). Moreover, this percentage has increased over the past decade and it is projected to continue to increase in the future (4). In other words, the primary care setting is serving as the de facto mental healthcare system in the United States (10). Primary care settings are the first point of contact and the ultimate treatment site of choice for many minority and low-income consumers. Mental health problems constitute more than 40% of patients' presenting complaints in the primary care setting (11,12). Unfortunately, these conditions are often misdiagnosed, not properly addressed, or simply treated incorrectly (8,10). Primary care is more available and easier to access than specialty mental health and many patients view mental health treatment in primary care settings as less stigmatizing than care received in specialty mental health settings. The growing recognition of the important role of primary care settings in the delivery of mental health services for minorities is noteworthy and is particularly evident in primary care settings that function within a system that integrates mental health specialists into overall healthcare. Making mental health services available and utilized by minorities with mental health or substance abuse disorders will require integrating mental health service and necessary supports into the primary care setting. Studies show, however, a substantial deficit in mental health education among primary care physicians during residency and postresidency training (11) and indicate a need for consistent supervision and clinical instruction in the primary care setting to optimize mental healthcare (13).

NON-MD CLINICIANS AND OTHER HUMAN SERVICE PROVIDERS FOR MENTAL HEALTH

Psychologists, social workers, master degree–level clinicians, and other therapists are traditionally seen as primary providers of psychotherapy. Training in psychology focuses on the understanding and treatment of mental health disorders with emphasis on theory and practice of psychotherapy. Within the profession of social work, the degree of emphasis on the provision of counseling and psychotherapy varies. However, the discipline of social work has traditionally emphasized a social justice approach which addresses health and mental health through intervention at various levels: individual, family, community, society.

   Much of the literature on disparities for the nonmedical mental healthcare provider sector has focused on differences in access to specialty mental health services, differential rates of treatment completion, and differential access to evidence-based treatments. In the frequently cited landmark report, *Mental Health: Culture, Race, Ethnicity*, the U.S. Surgeon General reviewed disparities in mental health and mental healthcare for ethnic minorities (14). A significant body of research supports the findings from this report suggesting that ethnic minorities are less likely to receive outpatient mental health services (15–18), more likely to dropout of psychotherapy and pharmacotherapy prematurely (19), and less likely to receive evidence-based psychotherapy (20–22).

USE OF COMPLEMENTARY AND ALTERNATIVE MEDICINE FOR MENTAL HEALTH

Complementary and alternative medicine describes a diverse group of medical and healthcare systems, practices, and treatments that are not part of the conventional medicine practiced by medical doctors and allied health professionals. It estimated that between $36 and $47 billion dollars were spent on CAM treatments in 1997 in the United States (23), and that Americans spend more money on out-of-pocket fees for CAM than they do for out-of-pocket fees for conventional medicine services (24). Sixty-two percent of Americans have used CAM within the last 12 months. CAM has become a pervasive although poorly characterized component of the American health-care landscape that includes ethnomedical systems and practices such as traditional Chinese medicine, Ayurvedic medicine, and shamanism. CAM therapies include prayer, meditation, chiropractic, yoga, massage, herbal medicine, high-dose vitamin therapy, and diet (25). Common reasons for using CAM treatments include wanting treatments to be based on a "natural approach"; wanting treatments to be congruent with the clients' own spirituality, values, and beliefs; past experiences in which conventional medical therapies had caused unpleasant side effects or had seemed ineffective; and lack of conventional medical treatments for the condition (26,27).

Use of CAM treatments by diverse communities is difficult to estimate given different methodologies and definitions used in survey studies as well as substantial intra-group variability. Barnes and colleagues (25) noted that for health problems, Asian Americans were more likely to use biologically based treatments than whites whereas African Americans were least likely to do so. African Americans had the highest use of CAM (70%) when prayer and megavitamin use was included. Latinos were also more likely than whites and Asian Americans to use prayer as a form of CAM treatment. Ma (28), in a small convenience sample, observed that nearly 95% of Chinese immigrants used self-treatment and home remedies. Keegan (29) noted that 44% and 30% of Latinos used herbal remedies and prayer or spiritual interventions, respectively.

Anxiety and depression are among the most common conditions for which CAM is used (25). In a national survey of over 2000 respondents conducted in 1997 to 1998, Kessler and colleagues (30) found that 57% of those with anxiety attacks and 54% of those with severe depression reported using CAM treatments, although only 20% and 19%, respectively, visited a CAM provider. Sixty-six percent of respondents seen by a conventional provider for anxiety and 67% for severe depression also used CAM treatments concomitantly. Communication between CAM providers and conventional practitioners appears limited however. A study by Simon and colleagues (31) suggests that most CAM provider visits for mental health reasons were self-referred and rarely do CAM providers communicate with a conventional medical provider about shared patients. Likewise, up to 77% of patients do not disclose use of CAM to their conventional medicine practitioners (32).

MEDICAL SERVICE, HUMAN SERVICE, AND CAM USE BY PERSONS WITH PSYCHIATRIC DISORDERS

Using the Collaborative Psychiatric Epidemiological Surveys (CPES) dataset, mental healthcare utilization estimates were calculated for persons with any 12-month DSM-IV disorder. (Disorders included depressive and other mood disorders, anxiety disorders, and alcohol or drug abuse or dependence.) Described in more detailed in Chapter 7, the CPES dataset is a merging of data from three national surveys: the National Latino and Asian American Study (NLAAS), the National Survey of American Life (NSAL), and the National Comorbidity Replication Study (NCS-R). Each of these surveys employed the World Health Organization Composite International Diagnostic Interview (WHO-CIDI) to determine diagnoses according to DSM-IV criteria and also service-use history (33). Restricting the analysis to those participants who took the full instrument (a sizeable proportion of those in NCS-R did not) yielded a total sample of 15,480 adults (aged 18 or older), of whom 3379 had a 12-month mental disorder.

Study participants were classified by ethnicity (non-Latino white, African American, Latino, and Asian) and nativity. Persons belonging to other ethnic categories were omitted as were foreign-born whites, since this group was too small to yield precise estimates.

As shown in Table 27.1, a large percentage of individuals with 12-month DSM-IV disorders reported seeing a medical doctor or being on medications for mental health reasons in the past 12 months. Non-Latino U.S.-born whites were the most likely (45%) to have received care under this medical care category, followed by U.S.-born Asian (42%). U.S.-born and foreign-born Latinos and U.S.-born African Americans had lower rates of utilization of medical services (38%, 32%, and 32%, respectively). The greatest disparity in utilization of medical services was among foreign-born African Americans (14%) and foreign-born Asians (20%), levels that are less than half that of their U.S.-born counterparts. Among those who reported using any medical service, the mix of service type (psychiatrists and hospitalizations, other medical doctors, or medications) was similar among the seven ethnicity by nativity groups shown in Table 27.1, although whites did report higher use of medications than other groups (82% of whites compared with 72% of nonwhites among those with any medical services use).

Utilization of non-MD clinicians or other human services revealed less variation with all groups reporting similar rates (19% to 25%) except for foreign-born African Americans who reported a lower rate (9%) and U.S.-born Asian Americans who reported a higher rate (34%; however, this difference compared with whites was not significant). Rates of service use for the four subcategories shown in Table 27.1—(i) psychologists, social workers, counselors, mental health hotline, nurses, occupational therapists, or other health professionals; (ii) religious or spiritual advisors; (iii) self-help groups; (iv) and internet support groups—did not significantly differ by ethnicity and nativity except for the lower rates for each subcategory for foreign-born African Americans and except for use of Internet support groups, which was highest among whites and Asians (regardless of nativity).

Almost 30% of individuals with 12-month DSM-IV disorders reported using prayer, spiritual healing, or other spiritual practices for their mental health problems. Because of the high endorsement of the use of this category, it is shown in Table 27.1 separately from other CAM categories. (Typically, under classifications of CAM, such as that of National Center for Complementary and Alternative Medicine (34), prayer or other spiritual practices are classified as Mind-Body Medicine, along with such techniques as hypnosis and meditation.)

Use of prayer, spiritual healing, or other spiritual practices was significantly lower among foreign-born Latinos (12%) and foreign-born Asians (13%). Foreign-born African Americans, however, reported a rate (28%) that was the same as that of U.S.-born groups (27% to 29%). It is important to note that in the WHO-CIDI, respondents are asked about the use of prayer and spiritual practices in the context of "alternative therapies" specifically for mental health problems. They were asked, "[This list] describes commonly used alternative therapies. Did you use any of these

TABLE 27.1	Past 12-Month Service Use[1] for Mental Health Problems[2] for U.S. Adults[3] with Any 12-Month DSM-IV Disorder[4]						
	White	**African American**		**Latino**		**Asian**	
	U.S. -born	**U.S. -born**	**Foreign -born**	**U.S. -born**	**Foreign -born[5]**	**U.S. -born**	**Foreign -born**
Sample size (N)	*1389*	*844*	*130*	*351*	*318*	*75*	*139*
Medical doctors or medications							
Psychiatrists and mental health hospitalizations	15 (1)	14 (1)	4 (3)	10 (2)	15 (2)	23 (9)	7 (2)
Other medical doctors	23 (1)	15 (2)	6 (2)	22 (3)	15 (3)	23 (8)	7 (2)
Medications[6]	37 (2)	21 (2)	11 (4)	29 (4)	26 (3)	24 (8)	14 (4)
Any of above 3 categories	45 (1)	32 (2)	14 (4)	38 (4)	32 (3)	42 (9)	20 (4)
Non-MD clinicians or other human services							
Psychologists, social workers, counselors, mental health hotline, nurses, occupational therapists, or other health professionals	19 (1)	15 (2)	4 (2)	20 (3)	14 (2)	31 (9)	14 (5)
Religious or spiritual advisors	7 (1)	9 (1)	4 (1)	7 (2)	6 (2)	15 (8)	3 (1)
Self-help groups[7]	5 (1)	3 (1)	3 (3)	3 (2)	5 (2)	2 (2)	6 (3)
Internet support groups	2.5 (0.4)	0.6 (0.4)	0.2 (0.2)	1.0 (0.5)	0.1 (0.1)	3.8 (3.1)	4.4 (3.2)
Any of above 4 categories	25 (1)	23 (2)	9 (3)	25 (3)	19 (3)	34 (8)	19 (5)
Prayer, spiritual healing, or other spiritual practices	*28 (2)*	*29 (2)*	*28 (5)*	*29 (2)*	*12 (2)*	*27 (5)*	*13 (4)*
Other complementary and alternative medicine (CAM)							
Herbal therapy, homeopathy, high-dose vitamins, or special diets	15 (1)	7 (1)	6 (2)	13 (2)	5 (2)	14 (6)	5 (2)

(continued)

TABLE 27.1	Past 12-Month Service Use[1] for Mental Health Problems[2] for U.S. Adults[3] with Any 12-Month DSM-IV Disorder[4] *(continued)*

	White	African American		Latino		Asian	
	U.S. -born	U.S. -born	Foreign -born	U.S. -born	Foreign -born[5]	U.S. -born	Foreign -born
Acupuncture, biofeedback, chiropractic, exercise or movement therapy, or massage	22 (1)	15 (2)	15 (5)	22 (3)	13 (3)	33 (8)	21 (4)
Hypnosis, imagery therapy, relaxation or meditation, energy healing, psychic, or any other nontraditional remedy or therapy	18 (1)	11 (1)	8 (3)	18 (3)	6 (1)	26 (11)	11 (3)
Any of above 3 categories	36 (1)	22 (2)	21 (6)	34 (3)	19 (3)	44 (11)	23 (4)
Any service use	71 (1)	56 (2)	45 (6)	62 (3)	51 (4)	72 (5)	46 (5)

[1]All data shown, except sample size, are weighted age-sex adjusted percentages with standard errors shown in parentheses.

[2]Questions on all types of service use were asked in the context of helping with "problems with your emotions or nerves or your use of alcohol or drugs."

[3]Ages 18 years or older.

[4]Disorders include depressive and other mood disorders, anxiety disorders, and alcohol or drug abuse or dependence.

[5]Foreign-born Latinos include persons born in Puerto Rico.

[6]Medications include sleeping pills or other sedatives, antidepressant medications, tranquilizers, amphetamines or other stimulants, and antipsychotic medications.

[7]Self-help group question omitted mention of alcohol or drugs: "Did you ever in your life go to a self-help group for help with your emotions or nerves?" However, 47% of persons responding yes to this question said that they had attended groups for people with substance problems such as Alcoholics Anonymous or Rational Recovery in the past 12 months.

therapies in the past 12 months for problems with your emotions or nerves or your use of alcohol or drugs?" Among the 15 specific items on the list, the 12th was "prayer or other spiritual practices" and the 15th was "spiritual healing by others." It is possible that participants did not consider prayer an "alternative therapy" and so did not carefully examine the list of choices.

There were significant differences in participants' usage of treatments and therapies in the other CAM categories especially by nativity. Differences by ethnicity were greatest for African Americans, who generally reported less use of these treatments and therapies. Among all groups, use of herbal therapy, homeopathy, high-dose vitamins, or special diets was the lowest among the categories of CAM shown in Table 27.1 compared with other categories of CAM. Rates for this category were particularly low among the foreign-born (5% to 6%) and also low among U.S.-born African Americans (7%) compared with other U.S.-born groups (13% to 15%).

Use of acupuncture, biofeedback, chiropractic, exercise or movement therapy, or massage was lowest among foreign-born Latinos (13%) and African Americans (15% for both U.S.-born and foreign-born) and similar among whites (22%) and Asians (33% for U.S.-born and 21% for foreign-born). Use of hypnosis, imagery therapy, relaxation or meditation, energy healing, psychic, or any other nontraditional remedy or therapy followed a similar pattern to that of the other CAM categories: it was low among foreign-born Latinos (6%), foreign-born African Americans (8%), U.S.-born African Americans (11%), and foreign-born Asians (11%), and higher among U.S.-born Latinos (18%), whites (18%), and U.S.-born Asians (26%).

Figure 27.1 plots the same service-use rates as in Table 27.1 for the three major categories described earlier: medical services (medical doctors and medications), non-MD clinicians and other human services, and CAM (including prayer and other spiritual practices). Also shown are the proportions of persons with a past 12-month disorder who had no service use of any kind. One might hypothesize that much of the differences between the ethnicity by nativity groups is caused by sociodemographic differences among the groups, such as differences in education, income, and insurance status. Other factors, such as comorbidity (i.e., multiple psychiatric disorders from more than one class: substance and nonsubstance disorders or mood and anxiety disorders) and functioning, may also affect service use and may differ by ethnicity and nativity.

Figure 27.2 plots the same service-use rates as in Figure 27.1, only here they are fully adjusted for sociodemographics (sex, age, education, marital status, and insur-

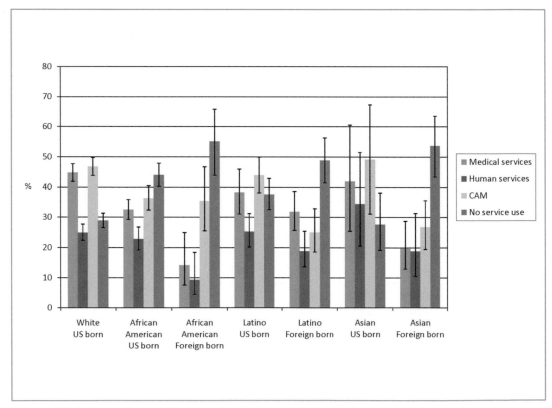

Figure 27-1. Percentages adjusted only for age and sex of any past 12-month use of medical services, human services, and CAM for mental health problems for U.S. adults with any 12-month DSM-IV disorder.

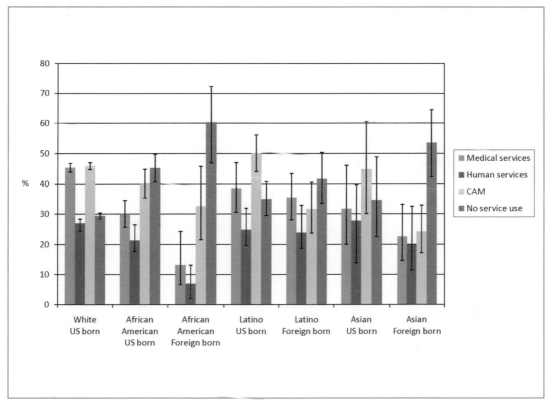

Figure 27-2. Percentages adjusted for sex, age, marital status, education, insurance, comorbidity, and functioning of any past 12-month use of medical services, human services, and CAM for mental health problems for U.S. adults with any 12-month DSM-IV disorder.

ance), comorbidity, and functioning (having one or more days out of the past 30 in which the respondent was totally unable to work or carry out normal activities). The adjustment was carried out by fitting logistic regressions, shown in Table 27.2, for each service-use category with the adjustment variables and ethnicity by nativity terms as independent variables. Figure 27.2 shows predicted probabilities by ethnicity and nativity with the adjustment variables set to their overall sample mean among all persons with 12-month disorders (and with the constant term in the model adjusted for the logistic transformation so that the predicted value at the mean of all independent variables coincides with the observed outcome frequency). Income was initially included in the models, but after controlling for the other adjustment variables, it was not significant, so it was dropped from the regressions.

What is remarkable about the fully adjusted Figure 27.2 is how similar it is to Figure 27.1, which is only adjusted for age and sex. Differences among the ethnicity by nativity groups remained essentially the same after adjustment by sociodemographics, comorbidity, and functioning. Comorbidity and functioning were found to be highly predictive of receipt of medical services and use of non-MD clinicians and other human services (Table 27.2). Comorbidity, but not functioning, was associated with an increased likelihood of using CAM. Comorbidity did not vary significantly by ethnicity or nativity, but functioning did, being significantly lower among U.S.-born African Americans compared with other groups, which were similar (data not shown).

TABLE 27.2	Logistic Regression Models of Past 12-Month Service Use for Mental Health Problems for U.S. Adults with Any 12-Month DSM-IV Disorder[1]			
	Medical Doctors or Medications	**Non-MD Clinicians or Other Human Services**	**CAM**	**No Service Use**
Female	1.7 [1.3, 2.2]***	1.2 [1.0, 1.5]*	2.0 [1.5, 2.5]***	0.5 [0.4, 0.6]***
Age (y)				
18–24	0.4 [0.2, 0.7]**	1.1 [0.7, 1.9]	0.7 [0.5, 1.1]	1.7 [1.0, 3.2]
25–34	0.4 [0.3, 0.6]***	1.0 [0.7, 1.4]	0.8 [0.6, 1.0]	1.6 [1.2, 2.2]**
35–44	0.9 [0.6, 1.3]	1.2 [0.9, 1.8]	0.8 [0.6, 1.0]	1.2 [0.8, 1.7]
45–54	1	1	1	1
55–64	1.1 [0.6, 1.9]	0.8 [0.5, 1.5]	1.0 [0.6, 1.6]	1.1 [0.7, 1.8]
≥65	0.4 [0.2, 0.8]**	0.3 [0.2, 0.7]**	0.7 [0.4, 1.2]	1.9 [1.0, 3.9]
Marital status				
Married	1	1	1	1
Divorced, separated, widowed	1.1 [0.8, 1.5]	1.7 [1.3, 2.4]***	1.0 [0.7, 1.3]	0.8 [0.6, 1.1]
Never married	0.9 [0.7, 1.2]	1.3 [0.9, 1.7]	1.0 [0.7, 1.3]	1.0 [0.7, 1.3]
Education				
Some high school or less	1.0 [0.7, 1.5]	0.8 [0.5, 1.2]	0.7 [0.6, 0.9]*	1.3 [0.9, 1.9]
High school graduate	1	1	1	1
Some college	1.3 [1.0, 1.6]	1.2 [0.9, 1.6]	1.8 [1.4, 2.2]***	0.7 [0.5, 0.9]**
College degree or more	1.2 [0.9, 1.6]	1.4 [1.1, 1.9]*	2.3 [1.7, 3.2]***	0.6 [0.4, 0.9]**
Ethnicity				
White, U.S.-born	1	1	1	1
African American, U.S.-born	0.5 [0.4, 0.7]***	0.7 [0.5, 1.0]	0.8 [0.6, 1.0]*	2.0 [1.6, 2.5]***
African American, foreign-born	0.2 [0.1, 0.4]***	0.2 [0.1, 0.4]***	0.6 [0.3, 1.0]	3.6 [2.1, 6.3]***
Latino, U.S.-born	0.8 [0.5, 1.1]	0.9 [0.6, 1.3]	1.2 [0.9, 1.6]	1.3 [1.0, 1.7]
Latino, foreign-born	0.7 [0.5, 1.0]*	0.9 [0.5, 1.4]	0.5 [0.4, 0.8]**	1.7 [1.2, 2.5]**
Asian, U.S.-born	0.6 [0.3, 1.1]	1.0 [0.6, 1.8]	1.0 [0.5, 1.8]	1.3 [0.7, 2.3]
Asian, foreign-born	0.4 [0.2, 0.6]***	0.7 [0.3, 1.3]	0.4 [0.2, 0.6]***	2.8 [1.7, 4.4]***

(continued)

TABLE 27.2	Logistic Regression Models of Past 12-Month Service Use for Mental Health Problems for U.S. Adults with Any 12-Month DSM-IV Disorder[1] *(continued)*			
	Medical Doctors or Medications	**Non-MD Clinicians or Other Human Services**	**CAM**	**No Service Use**
Insurance				
Private	1	1	1	1
Public	2.1 [1.6, 2.7]***	1.3 [0.8, 2.2]	0.9 [0.6, 1.4]	0.8 [0.5, 1.1]
None	0.5 [0.3, 0.7]***	0.8 [0.6, 1.1]	0.8 [0.6, 1.0]*	1.7 [1.3, 2.3]***
Comorbid with disorder of another class[2]	2.0 [1.6, 2.6]***	1.8 [1.4, 2.2]***	1.6 [1.2, 1.9]***	0.5 [0.4, 0.7]***
Unable to function 1 or more days out of past 30 days because of mental health problems	2.2 [1.7, 2.9]***	2.5 [1.8, 3.4]***	1.1 [0.7, 1.6]	0.5 [0.3, 0.7]***

[1]See footnotes 2–6 from Table 27.1.

[2]Person has 12-month substance and nonsubstance disorders or 12-month mood and anxiety disorders.

*$p < .05$

**$p < .01$

***$p < .001$

Insurance status was predictive of medical services, with those with public insurance being more likely to get services and those with no insurance less likely, but was not predictive of the use of non-MD clinicians and other human services or the use of CAM. Being divorced, separated, or widowed was strongly associated with use of non-MD clinicians and other human services, but marital status was not associated with other service-use categories. Interestingly, the effect of education was greatest on the use of CAM relative to other categories of service use. Persons with some college or a college degree or more had much greater use of CAM compared with persons with only a high school or less education.

DISCUSSION

Disparities were apparent among different ethnicity by nativity groups for persons with 12-month disorders in their use of any medical services (seeing a medical doctor or taking medications), non-MD clinicians and other human services, and CAM. Differences among the groups were greater for the receipt of medical services and CAM than they were for human services. (However, percentages were, in general, higher for medical service use and CAM than for human service use, so we had more power to detect disparities for medical services and CAM than for human services.) The most striking differences were between the U.S.-born and the foreign-born. Making a relative comparison and expressing the foreign-born level as a percentage of U.S.-born level, we found that for medical services, the foreign-born level of use was 65% of that of the U.S.-born; for human services, the foreign-born level was 74% of that of the U.S.-born; and for CAM, the foreign-born level was 57% of that of the U.S.-born. Hence, the *relative* disparity by nativity was not hugely different among these three categories of use.

Foreign-born African Americans had very low levels of use of medical and human service use, but their overall CAM use was similar to that of foreign-born Latinos and Asians. Foreign-born African Americans cited the use of prayer and other spiritual practices as "alternative therapy" for their mental health problems at levels similar to U.S.-born groups, which were higher than the levels of use of prayer and other spiritual practices acknowledged by foreign-born Latinos and Asians. However, one wonders whether endorsement of the use of prayer might be higher if the question were asked differently than as an item on a list of alterative therapies—for example, if they were asked whether they prayed for help for their mental health problems.

Consistent with other literature, CAM treatments and therapies were frequently used for mental disorders (4,23,25). Despite the popular conception that "unconventional" treatments are used with greater frequency by ethnic minority communities, our results show patterns of CAM use that are similar to that of the other service sectors, with the foreign-born reporting lower levels of CAM use. However, it is possible that the selection and wording of the CAM items in the WHO-CIDI used in the CPES studies affected this result. Respondents' choices for alternative therapies in the WHO-CIDI was a list of typical American "New Age" treatments and therapies: homeopathy, herbal therapy, high dose mega-vitamins, special diets, acupuncture, biofeedback, chiropractic, exercise or movement therapy, massage therapy, hypnosis, imagery techniques, relaxation or meditation techniques, and energy healing.

Only the NLAAS component of CPES asked specifically about seeing a doctor of oriental medicine (on a question about seeing a "healer" that was not highly endorsed). None of the questions asked about alternative therapies using terms, such as *curanderos, sobadores*, shamans, and ayurveda, that might be more familiar to less acculturated Latinos, Asians, and Caribbean immigrants. However, the Mexican American Prevalence and Services Survey (MAPSS), which surveyed Mexican-origin adults from Fresno, California in 1996, asked specifically whether the respondent had seen a "folk healer (*curandero*), natural healer (*naturista*), spiritualist (*espiritista*) or medium, *santero*(a), psychic, astrologist, or *sobador*(a)" for mental health problems, and found low rates of use of these providers among both the foreign-born (5.4%) and the U.S.-born (3.5%) (35). Hence, among Latinos at least, it seems unlikely that adding more culturally appropriate CAM choices to questionnaire would have appreciably altered our overall CAM results.

We also examined overlapping use among the different service-use categories. Persons using CAM typically also used other services for their mental health problems. Indeed, use of CAM, but not the use of prayer or other spiritual practices, was highly predictive of use of medical services. There was no evidence to suggest that CAM was used as a substitute for medical treatments. Awareness of the disorder may also play a role. Respondents who had a disorder, but who did not believe that they had a disorder, would naturally not seek out any treatments or services for it.

Awareness of a disorder, either self-awareness or a clinical diagnosis, may cause a person to seek out treatments and services from multiple care domains.

There was a large amount of overlap between the use of psychologists, social workers, and other non-MD clinicians and seeing psychiatrists: 42% of all persons who saw a non-MD clinician in the past 12 months also saw a psychiatrist in the past 12 months. It may be that many of the persons seeing non-MD clinicians are seeing them in a clinic setting where they regularly see the non-MD clinician for talk therapy and see a psychiatrist more infrequently but at routine intervals for medication maintenance or periodic assessment.

The evidence of overlapping service use underscores the importance of coordinating care across sectors—or, at least, having providers being aware of and understanding their patients' treatment seeking in other sectors. CAM is often considered by medical providers and public mental health systems as not being a valuable mode of treatment or therapy. However, being sensitive to the use of CAM and acknowledging that the patient may receive benefits from it may further the relationship between the traditional provider and the patient and enhance the effectiveness of the traditional therapy.

It is notable that non-MD clinicians and other human service providers were not used as frequently as medical services and CAM. Given the current findings as well as previous research that suggest a significant percentage of individuals with mental health problems do not obtain any services (14), non-MD service providers may be an underutilized resource for all persons in need of mental health services. Furthermore, because human service providers, such as psychologists and social workers, have a strong tradition of community and home-based work, these professions have great potential for addressing some of the institutional, geographic, cultural, and linguistic barriers to care experienced by ethnic minority persons with mental illnesses.

IMPLICATIONS FOR TRAINING AND EDUCATION

The results of this study have implications for workforce development and training. Ethnic-linguistic matching, whereby the ethnicity and language of client is matched with that of providers has been a mainstay of culturally and linguistically appropriate and have been associated with diminished rates of drop-out services (36,37). While our analyses suggest that a significant proportion of ethnic minorities use medical services for treatment of mental health, the numbers of physicians from ethnic minority backgrounds are limited. Of physicians in the workforce, African Americans, Latinos, Asians, and American Indians or Alaskan natives make up less that 25% of the total (38), despite these groups representing 33% of the general populations (Table 27.3). Likewise, minorities make up only 19% of psychiatrists. These numbers are even more disparate with regard to non-MD mental health clinicians. Minorities comprise less than 10% of all psychologists and less than 15% of all social workers (39). This reflects the importance of recruitment of minorities into both the medical and nonmedical provider workforce.

There is evidence, however, to suggest that ethnic minorities take on the values and perspectives of the profession and may perpetuate ethnic bias in assessment and treatment (40). Culturally and linguistic competence training is also an essential component and an important strategy for reducing ethnic health disparities (41), particularly given the shortage of ethnic minorities in the workforce. Cultural

TABLE 27.3	Percentage of Population: Physicians, Psychiatrists, Psychologists, and Social Workers by Race and Ethnicity[1]				
Race/ Ethnicity	**Population[2] 2005**	**Physicians[3] 2005**	**Psychiatrists[4] 2002**	**Psychologists[4] 2004**	**Social Workers[4] 2004**
White	67	77	81	93	92
African American	13	5	3	2	4
Latino	14	4	5	3	3
Asian	5	14	11	2	1
American Indian or Alaskan Native	1.5	0.1	0.1	0.3	0.2

[1]Adapted from Howard H. Goldman, personal communication, March 16, 2008, regarding the Fundamental Policy–Spotlight on Mental Health Conference.

[2]Population data from the U.S. Census Bureau.

[3]Physician data from the American Medical Association, Physician Characteristics and Distributions in the U.S., 2007. Percentages are for those with a designated race/ethnicity.

[4]Psychiatrist, psychologist, and social worker data from Mental Health, United States, 2004 SAMSHA. Percentages are for those with a designated race/ethnicity.

and linguistic competence is endorsed by multiple professional organizations (42,43,44), and there are many approaches to improving cultural competence (45). However, many training programs fail to address cultural competence adequately within their curricula (46), and many existing cultural competency workshops may have limited efficacy (47). Topics that emphasize content descriptions of ethnic differences have limited benefit, and risk promoting stereotyping and simplification of cultural issues (48,49). Efforts to implement cultural competence frequently use an additive approach in which cultural concepts, themes, and perspectives are added to the curriculum without changing its basic structure or approach. Rather than this approach, many experts suggest that curricula that integrate cultural competence into all years of professional education may have a more meaningful impact on trainees (50,51).

CONCLUSION

Disparities in service utilization are apparent across all sectors of service use, especially for foreign-born ethnic minorities, and in particular for foreign-born African Americans. These disparities do not appear to be caused by differences in basic sociodemographic factors between ethnic groups of differing nativity. Non-MD clinicians and other human service providers appear to be underutilized for mental health treatment in comparison to medical providers and CAM. Bolstering the role of non-MD clinicians and other human services providers may be an effective and cost-efficient strategy for addressing disparities in access to mental health services. However, on a proportional basis, there are fewer ethnic minority non-MD clinicians currently in the workforce than there are minority psychiatrists and other physicians. Hence, effective recruitment of minorities and effective cultural and linguistic competency training for all providers is essential.

References

1. Frank RG, Kamlet MS. Determining provider choice for the treatment of mental disorder: The role of health and mental health status. *Health Serv Res* 1989;24(1):83–103.
2. Kessler RC, Zhao S, Katz SJ, et al. Past-year use of outpatient services for psychiatric problems in the national comorbidity survey. *Am J Psychiatry* 1999;156:115–123.
3. Vega WA, Kolody B, Aguilar-Gaxiola S, et al. Gaps in services utilization by Mexican Americans with mental health problems. *Am J Psychiatry* 1999;156(6):928–934.
4. Wang PS, Demler O, Olfson M, et al. Changing profiles of service sectors used for mental health care in the United States. *Am J Psychiatry* 2006;163:1187–1198.
5. Etchason J, Armour B, Ofili E, et al. Racial and ethnic disparities in health care. *JAMA* 2001;285:883.
6. Wells K, Klap R, Koike A, et al. Ethnic disparities in unmet need for alcoholism, drug abuse, and mental health care, *Am J Psychiatry* 2001;158:2027–2032.
7. Wang PS, Berglund P, Kessler RC. Recent care of common mental disorders in the United States: Prevalence and conformance with evidence-based recommendations. *J Gen Intern Med* 2000;15:284–292.
8. Young AS, Klap R, Sherbourne CD, et al. The quality of care for depressive and anxiety disorders in the United States. *Arch Gen Psychiatry* 2001;58:55–61.
9. Schneider EC, Zaslavsky AM, Epstein AM. Racial disparities in the quality of care for enrollees in Medicare managed care. *JAMA* 2002;287:1288–1294.
10. Regier DA Narrow WE, Rae DS, et al. The de facto US mental and addictive disorders service system: Epidemiologic catchment area prospective 1-year prevalence rates of disorders and services. *Arch Gen Psychiatry* 1993;50(2):85–94.
11. Leigh H, Stewart D, Mallios R. Mental health and psychiatry training in primary care residency programs, I: Who teaches, where, when and how satisfied? *Gen Hosp Psychiatry* 2006;28:189–194.
12. Didden DG, Philbrick JT, Schorling JB. Anxiety and depression in an internal medicine resident continuity clinic: Difficult diagnosis. *Int J Psychiatry Med* 2001;31:155–167.
13. Unützer J, Schoenbaum M, Druss BG, et al. Transforming mental health care at the interface with general medicine: Report for the President's Commission. *Psychiatr Serv* 2006; 57:37–40.
14. Department of Health and Human Services. *Mental Health: Culture, Race, Ethnicity. Supplement to Mental Health: Report of the Surgeon General.* 2001.
15. Garland A. Racial/ethnic disparities in mental health service use among children in foster care. *Child Youth Serv Rev* 2003;25(5–6):491–507.
16. Garland AF, Lau AS, Yeh M, et al. Racial and ethnic differences in utilization of mental health services among high-risk youths. *Am J Psychiatry* 2005;162(7):1336–1343.
17. Wood PA, Yeh M, Pan D, et al. Exploring the relationship between race/ethnicity, age of first school-based services utilization, and age of first specialty mental health care for at-risk youth. *Ment Health Serv Res* 2005;7(3):185–196.
18. Snowden LR, Thomas K. Medicaid and African American outpatient mental health treatment. *Ment Health Serv Res* 2000;2(2):115–120.
19. Wang JL. Mental Health Treatment Dropout and Its Correlates in a General Population Sample *Med Care* 2007;45:224–229.
20. Chambless DL, Sanderson WC, Shoham V, et al. An update on empirically validated therapies. *Clin Psycholog* 1996;29:5–18.
21. Hall GNC. Psychotherapy with ethnic minorities: Empirical, ethical, and conceptual issues. *J Consult Clin Psychol* 2001;69:501–510.

22. Lau AS. Making the case for selective and directed cultural adaptations of evidence-based treatments: Examples from parent training. *Clin Psychol Sci Pract* 2006;13(4):295–310.

23. Eisenberg DM, Davis RB, Ettner SL, et al. Trends in alternative medicine use in the United States, 1990–1997: Results of a follow-up national survey. *JAMA* 1998;280(18): 1569–1575.

24. Center for Medicare and Medicaid Services. 1997 *National Health Expenditures Survey.* Available at http://www.cms.hhs.gov/statistics/nhe/.

25. Barne, PM, Powell-Griner E, McFann K, et al. *Complementary and Alternative Medicine Use Among Adults: United States, 2002.* CDC Advance Data Report #343, 2004.

26. Wu P, Fuller C, Lu X, et al. Use of complementary and alternative medicine among women with depression: Results of a national survey. *Psychiatr Serv* 2007;58(3):349–356.

27. Eisenberg DM. Advising patients who seek alternative medical therapies. *Ann Intern Med* 1997;127(1):61–69.

28. Ma GX. Between two worlds: The use of traditional and Western health services by Chinese immigrants. *J Community Health* 1999;24(6):421–437.

29. Keegan L. Use of alternative therapies among Mexican-Americans in the Texas Rio Grande Valley. *J Holistic Nursing* 1996;14(4):277–294.

30. Kessler RC, Soukup J, Davis RB, et al. The use of complementary and alternative therapies to treat anxiety and depression in the United States. *Am J Psychiatry* 2001;158(1):159–168.

31. Simon GE, Cherkin DC, Sherman KJ, et al. Mental health visits to complementary and alternative medicine providers. *Gen Hosp Psychiatry* 2004;26:171–177.

32. Robinson A, McGrail MR. Disclosure of CAM use to medical practitioners: A review of qualitative and quantitative studies. *Complement Therap Med* 2004;12(2–3):90–98.

33. Kessler RC, Üstün TB. The World Mental Health (WMH) survey initiative version of the World Health Organization (WHO) Composite International Diagnostic Interview (CIDI). *Int J Methods Psychiatr Res* 2004;13:93–121.

34. National Center for Complementary and Alternative Medicine (NCCAM). *What Is CAM?* 2008. Available at http://nccam.nih.gov/health/whatiscam/.

35. Vega WA, Kolody B, Aguilar-Gaxiola S. Help seeking for mental health problems among Mexican immigrants and Mexican Americans. *J Immigrant Health* 2001;3:133–140.

36. Ortega AN, Rosenheck R. Hispanic client–case manager matching: Differences in outcomes and service use in a program for homeless persons with severe mental illness. *J Nerv Ment Disord* 2002;190:315–323.

37. Karlsson R. Ethnic matching between therapist and patient in psychotherapy: An overview of findings, together with methodological and conceptual issue. *Cultur Diversity Ethnic Minority Psychology* 2005;11(2):113–129.

38. American Medical Association. *Physician Characteristics and Distributions in the US, 2007.*

39. Manderscheid RW, Berry JT. *Mental Health,* United States, 2004. DHHS Pub. No 06-4195. Rockville, MD: Substance Abuse and Mental Health Services Administration; 2006.

40. Loring M, Powell B. Gender, race, and DSM-III: A study of objectivity of psychiatric diagnostic behavior. *J Health Soc Behav* 1988;29:1–22.

41. Betancourt JR, Green AR, Carrillo JE, et al. Cultural competence and health care disparities: Key perspectives and trends. *Health Affairs* 2005;24(2):499–505.

42. American Psychological Association. *Guidelines for Providers of Psychological Services to Ethnic, Linguistic, and Culturally Diverse Populations.* 1993. Available at http://www.apa.org/pi/oema/guide.html.

43. NASW National Committee on Racial and Ethnic Diversity. NASW Standards for Cultural Competence in Social Work Practice. Washington, DC: National Association of Social Workers; 2001.

44. American Psychiatric Association. *Practice Guidelines for the Psychiatric Evaluation of Adults.* Washington, DC: American Psychiatric Publishing, 1995.

45. Betancourt JR, Green AR, Carrillo JE. *Cultural Competence in Health Care: Emerging Frameworks and Practical Approaches.* 2000. The Commonwealth Fund. Retrieved on October 10, 2008, from http://www.commonwealthfund.org/usr_doc/betancourt_culturalcompetence_576.pdf?section=4039.

46. Flores G, Gee D, Kastner B. The teaching of cultural issues in US and Canadian medical schools. *Academic Med* 2000;75(5):451–455.

47. Beagan BL. Teaching social and cultural awareness to medical students: "It's all very nice to talk about it in theory, but ultimately it makes no difference." *Academic Med* 2003;78: 605–614.

48. Kai J, Spencer J, Wilkes M, et al. Learning to value ethnic diversity: What, why and how? *Med Educ* 1999;33:616–623.

49. Kai J, Bridgewater R, Spencer J. "Just Think of TB and Asians, That's All I Ever Hear": Medical learners' views about training to work in an ethnically diverse society. *Med Educ* 2001;35:250–256.

50. Betancourt JR. Cross-cultural medical education: Conceptual approaches and frameworks for evaluation. *Academic Med* 2003;78(6):560–569.

51. Kagawa-Singer M, Kassim-Lakha S. A strategy to reduce cross-cultural miscommunication and increase the likelihood of improving health outcomes. *Academic Med* 2003;78(6): 577–587.

28 The Role of Education

Evaristo Akerele, Niru Nahar, and Ada Ikeako

INTRODUCTION

Education plays a significant role in socioeconomic status (1). Therefore, to improve the socioeconomic opportunities across the spectrum for women and ethnic minorities, education is of paramount importance. Fortunately, there is increasing diversity at our institutions in undergraduate, graduate and postgraduate education. Historically this has not always been the case. Women were not admitted to institutions of higher learning such as universities. Hence, the establishment of universities focused solely on the education of women such as Radcliffe College, chattered in 1894. Significant progress has been made in the integration of women into mainstream academic institutions. Radcliffe College for women recently announced its decision to become the Radcliffe Institute for Advanced Study, no longer serving as an undergraduate institution for women. It merged completely with Harvard College in 1999. Similarly, there is increasing ethnic diversity at all levels of education. Nonetheless, the disparity in educational opportunities for women and ethnic minorities continues to exist.

In this section, current status of this disparity will be examined. The disparity in gender, ethnicity, and place of primary education will be discussed. This chapter will focus on undergraduate, graduate, and postgraduate education.

UNDERGRADUATE EDUCATION

Ethnicity

African Americans and Hispanics graduate from high school at lower rates compared with whites (2). According to National Center for Education Statistics (NCES), 27% of 16- to 24-year-old students who dropped out of high school in 2001 were Hispanic. Moreover, the racial and ethnic minorities who do graduate from high school are not always ready for college-level work in mathematics, science, or English (3). In addition, only 39.9% of African American and 34% of Hispanic high school graduates (18 to 24 years old) enrolled in college from 2000 to 2002 compared with 45.5% of white high school graduates in the same years. When minorities do attend college, they are more likely to enter 2-year institutions. If they attend 4-year institutions, they are less likely to graduate than are whites.

Although there are encouraging numbers of minorities earning medical and other advanced degrees, gender, economic, and racial differences continue to persist at all levels of education. Despite significant progress over time, wide gaps remain in access to and success in college. Higher education for African Americans, Hispanics,

Chapter 28 ■ The Role of Education **291**

Asian/Pacific Islanders, and American Indian/Alaska Natives rose from 17% in 1976 to 32% in 2004. Nonetheless, underrepresented minority groups continue to lag behind their white and Asian peers in college attendance. By 2004, 60.3% Asian/Pacific Islanders 18 to 24 years old were enrolled in college, as were 41.7% of white, 31.8% of African Americans, 24.7% of Hispanics, and 24.4% of American Indian/Alaska Natives. These college enrollment percentages matched minority representation in the general population. However, the proportion of degrees awarded to most racial minority groups fell short of their representation in the population. Slightly less than 10% of all college degrees awarded by U.S. degree granting institutions in 2003 to 2004 and 9.3% of bachelor's degrees and 6% of doctorates went to African Americans, who make up 12% of the population. Hispanics fared worse, earning 7.3% of all degrees, 6.8% of bachelor degrees, and 3.4% of doctorates, despite making up 14% of the U.S. population (4).

Overall, 62% of beginning postsecondary students in 2003 to 2004 were white, 15% were Hispanic, 13% were African American, and 5% were Asian. The remaining students were American Indian (1%) and multiple or other races (4%). The racial/ethnic distribution of beginning postsecondary students varied by type of institution; at both public and private not-for-profit 4-year institutions; 70% were white, and at 2-year institutions, 60% were white. In contrast, at less-than-2-year institutions, 38% were white. Less-than-2-year institutions had proportionately more African American (22%) and Hispanic (33%) students than other institution levels. In contrast, at 4-year institutions, 11% of beginning postsecondary students were African American, and 10% were Hispanic; at 2-year institutions, the corresponding proportions were 15% and 16%.

Gender

In the student population, men have fallen far behind women. Between 1970 and 2001, women went from being the minority to the majority of the U.S. undergraduate population, increasing their representation from 42% to 56% of undergraduates (5). Projections to 2013 indicate that women's undergraduate enrollment will increase to 8.9 million or 57% of the undergraduate population (6). Consistent with these enrollment changes, women surpassed men in educational expectations and degree attainment over the last 30 years (5). While in the aggregate, women have made great progress in gaining access to and completing postsecondary education; gender differences are not uniform across all groups (7). For example, among all undergraduates enrolled in 1999 to 2000, women made up 63% of African American undergraduates, 62% of students age 40 or older, and 70% of single parents (8). Women constituted a majority of beginning postsecondary students overall (57%), but the distribution of men and women varied by type of institution. Women made up 56% of the beginning student population at both 2- and 4-year institutions, but they accounted for 73% at less-than-2-year institutions. Proportionately more students 30 years or older were female (66%) than in any other age group. A greater percentage of African American and Hispanic beginning postsecondary students (62% and 61%, respectively) were women than were white or Asian (56% and 52%). African Americans and Hispanics have indeed increased their numbers among bachelor's degree recipients. However, it has been African American and Hispanic women who have made the greatest gains. Currently, African American and Hispanic women earn 66% and 60% of all bachelor's degrees awarded to African Americans and Hispanics, respectively (7).

Other factors positively influencing the percentage of students enrolling at a 4-year college included parents' education, income, college admissions test scores, and level of high school mathematics completed. Eighty-seven percent of beginning postsecondary students scoring in the highest 25% on college admissions tests and 84% of those who took calculus in high school enrolled first at the 4-year level (9). Persistence and attainment were correlated with program type, enrollment intensity, dependency status, and employment while enrolled. In 2005 to 2006, students in certificate programs had higher rates of completion than those in associate's degree programs; students who were enrolled full-time completed degrees at higher rates than those enrolled part-time; and independent students had higher completion rates than dependent students, although larger percentages of dependent than independent students were still enrolled. Students who worked full-time left postsecondary education without completion at higher rates and remained enrolled at lower rates than those who did not work or worked part time (9).

GRADUATE EDUCATION

Although recent increases in the numbers of ethnic and racial minority applicants, accepted applicants, and matriculants to medical school are promising, it is important to note that there remain fundamental structural problems in our nation's education system that impede efforts to increase diversity in medical education. These problems in the medical education pipeline, often at the K–12 levels, play an essential role in limiting the number of racial and ethnic minorities applying and being accepted to a medical school (2).

Ethnicity
Master's and Doctoral Degrees African Americans compose roughly 12% of the U.S. population and are represented among associate degree recipients at this same level (10). The level of African American representation declines to just over 9% for bachelor's degree recipients but increases to more than 10% among master's degree recipients. The downward trend is then notable in the first professional (7%) and doctoral degrees (6.1%). Hispanics showed a consistent downward trend, ranging from just under 12% among associate degree recipients to just over 3% for doctoral degree recipients (11).

African American students are far more likely to receive a master's degree from a "single degree doctoral" institution than are non-Hispanic whites. Specifically, 17% of master's degrees awarded to African Americans were conferred by institutions that award a doctoral degree in only one discipline, compared with only 10% of master's degrees conferred to white students. At the same time, African American students were much less likely than whites to receive a master's degree from institutions that award doctoral degrees across a comprehensive set of disciplines (i.e., the traditional, large public and private research universities). In contrast, Asian Americans were far more likely to receive master's degrees from the comprehensive doctoral universities than whites. Hispanics were somewhat less likely than whites to receive a master's degree from a comprehensive doctoral university but more likely than any other group to receive a master's degree from a doctoral institution with a focused doctoral program mix (11).

Approximately 60% of American citizens/permanent residents are white (10,11). In academic year 2006 to 2007, 55% of doctoral degree recipients were in that group. Only 15% of doctoral degree recipients were persons of color, either U.S. citizens or permanent residents.

Medical Doctoral Degree   The Association of American Medical Colleges (AAMC) data indicate that the number of whites applying to medical schools dropped from approximately 35,000 in 1974 to 20,000 in 1992 and gradually rose again to 30,000 in 1997 (12). It has since dropped to the 1992 levels in 2004. The number of minority applicants has increased overall for all groups from 1974 to 2004. The increase has been from 1217 to 6734 for Asians, 2295 to 2802 for African Americans, 837 to 2545 for Hispanics, and 127 to 145 for Native Americans. In 2004, African Americans constituted 7.8% and Hispanics constituted 7.1% of all applicants. Of all minority applicants in 2004, Asians were the largest group (19%). African Americans, Hispanics, Native Americans/Alaska Natives, and Native Hawaiians/Other Pacific Islanders comprised 15.3% of the applicant pool. An examination of applicants from Hispanic and Asian groups revealed variation in the number of applicants by subgroup. For example, the numbers of applicants from some Hispanic subgroups have been increasing steadily. Mexican American applicants, in particular, have increased by 9.8% from 2002 to 2004. Puerto Rican applicants, however, have declined by 20.3% from 2002 to 2004. Asian Indians accounted for 32.1% of all Asian applicants in 2004, and Chinese followed at 20.1%. The highest increases were in the Asian and Hispanic groups; they experienced a threefold increase in number of applicants. The percentage of applicants accepted into medical school in 2004 was as follows: 52% for whites, 48% for Asians, 41% for African Americans, 49% for Hispanics, and 37% for Native Americans (Fig. 28.1).

Within each ethnic group, every applicant has a 52% or less chance of being accepted to a medical school. Across ethnic groups the odds are as follows: whites are twice, thrice, and four times as likely to be accepted to medical school as Asians, African Americans, and Hispanics, respectively. The number of white individuals graduating from medical school has decreased from 12,788 in the early 1980s to

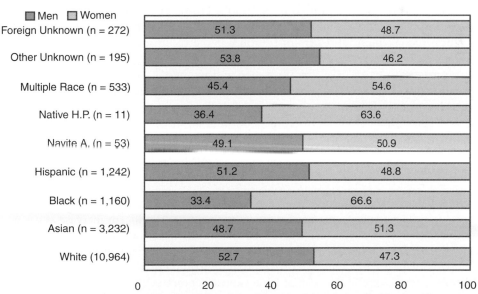

Figure 28-1. Percentage of accepted medical school applicants by race and gender. (From Castillo-Page L, Zhang K, Steinecke A, et al. *Minorities in Medical Education: Facts & Figures 2005.* Retrieved October 21, 2008, from https://services.aamc.org/Publications/showfile.cfm?file=version53.pdf& prd_id=133&prv_id=154&pdf_id=53, with permission.)

10,120 in 2004. Nonetheless, in 2004, 64% of medical school graduates were white. Asians represented 20% in the same year, with African Americans, Hispanics, and Native Americans representing 6.5%, 6.4%, and 0.6%, respectively. Overall, minority graduates have increased. Since 1980, Hispanic graduates have doubled from 462 to 1007, and African American graduates have increased from 768 to 1034. Among all Hispanic graduates, Mexican American graduates doubled from 1980 to 2004, still significantly off their representation in the general population. African Americans, for example, represent more than 12% of the U.S. population. African American and Hispanic enrollment has remained steady at 10% of total enrollments within the same time frame.

In 2003 and 2004, Hispanic matriculants to medical school increased from 6.6% (1089) in 2003 to 7.0% (1175) in 2004 of the total pool of matriculants (12). This increase was largely caused by an increase in the number of Mexican American matriculants. In the same year, the number of African American matriculants also increased, raising their percentage within the overall matriculant pool (from 6.4% [1060] in 2003 to 6.5% [1086] in 2004).

It is noteworthy that the medical school faculty in 2004 was 72% white, 12.6% Asian, 4% Hispanic, 3% African American, and 0.1% Native American. Hispanics, African Americans, Asians, and Native Americans/Alaska Natives and Native Hawaiians/Other Pacific Islanders were primarily concentrated at the rank of assistant professor.

Gender

Master's and Doctoral Degrees   Women continue to outnumber men at the graduate and doctoral levels; however, women are concentrated in specific areas of study (11). At the master's level, women triple the number of men in education, whereas men triple the number of women in engineering and computer and information science. African American women in education exceed men by a ratio of 4 to 1; in psychology, the ratio is 5 to 1 (11). However, men are twice as many as women in engineering. Similarly, among Hispanics, women exceed men by 4 to 1. Business management and administration was the top discipline for men in general and for each ethnicity. Business management and education are the top two fields at the master's degree level for both men and women. However, interestingly, international women received vast majority of doctoral degrees in math, engineering, and law—more than 60% of degrees in those fields. African American women earned a significant share of doctorates, more than 20%, in ethnic and cultural programs, as well as in technological studies and religious vocations (11). For Hispanic women, foreign language and literature are the most popular at the master's and doctoral levels.

Medical Doctoral Degree   The AAMC report indicates that there has been an increase in number in both men and women, with a more significant increase in women graduates being awarded first degrees in the health fields between 1992 and 2001 (12). In 1992, 17,694 men were awarded first professional degrees in the health field compared with 19,340 men in 2001 representing an increase of 1646 men. In 1992, 10,609 women were awarded first professional degrees in the health field compared with 17,294 in 2001, representing an increase of 6685 women.

The number of women applicants to medical schools was about 8700 in 1974 and men about 34,000. That number decreased steadily for men, having its lowest point in 1988 about 15,000. The numbers for women applicants increased and reached just over 10,000 in 1988. By 2004, the number of women applying to medical school was slightly higher than men, 18,018 and 17,717 respectively. There are more women matriculating in the African American and Native American groups than men. However, the men still outnumber women in the white (53%) and Hispanic (51%) groups. While the number of men graduating from medical school has gradually decreased from about 11,600 in 1980 to 8565, in 2004, women have more than doubled their numbers over the same period, reaching 7256 (12). In 2004, a total of 15,821 students graduated from medical school. Women were nearly 46% of all those graduates. Overall, there are still more men graduating from medical school than women.

Today, more African American and Hispanic women apply to medical school than men. Additionally, women comprise the majority of African American and Hispanic first-time applicants. In 2003, women for the first time surpassed men in medical school applicants. In 2004, women comprised 50.4% of all applicants. In most racial and ethnic groups, women made up more than 50% of first-time applicants. In particular, African American women made up 69.5% of all African American first-time applicants. As the number of women applicants has grown, racial and ethnic minority women applicants have also steadily increased their numbers. Among minority women applicants, African American women have made the greatest gains. In 2004, African American women were nearly 70% of all African American applicants to medical school. Within Hispanic applicant subgroups, the number of women applicants has surpassed that of their male counterparts, with the exception of Cuban Americans, where men outnumber women (12).

In 2004, the acceptance rates for women in most racial and ethnic groups surpassed those of their male counterparts. African American women were nearly 67% of all African Americans accepted in 2004 (12). In 2004, for most ethnic and racial groups, women were either nearly 50% of all matriculants or they surpassed the matriculation rates of men. The difference in matriculation rates for African American men and women was similar to their acceptance patterns. In 2004, African American women made up 66.1% of all African American matriculants, only slightly less than the percentage of African American women accepted.

The fluctuations in women and minority applicants can to some extent be attributed to (i) anti–affirmative action court rulings and state ballot initiatives such as *Hopwood v. University of Texas* in 1995, and *California Proposition 209* in 1996 (13) and (ii) two recent pro–affirmative action Supreme Court rulings (14,15) in 2003/2004.

At all levels from assistant professor upward, there are more men than women. However, full professors were primarily men, ranging from 80% to 83% of the total number in 2004. Approximately 70% of women faculty were at the instructor and assistant professor levels.

POSTGRADUATE EDUCATION IN PSYCHIATRY

Ethnicity

Whites accounted for the largest percentage of psychiatry residents (51.7% in 2006 to 2006 vs. 49.7% in 2004 to 2005), with the percentage of ethnic minorities staying relatively constant. There is also an increase of residents identifying themselves as "other." The GM Track separately asked for the residents' Hispanic or Latino identification, with 8.4% of the residents identifying themselves as having Hispanic identity, an increase from previous years (16). African Americans constituted 7.4% in 2006 to 2007 and 7.2% in 2004 to 2005. Native Americans are decreasing in percentage (0.3% to 0.2%) (16).

Gender

According to American Medical Association Master File diversity data of January 2006, there are 37,556 active psychiatrists; among them, 33% are women. The Graduate Medical Education (GME) indicates that in 2005 there were 1250 first-year residents and fellows (17). Furthermore, 53% of the psychiatry residents were women, 8% Hispanic, and 7% African American (17). The American Psychiatric Association (APA) data indicate that the number of all residents and fellows has been slowly going up since the decline in the early to mid 1990s (18). The number of psychiatry residents continues its steady increase except for a small decrease in 2008. The data indicate that the percentage gap between women and men residents has now increased to 6.2%, favoring women (18). The last time men outnumbered women in psychiatry residency was in 2001 to 2002, in which 49.9% of residents were men and 49% were women. Across medicine, women residents make up 43.6% of all residents and fellows (19). Combined programs show a higher percentage of men except for the triple board programs, where 67% of residents are women (18).

U.S. AND INTERNATIONAL MEDICAL GRADUATES

In 2008, a total of 1013 medical graduates will enter first-year psychiatry residency programs in 2008, a small increase over the previous year's total of 1000 (20). The number of graduates from U.S. medical schools choosing psychiatry has dropped slowly but steadily for several years. The current number (595) in 2008 represents a drop of 6% from 2007 and 8.8% from 2005. Psychiatry continues to rely on international medical graduates to fill many of its residency training slots. This year a total of 1069 positions were offered, with 94.8% of those being filled. U.S. medical school graduates accounted for 55.7% of the filled positions.

With insufficient numbers of students in the pipeline, the competition for residents will be brisk. Some medical specialties are already looking for ways to increase their training capacity, either by attempting to roll back the restrictions in the Balanced Budget Act of 1997 or by decreasing the duration of residency training and thereby increasing the number of residents who can be trained (21). As students search for the best path to their future, it seems inevitable that most will gravitate to specialties that demand their level of education. While some may be dissuaded from choosing psychiatry because of its strong overlap with nonphysician therapists, or because of managed care's strictures (22), or simply because psychiatry is seen as too distant from "real" medicine (23), others will be attracted to psychiatry because of its biological paradigm and the intensity of patient contact that it affords (24). Yet some may wonder what became of the profession's antecedent paradigms and of the practitioners who trained under them—and what might be its next (25). These concerns do not appear as great for International Medical Graduates (IMGs), who, in 1975, accounted for 25% of psychiatrists, who fill 40% of psychiatry's residency positions in 1979, and currently account for 31%. Cultural differences may exist, but IMGs contribute a great deal to the profession, often in ways that differentiate them from U.S. medical graduates. When assessed in 1996, IMG psychiatry residents tended to be older than U.S. graduates, and many more were women. After residency, they practiced more hours, worked more often in public institutions, and cared for more psychotic patients than their U.S.-educated peers (26). Indeed, in 2000, one-third of IMG psychiatrists who were involved in patient care worked as staff physicians, double the percentage of U.S. grads, and they accounted for almost one-half of these positions. That such differences should exist between U.S. and international grads tells something of the priorities and expectations that U.S. students have on entering the profession and of the jurisdictional boundaries that they are most likely to defend (27). The number of international medical graduates continues to decline, down by 8.8% from 2000 (18). This is important because International Medical Graduates constitute approximately 33% of all psychiatrists (average 23.5% among all physicians) (28). If both the U.S. graduates and International Medical graduates entering psychiatry continue to decline, there is a potential for a shortage of psychiatrists in the near future.

CONCLUSION

Clearly, disparity exists in the education of Americans. It does appear that the root of the problem is multifaceted; primarily socioeconomic status, high school educational opportunities, race, and gender. At the college enrollment level, all ethnic groups are proportionally represented. The disparity seems to begin with graduation from college, with minorities showing a significant drop in percentage at graduation from college.

Since 2001, college enrollment of women has exceed that of men. The gap is significantly wider among minorities. Especially, among African Americans there are significantly more women than men graduating from medical school. In contrast, women of all ethnic backgrounds are underrepresented in engineering and computer science. Medical school acceptance and graduation are also correlated to gender.

The low representation of women in the upper echelons of faculty does not seem to have affected women medical school graduates. The same cannot be said for ethnic minority groups. Nonetheless, it is important that we identify the root causes of this disparity and address them appropriately.

The importance of a diverse student and professional body cannot be understated. In psychiatry, women outnumber men, and U.S. medical graduates outnumber international graduates. It is essential to improved quality of care, economic development, and access to healthcare that proportional representation is achieved in our educational institutions.

FUTURE DIRECTIONS

The data indicate that minorities are more likely to complete 2-year colleges rather than 4-year colleges. They are more likely to get a doctorate at an institution that has only one doctoral specialty. These types of institutions are less likely to be Ivy League colleges/universities. It is possible to hypothesize that the disparity in education would be even greater in Ivy League schools. This is the subject of future research and beyond the scope of this chapter.

The area of greatest disparity is at the academic level of full professor for both women and ethnic minorities. It may be helpful to examine the impact of this potentially on both diversity and proportional representation at our educational institutions.

References

1. Bérengera V, Verdier-Chouchaneb A. Multidimensional measures of well-being: standard of living and quality of life across countries. *World Dev* 2007;35(7):1259–1276

2. Cooper RA. Medical schools and their applicants: an analysis. *Health Aff (Millwood)* 2003;22(4):71–84.

3. ACT. Crisis at the core: preparing all students for college and work. *Activity* 2005;43(1).

4. Lederman D. *The Postsecondary Picture for Minority Students (and Men). Analysis of the Data of the National Center for Education Statistics, "Status and Trends in the Education of Racial and Ethnic Minorities."* Higher Education, 2007. Available at http://www.insidehighered.com. Accessed August 12, 2008.

5. Freeman CE, ed. *Trends in Educational Equity of Girls & Women: 2004.* NCES 2005–016. Washington, DC: U.S. Department of Education, 2004.

6. Gerald DE, Hussar WJ, eds. *Projections of Education Statistics to 2013.* NCES 2004–013. Washington, DC: U.S. Department of Education, 2004.

7. Horn KP, et al, eds. *Gender Differences in Participation and Completion of Undergraduate Education and How They Have Changed Over Time. Postsecondary Education Descriptive Analysis Reports.* NCES 2005-169. Washington, DC: U.S. Department of Education, 2005.

8. Horn L, Peter K, Rooney K, eds. *Profile of Undergraduates in U.S. Postsecondary Institutions: 1999–2000.* NCES 2002-168. Washington, DC: U.S. Department of Education, 2002.

9. Berkner L, Choy S, Hunt-White T, eds. *Descriptive Summary of 2003–04 Beginning Postsecondary Students: Three Years Later.* NCES 2008-174. Washington, DC: U.S. Department of Education, 2008:iii-xii.

10. U.S. Bureau of Census: U.S. Census, 2000.

11. Borden VMH. Top 100 graduate and professional degree procuders—interpreting the data. *Diverse* 2008. Available online at http://www.diverseeducation.com/artman/publish/article_11384.shtml. Accessed December 16, 2008.

12. Association of American Medical Colleges. *Minorities in Medical Education: Facts & Figures 2005.* Washington, DC: Center for Workforce Studies, 2005.

13. *Hopwood v. Texas, 78 F.3d 932 (5th Cir. 1996),* 1996.

14. *Grutter v. Bollinger, 539 U.S. 306 (2003).* 2003 United States Supreme Court: U.S. 32.

15. *Gratz v. Bollinger, 539 U.S. 244 (2003).* 2003 United States Supreme Court.

16. Brotherton SE, Etzel SI. AMA and AAMC data from the National Survey of GME Programs. *JAMA* 2006;296:1154–1169.

17. American Association of Medical Colleges. *Graduate Medical Education.* Washington, DC: Center for Workforce Studies, 2006:15–18.

18. American Psychiatric Association. *Resident Census: Characteristics and Distribution of Psychiatry Residents in the U.S.* Arlington, VA: American Psychiatric Association, 2007.

19. Brotherton SE, Etzel SI. Graduate medical education, 2006–2007. *JAMA* 2007;298(9):1081–1096.

20. Moran M. Match shows slight increase in graduates going into psychiatry. *Psychiatry News* 2008;43(9):1.

21. Johns MM. The time has come to reform graduate medical education. *JAMA* 2001;286(9):1075–1076.

22. Tamaskar P, McGinnis RE. Declining student interest in psychiatry. *JAMA* 2002;287(14):1859.

23. Rao NR. Recent trends in psychiatry residency workforce with special reference to international medical graduates. *Acad Psychiatry* 2003;27(4):269–276.

24. Sierles FS, Yager J, Weissman SH. Recruitment of U.S. medical graduates into psychiatry: Reasons for optimism, sources of concern. *Acad Psychiatry* 2003;27(4):252–259.

25. Double D. The limits of psychiatry. *BMJ* 2002;324(7342):900–904.

26. Pasko T, ed. *Physician Characteristics and Distribution in the US, 2002–2003 Edition.* American Medical Association: Chicago, 2002.

27. Cooper RA. Where is psychiatry going and who is going there? *Acad Psychiatry* 2003;27(4):229–234.

28. American Association of Medical Colleges. *Physician Specialty Data: A Chart Book.* Washington, DC: Center for Workforce Studies, 2006:3–11.

29 The Role of Continuing Medical Education

Carlyle H. Chan and Joseph B. Layde

INTRODUCTION

Disparities in access to psychiatric care and in the quality of mental healthcare patients receive are problems that require intervention by practicing psychiatrists, other physicians, and nonphysician healthcare providers. Continuing education has an important role in calling professionals' attention to the issue of care disparity and in giving those professionals the information they need to help improve the quality of care delivered to all their patients with mental health issues.

In this chapter, we shall first present an overview of the system of continuing medical education and how it can be used to help physicians address issues of disparity in mental healthcare; we shall then present a brief discussion of current disparities in the care of patients with depression in the United States as an example of information physicians and other clinicians should learn as continuing education programs strive to heighten awareness of healthcare disparities.

THE STRUCTURE OF CONTINUING MEDICAL EDUCATION IN THE UNITED STATES

> *A residency director was concerned about residents appreciating the difficulty that some low income patients had in keeping or arriving on time for clinic appointments. As part of residency orientation, he organized a scavenger hunt to obtain culturally relevant products from various ethnic neighborhoods in the community. The caveat was that residents had to reach all their destinations via public transportation. The program director heard fewer complaints about no shows and late arrivals after instituting this learning experience.*

Once graduate medical education is completed, there is no longer a program director to guide the development of new knowledge, skills, and attitudes. The concept of lifelong learning is intertwined with that of self-assessment. The challenge of achieving cultural awareness in continuing medical education is fourfold. First, a clinician must self-assess the need for further or continued training. Second, the clinician must allocate time away from a busy clinical practice and among competing offerings in continuing medical education (CME), particularly ones providing updated data on new clinical research treatment findings. Third, few sources of external funding are available to support CME offerings related to cultural issues. Finally, there is also a need to recognize that cultural competency is not unlike other competencies. It is a developmental process that requires years of active learning to progress to the proficient and expert stages of practice.

Developing cultural sensitivity is not easily accomplished by lectures, a passive learning technique. Active learning exercises like the one in the introduction enrich training and expand the appreciation of cultural awareness.

Life after residency and fellowship training falls in the province of the American Board of Medical Specialties (ABMS), the Federation of State Medical Boards, the Accreditation Council for Continuing Medical Education, and specialty societies such as the American Psychiatric Association (APA).

Board certification has evolved from lifetime certification to 10-year, time-limited certification to maintenance of certification (MOC). The ABMS MOC program consists of four parts: professional standing, lifelong learning and self-assessment, cognitive expertise, and practice performance assessment.

Professional standing ties board certification to medical licensure, that is, a license to practice medicine is required to maintain certification. Lifelong learning maintains the traditional CME process but adds the expectation of self-assessment. The expectation for self-assessment places a new responsibility for clinicians to determine their own areas to improve. Demonstrating one's cognitive expertise (the third part of MOC) will mean continuing to take and pass written certification exams every 10 years.

The fourth part of MOC, practice performance assessment, is the biggest change in the certification process. This section is intended to link lifelong learning with clinical outcomes. Psychiatrists (and physicians in general) will be expected to review their own clinical practices and identify an area where clinical results could be improved. Physicians will be expected to select several patients and document an outcome, comparing that outcome with that of a reference group. They will then be expected to research and select a change in clinical practice that will affect the outcome. Finally, they will select another group of patients to monitor and document whether the practice change actually had its intended effect. Five CME credits can be awarded for the initial practice assessment, five more for the practice change, and a further five for the follow-up practice assessment. Psychiatrists who complete all three portions can be awarded a bonus of five credits, but they need to work with an accredited CME sponsor to develop an individualized program.

The ABMS has also adopted the six competencies that are an integral part of graduate medical education, including patient care, medical knowledge, interpersonal and communication skills, professionalism, systems-based practice, and practice-based learning and improvement. If one closely examines cultural competency, one quickly realizes that this particular competency transcends all six core competencies. Knowledge and appreciation of cultural issues can have an immediate effect on patient care and influence communication and interpersonal skills as well as medical professionalism.

In addressing the challenges listed at the start of this chapter, psychiatrists can utilize the APA's Online Self-Assessment (which has a limited number of culturally based questions) to check on their cultural awareness. CME credits are awarded for this activity. Involvement with a hospital- or practice-based quality improvement program might also identify a clinical need for more culturally based training.

Finding course offerings in this area will remain a challenge. However, several fine texts and videos have been created that could fill a content need. The fourth part of MOC, practice performance assessment, provides an opportunity to develop an individual or group practice approach to a culturally relevant clinical issue. For example, a practitioner may notice several incidences in which members of a particular ethnic group appeared overmedicated on a standard dose of antipsychotic medication. By documenting these occurrences, researching the medical literature to discover that particular ethnic groups may indeed require lower doses of an antipsychotic, developing a new dosing protocol when treating individuals of this ethnic group, and then monitoring the results of a subsequently treated group of patients, a psychiatrist's newfound awareness could be demonstrated in an improved clinical outcome. This activity (if approved by an accredited CME provider) would not only provide documentation of fulfilling the fourth part of MOC but also 20 new CME credits that could be applied toward licensure.

While competency has been the goal of residency education for the past several years, postgraduate clinicians ought to view it as a minimum standard and consider developing their specialized expertise. Brothers Herbert Dreyfus, a philosopher, and Stuart Dreyfus, a computer scientist, have been thinking and working on artificial intelligence and have written about the acquisition of knowledge and expertise in humans (1). They note that there are at least five developmental stages: novice, advanced beginner, competent, proficient, and expert. (Others have written about a sixth stage, master.) The stages appear true in any type of learning endeavor, be it medicine or sports or chess.

The initial stages of learning a skill or task are rules based. A novice follows guidelines or instructions on how to proceed. For example, the beginning medical student memorizes diagnostic criteria and must seek guidance for medication selection and specific dosing. Through exposure, repetition, and practice a physician advances from novice (beginning medical student) to advanced beginner (entering residency) to competent (completion of residency). As physicians advance along this path, they no longer simply follow rules but are able to diagnose patients without the classic textbook symptoms and use their clinical experience to adapt treatments for those patients who are more complex in their clinical presentation or who have failed to respond to initial treatments or had side effects. The advanced physician is able to prioritize decision-making to account for new and increasing complexities.

How does the practicing clinician move beyond competency? The Dreyfus brothers point out that experts, rather than use rules to make decisions, tend to use "intuition" (1). By "intuition" they do not mean a hunch. Rather, they are referring to a nonverbal process of utilizing accumulated knowledge and experience, or "knowhow," partly akin to pattern recognition. Studies of master chess players reveal that they do not think through their moves or plan three moves ahead. They just "know" the correct move. Driving an automobile is another example. Parents who teach their children how to drive quickly realize that they need to deconstruct the techniques they no longer think about, for example, turning a corner. Trying to verbalize how to keep your balance while riding a bike is yet another example.

Studies have also shown that across a variety of fields and professions, including chess and sports, it consistently seems to take about 10 years to become an expert in a field (2). Now, repeating a task for 10 years does not automatically qualify one as an expert. Weekend golfers are testimony to that. Conversely, not practicing a task can cause an expert's skills and abilities to deteriorate. The Dreyfuses cite the example of an experienced pilot who had not flown a particular plane in years who encountered a problem to which normally he would have responded automatically (1). However, because he was rusty in his flight skills, he had to think about his response rather than react, and this led to almost disastrous consequences.

It takes a combination of practical experience plus study and application of that study to the task(s) at hand to progress beyond competency. This ability to intuit the correct diagnosis or treatment, while masterful, can also be fraught with the possibility of errors of bias. Groopman's book *How Doctors Think* delves into this process. Groopman warns doctors to guard against these errors and be ever vigilant and aware of individual biases (3).

DISPARITIES IN CARE FOR DEPRESSION: A CHALLENGE FOR CONTINUING EDUCATION

A psychiatrist 10 years out of training moved her practice from a small town in New England to a large city in Texas. She found that she was ill-equipped to deal with many of the cultural issues that the patients in her new practice presented. Many of them spoke Spanish as their first language, and their beliefs about mental health were quite different from those of her patients in New England. Fortunately, she found that the continuing medical education programs offered in her new hometown included a variety of courses on cultural issues relevant to Hispanic mental health patients. After taking a series of the courses and brushing up on her college Spanish through a medical Spanish class, she felt much better able to serve her new patients well.

Mental health workers face challenges in their practices as they encounter patients who come from a different background than their own. Psychiatrists, nonpsychiatric physicians, psychologists, social workers, physician assistants, nurse practitioners, and others who provide mental healthcare to patients from a variety of ethnic and cultural backgrounds need to keep abreast of information regarding optimal mental health treatments for all their patients. Continuing education carried out over the professional lifetimes of caregivers should include descriptions of cultural and ethnic differences in the presentation of psychiatric disorders, as well as up-to-date information on the differences in the sort of care patients from varied backgrounds receive for their mental health problems. A brief discussion of disparities in the care of patients with depression is presented here as an illustrative example of what caregivers should learn in continuing education about mental health disparities so that future generations of Americans will experience less inequality in mental healthcare.

The purpose of continuing medical and allied health education should be the provision of better care to patients, which requires that practitioners understand things that get in the way of their patients getting optimal care. Accordingly, a goal of continuing education for all those groups should be the familiarization of healthcare providers with what is known both about those factors which reduce the detection of mental health problems in minority patients and those which reduce the likelihood of successful treatment of mental health problems in such patients.

Because most patients with mental health problems are more likely to seek help from their primary healthcare provider rather than from a psychiatrist, it is particularly important that some continuing education on mental health treatment disparity be targeted to those primary care providers. Nondetection of mental health problems, particularly depression, in primary care clinics leaves millions of Americans with serious, treatable illness at increased risk for absenteeism from work, lower quality of life, and even suicide. A decade ago, internists and family practitioners in a large, multi-center study conducted in Boston, Chicago, and Los Angeles were found to be less likely to detect a mental health problem in African American patients than in white patients (4). Because African American and Hispanic patients underutilize specialty mental healthcare, those groups, even more than others, count on their primary care providers for detection of serious mental health problems.

As a result of reports like Borowsky's, considerable attention has been given in recent years to increasing the sensitivity of primary care providers to the unmet mental health needs of their African American and Hispanic patients (4). The Quality Improvement for Depression Project has conducted randomized clinical trials of various quality improvement strategies aimed at improving the management of major depression in primary care settings. Encouragingly, African American and Hispanic patients taking part in the trials reported that their primary care providers recommended depression treatments at roughly the same rate as white patients reported. However, African American and Hispanic patients in the trials were less likely than white patients to report that they took prescribed antidepressant medications or followed through with recommended mental health specialty care (5). Continuing education of both mental health and primary care providers needs to highlight this lower adherence to prescribed mental health treatment among African American and Hispanic patients to encourage practitioners to redouble their efforts to ensure that their patients follow through with essential components of their mental healthcare.

The degree of disparity in treatment of depression in Asian Americans from that in the majority population is controversial, with one study finding Asian Americans more likely than whites to receive antidepressant treatment for depression and another study finding Asian Americans less likely than whites to receive effective treatment of depression after hospitalization (6,7). A recent review (8) hypothesizes that whites may be particularly susceptible to disparities in care associated with low socioeconomic status, noting that the Strothers et al. study (6), which used a sample with an overall lower socioeconomic status than the Virnig et al. study (7), may have exposed the particularly high risk of poor whites to receive disparately poor care for depression.

Although depression is the mental health condition most commonly treated by both primary care providers and mental health specialists, it is not the only disorder that should be a focus of continuing education on disparities in care. As further research becomes available on treatment disparities among Americans with other diseases, such as schizophrenia and bipolar, anxiety, and substance use disorders, it also should be widely disseminated to practitioners through continuing education.

Written materials can be used as a useful part of continuing education of mental health practitioners on how to alleviate disparities in patient care. The APA provides several resources which are useful for the continuing education of psychiatrists on issues regarding care for disadvantaged groups of patients.

FOCUS—The Journal of Lifelong Learning in Psychiatry, is the APA's journal specifically aimed at psychiatrists seeking continuing education. The Winter 2006 issue of *FOCUS*, entitled "Gender, Race, and Culture," is a particularly useful resource providing information on appropriate mental health treatment for Hispanics, American Indians, and Chinese Immigrants (9).

A series of residency training curricula published by members of the APA's minority and underrepresented component committees can also be used as tools for continuing education. Curricula have been published in the APA journal *Academic Psychiatry* on the care of gay men and Lesbians (10), women (11), American Indians and Alaska Natives (12), Hispanics (13), Asian Americans (14), and African Americans (15). These curricula provide information on clinically relevant cultural and ethnic issues in underserved groups of patients.

CME courses on DSM-IV-TR Cultural Formulation and Clinical Applications for Cultural Psychiatry have been given at the APA Annual meeting. The APA Office of Minority and National Affairs publishes a guide to the annual meeting's CME offerings each year including workshops by the APA Minority Fellows, and the APA Component's Minority and Underrepresented Groups that are about diversity issues. The Society for the Study of Culture and Psychiatry's annual meeting in June (http://www.Societyandculture.org/cms) is devoted to cultural issues. There are also many excellent regional conferences, such as the annual Cultural Competence and Mental Health Summit in California (http://www.cimh.org), and the Quality Healthcare for Culturally Diverse Populations, biannually (http://www.diversityrx.org). While not CME, Dr. Russell Lim's *Clinical Manual of Cultural Psychiatry* (16) is an excellent starting point for the busy clinician and a DVD is being prepared for CME credit. California and New Jersey have State legislation requiring CME sessions to address issues of Cultural Competence.

CONCLUSION

Continuing medical education means recognition of this developmental model of how individuals acquire expertise and places the concept of lifelong learning into context. Incorporating cultural sensitivity and awareness into specialty practice requires an appreciation that learning has not ended with residency training. Achieving expert status in a discipline requires self-assessment not only of knowledge, skills, and attitudes but also of clinical outcomes. It then requires the active searching for new knowledge and experience and, finally, application to patient care to reinforce the new learning.

The responsibility to educate ourselves about cultural diversity is part of our social contract with society. If we do not fulfill this responsibility on our own, then society will respond, usually in the form of legislation. In fact, this has already happened. California and New Jersey have mandated cultural competency CME and Ohio is considering such legislation (17).

There is a need for new vehicles of CME as well as new sources of content. Online Internet-based teaching programs could be universally available, 24 hours a day, 7 days a week and could provide relevant educational materials for all psychiatrists regarding cultural issues specific to individual cultures and minority groups. In addition, there is a need to develop curriculum for the growing number of International Medical Graduate psychiatrists to assist them not only in meeting the challenges of practicing with America's melting pot of citizens in need of mental health services but also in appreciating the nuances of the American healthcare system (18).

References
1. Dreyfus HL, Dreyfus SE, Athanasiou T. *Mind Over Machine: The Power of Human Intuition and Expertise in the Era of the Computer*. New York: Free Press, 1988.
2. Ross PE. The expert mind. *Sci Am* 2006;295:64–71.
3. Groopman JE. *How Doctors Think*. Boston: Houghton Mifflin, 2007.

4. Borowsky SJ, Rubenstein LV, Meredith LS, et al. Who is at risk of nondetection of mental health problems in primary care? *J Gen Intern Med* 2000;15:381–388.

5. Miranda J, Cooper LA. Disparities in care for depression among primary care patients. *J Gen Intern Med* 2004;19:120–126.

6. Strothers HS 3rd, Rust G, Minor P, et al. Disparities in antidepressant treatment in Medicaid elderly diagnosed with depression. *J Am Geriatr Soc* 2005;53:456–461.

7. Virnig B, Huang Z, Lurie N, et al. Does Medicare managed care provide equal treatment for mental illness across races? *Arch Gen Psychiatry* 2004;61:201–205.

8. Simpson SM, Krishnan LL, Kunik ME, et al. Racial disparities in diagnosis and treatment of depression: A literature review. *Psychiatr Q* 2007;78:3–14.

9. Primm AB. Gender, race, and culture. *Focus* 2006;4(1):1–149.

10. Stein TS. A curriculum for learning in psychiatric residencies about homosexuality, gay men, and lesbians. *Acad Psychiatry* 1994;18:59–70.

11. Spielvogel AM, Dickstein LJ, Robinson GE. A psychiatric residency curriculum about gender and women's issues. *Acad Psychiatry* 1995;19:187–201.

12. Thompson JW. A curriculum for learning about American Indians and Alaska Natives. *Acad Psychiatry* 1996;20:5–14.

13. Garza-Treviño ES, Ruiz P, Venegas-Samuels K. A psychiatric curriculum directed to the care of the Hispanic patient. *Acad Psychiatry* 1997;21:1–10.

14. Lu FG, Du N, Gaw A, et al. A psychiatric residency curriculum about Asian American issues. *Acad Psychiatry* 2002;26:225–236.

15. Harris HW, Felder D, Clark MO. A psychiatric residency curriculum on the care of African American patients. *Acad Psychiatry* 2004;28:226–239.

16. Lim RF, ed. *Clinical Manual of Cultural Psychiatry*. Arlington VA: American Psychiatric Publishing, 2006.

17. Croasdale M. States, CME Incorporating Cultural Competency Training. *AMA News* July 1, 2007.

18. Glazer N, Moynihan DP. *Beyond the Melting Pot: The Negroes, Puerto Ricans, Jews, Italians and Irish of New York City*. 2nd ed. Cambridge: MIT Press, 1970.

30 Ethnic and Racial Group– Specific Considerations

Margarita Alegría, Meghan Woo, David Takeuchi, and James Jackson

INTRODUCTION: DEFINITION OF THE POPULATIONS

The racial and ethnic composition of the United States is rapidly changing, spurred by an influx of immigrants from South and Central America, Asia, and the Caribbean. Latinos (defined as persons of Mexican, Puerto Rican, Cuban, South or Central American, or other Spanish cultural or origin regardless of race) are currently the largest ethnic minority population, totaling 45.5 million, or 15% of the estimated total U.S. population (1). Black Americans (defined as people having origins in any of the black race groups of Africa) are the second largest racial minority population and currently comprise 13% of the U.S. population (or 36.2 million people) (2). Although black immigrants have arrived in the United States in smaller numbers, they have contributed to an increasingly diversified U.S. black population. Caribbean blacks are the largest subgroup of black immigrants, comprising 60% of the foreign-born black population and more than 4% of the national black population. Totaling nearly 12 million people, Asian Americans (defined as people having origins in any of the original peoples of the Far East, Southeast Asian, or the Indian subcontinent) have grown at the fastest rate of any major racial group, making up nearly 4% of the U.S. population.

Despite the increasing public prominence of Latino, Asian, and black populations in the United States, there is limited knowledge about their mental health. This lack of mental health data has emerged as a critical issue over the past two decades as community organizations seek to address the pressing and complex health and mental health needs of racial/ethnic minority groups who have different cultural norms and who often have low levels of English language proficiency. Understanding the patterns of mental health needs and effectively planning services for this growing and extremely diverse population is especially critical to effectively respond to the distinct service needs of these groups.

To address this lack of data, the Collaborative Psychiatric Epidemiological Studies (CPES) is the first of its kind to provide comprehensive, epidemiological data regarding the distributions, correlates, and risk factors of mental disorders among the general U.S. population with special emphasis on minority groups. The CPES joins together three nationally representative surveys of household residents (18 and older) in the noninstitutionalized populations of the coterminous United States; the National Latino and

Asian American Study (NLAAS), the National Survey of American Life (NSAL), and the National Comorbidity Study Replication (NCS-R). The studies include separate national probability samples of Latinos and Asians (NLAAS), African Americans and Caribbean blacks (NSAL), and the U.S. population (NCS-R).

The CPES dataset provides the first national data with sufficient statistical power to investigate cultural and ethnic influences on mental disorders as well as an in-depth examination of factors contributing to psychopathology and service use disparities. The CPES data, now available to the general public, have already yielded substantial and influential findings that shed light on racial/ethnic differences in psychiatric disorders and service use. However, to date there has not been a comprehensive review of these study findings. To fill this gap, this chapter presents a summary of published findings focused on the distributions, correlates, and risk factors of mental disorders and service use outcomes among the primary racial/ethnic minority groups of the CPES data set.

Providing a comprehensive review of the published findings from the CPES will allow us to compare similarities and differences between Latinos, Asians, African Americans, and Afro-Caribbeans, thereby providing a broad picture of the mental health status of racial/ethnic minority groups in the United States. We then compare study findings across the samples by focusing on similarities and differences across the racial/ethnic groups. Finally, we examine contextual and service use characteristics associated with mental health disorders among racial/ethnic minorities in the United States. We conclude with recommended areas for future research focusing on diagnostic, treatment, and preventive considerations. It is important to note that rates cited in this review may vary slightly from earlier published results because the diagnostic algorithms of the World Mental Health Survey Initiative Version of the Composite International Diagnostic Interview (WMH-CIDI) have changed since the original release of the data.

GROUP-SPECIFIC CONSIDERATIONS

Sociodemographic Characteristics

Not surprisingly, the sociodemographics of Latinos, Asians, African Americans, and Afro-Caribbeans differ dramatically when compared with each other as well as when compared with the general U.S. population. This is supported by findings from the 2000 Census (2) as well as descriptive data from the CPES datasets (data not shown). For example, in 2000, the median age of the U.S. population was 35.4 years. Comparatively, the median age for Asians was 33 years, followed by 30.4 years for blacks. Latinos were the youngest, with a median age of 26.0 years.

The socioeconomic status of these groups also varied. Regarding educational attainment, the percentage of Asians (aged 25 and older) who did not graduate from high school was comparable to the general U.S. population (19.6%), whereas this number was much higher for Latinos (47.6%) and blacks (27.7%). Asians (44%) were most likely to earn at least a bachelor's degree compared with the general population (24%), blacks (14.3%), and Latinos (10.4%). A common theme in examining the demographic characteristics is the vast heterogeneity that exists within the racial groups. For example, among Asians, Asian Indians had the highest percentage with a bachelor's degree (64%), whereas more than half of the Hmong and Cambodians had less than a high school education. Income level followed a similar pattern, with Asian families reporting a higher median income than the median for all families in the United States ($59,300 versus $50,000). Comparatively, Latinos and blacks reported much lower median family incomes ($34,400 and $33,300, respectively). Poverty rates were also similar, with blacks reporting the highest percentage in poverty (25%) followed by Latinos (22.6%). Asians reported poverty rates similar to those of the general U.S. population (12.6% and 12.4%, respectively). These rates again varied dramatically by subethnic group. For example, among Latinos, poverty rates ranged from 27.5% for Dominicans to 14.6% for Cubans, whereas among Asians these rates ranged from 37.8% for the Hmong to 6.3% for Filipinos.

Household composition also differed across these groups, with Asians reporting the highest rate of being married (60%) compared with the general population (54%), Latinos (51.3%), and blacks (36%). The percentage of female-headed households with no husband present was similar for black households (31.7%) and the general population (31.5%), but much lower among Latino (17.3%) and Asian (8.8%) households (2).

DIAGNOSTIC CONSIDERATIONS: MENTAL DISORDERS AMONG RACIAL/ETHNIC MINORITY GROUPS IN THE UNITED STATES

Depressive, Anxiety, Substance Use, and Any DSM-IV Disorders

Table 30.1 presents lifetime and 12-month prevalence estimates of DSM-IV disorders for each of the major racial/ethnic subgroups included in the CPES dataset. Consistent with published results from the CPES (3,4), non-Latino whites reported the highest rates of lifetime and 12-month disorders compared with all other racial/ethnic subgroups, whereas Asians reported the lowest rates. These results are most striking for the any disorder category, where over 40% of non-Latino whites and less than 17% of Asians reported a lifetime prevalence of any disorder. All other groups fell in between, with approximately 30% of African Americans and Latinos and 24% of Afro-Caribbeans reporting any lifetime disorder. The rates for the racial/ethnic minority groups were all significantly lower than for non-Latino whites ($p \leq .001$). Lifetime prevalence of any anxiety disorder was the most common disorder category, with 24.3% of non-Latino whites, 18.4% of African Americans, 16.5% of Latinos, 15.1% of Afro-Caribbeans, and 10.3% of Asians meeting criteria. For a lifetime prevalence of any depressive disorder, non-Latino whites reported the highest rate (21.4%) followed by Latinos (16%), Afro-Caribbeans (12.8%), African Americans (11.5%), and Asians (9.1%). Finally, non-Latino whites reported a significantly higher lifetime prevalence rate for substance use disorders (15.4%) as compared with African Americans (11.8%, $p \leq .01$), Latinos (10.6%, $p \leq .01$), Afro-Caribbeans (8.4%, $p \leq .01$), and Asians (3.6%, $p \leq .001$). Rates followed a similar pattern for 12-month prevalence of DSM-IV disorders (see Table 30.1).

One of the most significant contributions of the CPES dataset is the ability to conduct subgroup analyses within each of the major racial/ethnic subgroups. Rather than consider each racial/ethnic category as a monolithic and uniform group, published results from the CPES have found vast differences in rates of disorders by ethnicity and sociodemographic characteristics.

Moreover, consistent with the immigrant paradox (where foreign nativity seems protective against psychiatric disorders despite the stressful experiences and poverty often associated with immigration), in aggregate, U.S.-born Latinos report higher risk

TABLE 30.1 Age and Gender Adjusted Lifetime and 12-Month Prevalence Estimates of DSM-IV Disorders by Racial/Ethnic Group

	NCS-R Non-Latino Whites (n = 4180)		NLAAS Latinos (n = 2554)			NLAAS Asians (n = 2095)			NSAL African Americans (n = 3570)			NSAL Afro-Caribbeans (n = 1438)		
	Weighted Percent/Mean	SE	Weighted Percent/Mean	SE	p Value[†]	Weighted Percent/Mean	SE	p Value[†]	Weighted Percent/Mean	SE	p Value[†]	Weighted Percent/Mean	SE	p-Value[†]
I. Lifetime prevalence														
Any depressive disorder	21.36%	0.87%	15.98%	0.87%	***	9.07%	0.95%	***	11.49%	0.62%	***	12.80%	2.27%	***
Any anxiety disorder	24.34%	0.87%	16.48%	0.94%	***	10.27%	0.92%	***	18.38%	0.84%	***	15.10%	1.67%	***
Any substance disorder	15.42%	0.68%	10.56%	1.36%	**	3.61%	0.60%	***	11.82%	0.76%	**	8.40%	2.33%	**
Any disorder	40.57%	1.20%	29.99%	1.60%	***	16.99%	1.26%	***	30.25%	1.13%	***	24.23%	2.22%	***
II. 12-month prevalence														
Any depressive disorder	19.08%	0.44%	8.79%	0.66%	NS	4.50%	0.73%	***	6.34%	0.49%	***	7.63%	1.72%	NS
Any anxiety disorder	13.85%	0.54%	9.55%	0.84%	***	6.51%	0.70%	***	10.23%	0.68%	***	9.51%	1.78%	*
Any substance disorder	4.23%	0.44%	2.37%	0.32%	**	1.11%	0.24%	***	2.94%	0.39%	*	2.84%	2.20%	NS
Any disorder	20.57%	0.79%	15.70%	1.08%	***	9.03%	0.79%	***	14.91%	0.76%	***	14.68%	2.12%	**

[†]Test of significance for each racial/ethnic group compared with non–Latino whites.
*p <.05, **p <.01, ***p <.001.
NS, nonsignificant (p >.05).

309

for most lifetime and past-year disorders than Latino immigrants (3). However, when disaggregated by subethnic group, the paradox was only consistently observed for depressive, anxiety, and substance use disorders among Mexican respondents, whereas no evidence for the immigrant paradox was found among Puerto Rican respondents. Interestingly, the paradox was consistently observed among Mexican, Cuban, and other Latino subjects for substance disorders (3).

Published results from the Asian sample of the NLAAS have also shown variation in rates of disorder by sociodemographic characteristics (4). Although in aggregate, lifetime rates did not differ by gender, English-language proficiency, or subethnic group, once disaggregated by nativity, variation in disorder status was found. In support of the immigrant paradox, U.S.-born Asian Americans reported the highest lifetime and 12-month rates of any disorder when nativity status, years in the United States, age at time of immigration, and generational status were considered (4). However, this association was quite complex, particularly when comparing risk for disorders by gender. For example, nativity and generational status were found to be the most stable predictors of mental disorders for women, with the U.S.-born and second-generation women at higher risk for lifetime and 12-month disorders compared with immigrant and first-generation Asian women. However, among Asian men, nativity and generational status were only associated with risk for any lifetime substance use disorder, with U.S.-born men and second generation men at higher risk for any substance use disorder compared with immigrant and first generation men.

Overall, epidemiological studies have also found lower prevalence of psychiatric disorders among U.S. blacks compared with the general population (5). This finding has remained in aggregate for African Americans and Afro-Caribbeans in analyses using the NSAL (11). However, after conducting subgroup analyses, evidence in support of the immigrant paradox has again been demonstrated using the Caribbean sample of the NSAL. Specifically, Afro-Caribbean immigrants reported lower rates of psychiatric disorders compared with U.S.-born Afro-Caribbeans (6). Moreover, increasing years of U.S. residency and increasing generational status were also associated with greater risk for mental health disorders. This relationship was particularly pronounced for substance use disorders, with first-generation Caribbean blacks significantly less likely but second-generation Caribbean blacks significantly more likely to meet criteria for any substance use disorder compared with African Americans (7). Timing of immigration was also associated with risk for mental illness, with immigration as a young adult (aged 18 to 34) found to be protective against disorders. However, once again, this pattern was found to vary on further examination of subgroups. For example, among women, this pattern was only evident for substance use disorders whereas among men the pattern existed for a broader range of mental disorders (6).

Eating Disorders

Analyses using the CPES dataset have also examined prevalence of eating disorders among racial/ethnic minority groups. For the NLAAS Latino population, anorexia and bulimia nervosa were found to be very uncommon. However, Latinos were found to have elevated rates of any binge eating and binge eating disorders (8). In particular, the U.S.-born Latinos and Latinos living a greater percentage of their lifetime in the United States were at higher risk for eating disorders. Diagnoses of anorexia nervosa were also extremely rare for black respondents of the NSAL, with no cases of 12-month anorexia reported for the Afro-Caribbean respondents (9). Instead, binge eating was the most prevalent eating disorder found among black respondents (9). Asian American men and women also reported low lifetime and 12-month prevalence rates of eating disorders although in general prevalence estimates were higher for women compared with men. Younger age in Asians as well as higher current BMI was also found to be strongly associated with binge eating disorder. Level of acculturation was not found to be associated with risk for eating disorders among Asian Americans.

Suicide Ideation and Suicide Attempts

The lifetime prevalence of suicidal ideation and suicide attempts among Latinos was 10.1% and 4.4%, respectively (10). Puerto Ricans were found to be at increased risk for reporting suicide ideation as compared with other Latino subgroups. Yet this difference was not observed once adjustments for demographic and sociocultural factors were taken into account. Again, acculturation level (e.g., being U.S.-born or English-speaking) was found to be independently and positively associated with augmented risk for suicide attempts among Latinos, even among those without any psychiatric disorder. African Americans and Caribbean blacks reported a lifetime prevalence of 11.7% for suicidal ideation and 4.1% for suicide attempts (11). Risk for attempted suicide was highest among the youngest age group, younger generations, and, surprisingly, among Caribbean black men. Suicidal ideation/attempts have not been examined using the Asian NLAAS sample.

TREATMENT CONSIDERATIONS: MENTAL HEALTH SERVICE USE AMONG RACIAL/ETHNIC MINORITY GROUPS IN THE UNITED STATES

Recent studies have documented disparities in the utilization of mental health services for Latinos, African Americans, and Asian Americans (12,13). Disparities in access to mental health services continue to pose significant concerns regarding equity among these groups. Although the prevalence rates of mental disorders for racial and ethnic minorities in the United States are similar or lower than those for non-Latino whites (3), minorities have less access to mental healthcare, are less likely to receive needed services, and receive lower quality of care.

Despite a clear need for mental health services, particularly for certain segments of the Latino population, researchers and practitioners have reported substantial difficulty in engaging ethnic and racial minorities to enter and remain in mental healthcare. Findings from the NLAAS indicate that U.S.-born Latinos are less likely to receive mental health services than non-Latino whites (14). However, rates of mental health service use are not consistent across Latino subethnic groups. Puerto Ricans (19.9%) are far more likely to receive past-year mental health services than Mexicans (10.1%), Cubans (11.49%), and other Latinos (11.0%) (15). Cultural factors such as nativity, language, and number of years in the United States have also been associated with use of mental health services for Latinos, with those who are U.S.-born, speak English, and have the most number of years in the United States reporting higher rates of both specialty and any mental health service use (15). When stratified across those with a DSM-IV diagnosis and those without, these cultural differences only remain for those without a mental health diagnosis. Thus, the area where Latinos appear to be most vulnerable in accessing care falls in preventive or discretionary use of mental healthcare. Access to mental healthcare among Latinos, particularly recent immigrants, also appears to be strongly related to policy restrictions regarding insurance coverage.

Latinos in general are disproportionately uninsured compared with the overall U.S. population, with Mexicans reporting the lowest rates of insurance (14).

Although rates of mental illness are relatively low among Asian Americans, rates of mental health service use are even lower, even among those with a probable diagnosis. Overall, Asian Americans have been found to have lower rates of mental health service use compared with the general population. For example, only 8.6% of Asian NLAAS respondents sought any mental health services in a 12-month period (compared with 17.9% of the general population in the NCS-R) (15). Moreover, only 34.1% of respondents who had a probable diagnosis sought any services (16). Asian respondents who met diagnostic criteria for an eating disorder also reported very low rates of treatment utilization. Similar to findings from the Latino sample, this study also found that mental health service use among Asians varied by nativity and generational status. Specifically, U.S.-born Asian Americans reported higher rates of service use than their immigrant counterparts, whereas third-generation or later Asian Americans reported higher rates than second- and first-generation immigrants. Surprisingly, these low rates of mental health service use persist despite relatively high rates of insurance coverage among Asian Americans, particularly compared with Latinos. Comparisons of insurance coverage between Asian Americans and Latinos using data from the NLAAS demonstrate that Asians report much higher rates of health insurance compared with Latinos, partly because of differences in occupational distributions where Asian Americans are more likely to work in jobs that offer private insurance (14). However, rates of insurance coverage are not consistent across all Asian subgroups. In particular, Vietnamese Americans reported high rates of uninsurance comparable to that of Latinos (14).

Consistent with the findings from both samples of the NLAAS, African Americans and Caribbean blacks use formal mental healthcare services at relatively low rates. Overall, only 10.1% of NSAL respondents used some form of mental healthcare in the past year, although service use was much higher among those who met criteria for a 12-month DSM-IV disorder (31.9%) (17). Furthermore, less than half of African Americans (45.5%) and less than a quarter (24.3%) of Caribbean blacks who met criteria for major depressive disorder received any form of therapy for the disorder. However, no overall differences have been found between Caribbean blacks and African Americans in formal mental health service use (18). Differences in rates of mental health service use have been found within the black Caribbean sample, once again in regards to immigration status, generational status, length of U.S. residence, and age at immigration. Specifically, first-generation Caribbean immigrants were less likely to use services than the U.S.-born and African Americans. However, among immigrants, longer time in the United States and younger ages at the time of immigration were linked to higher rates of mental health service use (18). Furthermore, third-generation Caribbean blacks reported higher rates of mental health service use than first- and second-generation Caribbean blacks as well as African Americans.

PREVENTIVE CONSIDERATIONS: THE ROLE OF LANGUAGE, RELIGION, AND OTHER CORRELATES OF MENTAL HEALTH DISORDERS AMONG U.S. RACIAL/ETHNIC MINORITIES

English language proficiency, religious attendance, family conflict, and reports of discrimination are correlates of mental health disorders for various racial/ethnic subgroups of the CPES. Exploration of these correlates will provide clues toward the prevention of mental disorders among these groups. For example, positive correlates of last-year psychiatric disorders for Latinos include family burden and family cultural conflict, perceived low neighborhood safety, exposure to discrimination, disrupted marital status, being out of the labor force, and low social standing. To varying degrees, these correlates figure as risk factors for psychiatric disorders and should be considered when developing preventive programs for Latinos. Positive correlates of last-year psychiatric disorder also included English language proficiency (19). English language dominance represents a strong cultural anchor for socially constructed meaning that may lead to immigrants joining certain peer networks and not others, putting them at risk for substance disorders but allowing for social mobility. On the other hand, religious attendance, common among low-income Latino groups, appears to help minorities cope with the hardship of disadvantageous circumstances by establishing socially protective ties that buffer negative stressors.

Findings from the Asian sample of the NLAAS have found an association between self-reports of discrimination and mental health among Asian Americans. In one study, self-reported racial discrimination was associated with greater odds of having any DSM-IV disorder, depressive disorder, or anxiety disorder within the past 12 months, even after controlling for several sociodemographic characteristics including acculturative stress, family cohesion, poverty, and social desirability (20). Furthermore, those who reported discrimination had a twofold greater risk of having one disorder within the past 12 months and a threefold greater risk of having two or more psychiatric disorders. In another study, experiences of unfair treatment and racial/ethnic discrimination were found to be a risk factor for smoking among Asian Americans (21). However, high levels of ethnic identification moderated this relationship, with high levels of ethnic identification associated with lower probability of current smoking among study respondents who reported high levels of discrimination. English-language proficiency was also a significant correlate of lifetime and 12-month disorders among Asian American men with those who spoke English proficiently (compared with nonproficient speakers) reporting lower rates of lifetime and 12-month psychiatric disorders. This association was not found among Asian American women.

Findings from the NSAL have also demonstrated a link between sociocontextual factors and mental health. In one study, correlates of depressive symptoms were examined among two classes of NSAL respondents: those who reported low and high levels of depressive symptoms (22). Among respondents in the high depressive symptoms class, lower socioeconomic status, female gender, experiences of negative interaction within the individual's social network (e.g., conflict, demands, criticism), and low social support were associated with higher depressive symptoms. In contrast, older age, male gender, and fewer experiences of negative interaction and of racial discrimination were associated with lower depressive symptoms. Interestingly, ethnicity and nativity were not found to be associated with depressive symptoms among blacks. Although there is mounting scientific evidence of a positive association between religious involvement and health among African Americans, this association has yet to be published using the NSAL data.

CONCLUSION

This summary of findings shows that the prevalence of disorders for all racial/ethnic minority groups appears to be lower compared with the general U.S. population and with non-Latino whites. However, the CPES study results also reveal the great subgroup variability present within each of these larger minority aggregate categories. We therefore caution against grouping together these subethnic groups to avoid masking wide differences in risk for psychiatric disorders within each of these sub ethnic groups.

Findings indicate that although in the aggregate, the U.S.-born are at higher risk for disorders than immigrants (providing evidence in support of the immigrant paradox); there is a more limited application of the immigrant paradox for several subgroups. For example, the paradox holds up for Mexicans and Afro-Caribbeans but not for Puerto Ricans. This implies that demonstrated differences in prevalence of psychiatric disorders among ethnicity by nativity subgroups are a function of multiple factors beyond foreign nativity. However, we also found that greater time in the United States for immigrants increased the risk of last-year psychiatric disorders (23). These results help explain the inconsistent findings of other studies regarding whether foreign nativity is protective against psychiatric disorders, given that type of disorder, subethnic groups studied, and variables included in adjustments might produce different results across studies.

Nonetheless, the risk for substance disorders seems to be substantially lower for racial and ethnic minority immigrants who arrive to the United States as adults, revealing the strong role of context and the neighborhood environment in increasing the risk for substance disorders. For younger immigrants, availability of alternative social networks in immigrant enclaves might protect them from substance disorders. Coming to the United States as an adult might protect against exposure to risky social networks linked to drug use. Consistent with other research (24), perceived level of neighborhood safety seemed associated with lower risk for substance-use disorders. This underlines the significance of the receiving context, chiefly early experience with neighborhood disadvantage as a risk factor for psychiatric illness, even after adjusting for individual-level socioeconomic status. Ethnographic studies are sorely needed to examine how regional differences in the United States for ethnic/racial minorities might relate to increased/decreased risk of psychiatric disorders.

These findings also emphasize the resiliency of racial and ethnic minority populations. The fact that levels of mental illness are consistently lower among immigrant minority groups despite persistent experiences of disadvantage, discrimination, and limited service use demonstrates the importance of understanding the dynamics of minority status linked to resiliency and improved coping. Our results suggest that protective mechanisms from the country of origin (e.g., family harmony, lower expectations for personal success) may buffer the negative impacts of hardship. Yet, these strategies may erode over time because of the additional demands of having to negotiate different cultural contexts in the United States. Sustaining family harmony, integrating in employment and developing a self-perception of high social standing appear to be central to decreased risk of depressive and anxiety disorders for Latinos, and possibly other ethnic and racial minority groups. Clinicians may need to consider these sociostructural factors when assessing the well-being and potential risk for mental disorders of ethnic/racial minorities.

However, decreased access to mental health services remains a crucial problem for all racial/ethnic minority groups. Unconventional means of delivering mental health services need to be developed for minority populations that have historically been unwilling to seek care. There is an imperative need to improve public systems of care that might not have the necessary resources to conduct community outreach, or to provide additional services (e.g., transportation, child care, patient advocacy) to facilitate attendance to mental healthcare. Strategies to improve detection of underlying mental health and substance abuse problems among ethnic and racial minorities are critical within community settings. Realigning provider incentives for increased screening and ancillary supports to counsel ethnic and racial patients into mental health and substance abuse treatments seems urgently needed if we are to reduce ethnic and racial service disparities.

Our findings also draw attention to the low levels of recognition of mental health problems among ethnic and racial minorities, highlighting the need for social marketing campaigns to generate awareness and problem recognition as well as broadcasting the benefits of mental healthcare. Efforts may be particularly necessary to bring ethnic and racial minorities up to date about mental health conditions that can lead to negative outcomes. Programs and activities, like dominoes and coffee groups, may help to diminish isolation and help preserve social connections for ethnic and racial minorities. An emphasis on mental wellness rather than illness needs to be adopted if we are to engage communities in improving their mental health despite economic and social issues. Establishing community agents that serve as support sources and patient liaisons to help minorities navigate the healthcare system should be tested as a promising approach.

AREAS FOR FUTURE RESEARCH

Diagnostic Considerations

National surveys restricted to English eliminate large segments of racial/ethnic categories, and require respondents to answer sensitive and complex questions in a language they poorly understand. For example, in the NLAAS, 50% of Latinos and 35% of Asian Americans in the NLAAS rated their English proficiency as fair or poor, which would have potentially excluded them from an English-only diagnostic assessment (25). Measurement artifacts caused by language may have profound implications for clinical practice. When recent Asian American and Latino immigrants with a mental health disorder contact U.S. health providers, they confront linguistic and symbolic distance that can affect diagnostic assessment. In the absence of sufficient numbers of bilingual and bicultural mental health service providers, little is known about how linguistic distance affects diagnosis and what additional data could help guide the nonbilingual/bicultural health provider evaluating a non–English-speaking immigrant. Some literature raises concerns about bias and misdiagnoses as a result of language of interview even for bilingual Latinos interviewed in English by non-Latino clinicians (26). And, some research (27) speculates that misdiagnosis and miscommunication in the clinical encounter between patient and provider stemming from language discordance may be responsible for the high dropout rate of ethnic minorities from mental health services. Additional work in this area is urgently needed.

Acculturation and cultural factors may cause differences in the presentation of psychiatric illness. Construct bias might explain the variations in the prevalence rates across ethnic minority immigrants and migrants. Current constructs for defining symptoms and mental health disorders are usually based on mainstream U.S. culture and DSM-IV criteria, and despite recent efforts to include culturally specific disorder and symptom expression, these constructs have not been fully integrated into DSM-IV. For example, standard criteria for eating disorders may not be appropriate for understanding psychological morbidity of eating disorders for Latinos or Asians, particularly the less acculturated, because of cultural differences in the presentation of eating disorder symptoms. Our results suggest areas of category fallacy, where nosological criteria developed for Western populations do not effectively map as illness expressions for Latinos (28). For example, in lifetime bulimia, requiring that binge eating and inappropriate compensatory behaviors both occur at least twice a week for several months (Criterion C) dramatically reduces the pool of possible cases for the Latino sample. The cognitive difficulty of these queries or the absence of these compensatory behaviors might minimize the detection of eating disorders in minority populations. Consideration should be given to how ignoring cultural expression of psychiatric illness could bias diagnostic assessment.

Treatment Considerations

In the Surgeon General's ground-breaking report on mental health needs of ethnic minority groups, the central argument was that the culture and context of the patient was relevant to the provision of quality services. Geller found that psychiatrists characterized minority patients who were indistinguishable from white patients in sociodemographic and clinical data (except for race) as less psychologically minded, less knowledgeable about mental health, and consequently less able to profit from psychotherapy. At the same time, clinical uncertainty appears to be accountable for the finding that minorities are more likely to have non-concordant psychiatric diagnoses in psychiatric emergency services and to have mental health disorders go undetected in primary care (29).

Additionally, ethnic minorities' cultural norms and expectations affect the level of disclosure as well as the manifestations of symptoms. Our recent study (30) emphasizes the problem of missing information and how clinicians base their judgments on the most generalized statement of illness, patient's past history of treatment, and, to a lesser degree, on family history of disorder. As a result, we found ethnicity/race to be a modifying factor of the association between patient's symptom reports and likelihood of receiving a diagnosis. Differential discussion of symptom areas, depending on patient's ethnicity or race, appeared to lead to differential diagnosis and increased likelihood of diagnostic bias (30). Future studies should consider how to deal with the problem of clinician's differential collection of diagnostic information depending on the ethnicity or race of the patient. Additional work is needed to better address how to enhance the patient provider interaction in mental healthcare.

Preventive Considerations

Adoption of preventive interventions to improve engagement in mental health services should be evaluated for ethnic and racial minorities who do not recognize and attend to their psychiatric illness, but are in need of preventive treatment, before they become disabled or impaired. Public mental health recognition campaigns should be evaluated, as well as antistigma social marketing campaigns, in communities with high unmet need.

In closing, the findings from the Collaborative Psychiatric Epidemiology Surveys (CPES) provide the most comprehensive data available on the mental health of racial and ethnic minority groups in the United States. As a further contribution, this chapter provides the first review of published findings focused on the distributions, correlates, and risk factors of mental disorders and service use outcomes among the primary racial/ethnic minority groups of the CPES dataset. Together, these findings illustrate a complex picture of racial/ethnic minority mental health and service use with great variation by subethnic group, nativity, gender, and other sociodemographic factors. However, these findings also provide important clues for how to best intervene and prevent mental illness for these groups. Therefore, it is our hope that these findings will be used as a roadmap by future researchers and practitioners alike as we continue to work toward the elimination of racial/ethnic disparities in mental health.

ACKNOWLEDGMENTS

The NLAAS data used in this analysis were provided by the Center for Multicultural Mental Health Research at the Cambridge Health Alliance. The project was supported by NIH Research Grant No. U01 MH 06220, funded by the National Institute of Mental Health. This publication was also made possible by Grant No. P50 MH073469-04 from the National Institute of Mental Health. The NSAL is supported by the National Institute of Mental Health (NIMH; U01-MH57716) with supplemental support from the Office of Behavioral and Social Science Research (OBSSR) at the National Institutes of Health (NIH), and the University of Michigan. The NCS-R is supported by grant U01-MH60220 from the National Institute of Mental Health, with supplemental support from the National Institute on Drug Abuse, the Substance Abuse and Mental Health Services Administration, the Robert Wood Johnson Foundation Grant No. 044708, and the John W. Alden Trust.

References

1. U.S. Census Bureau. U.S. hispanic population surpasses 45 million: now 15 percent of total. In: U.S. Census Bureau News. Washington, DC: 2008.
2. McKinnon JD, Bennett CE. *We the People: Blacks in the United States in Census 2000 Special Reports.* Washington, DC: U.S. Census Bureau, 2005.
3. Alegría M, Canino G, Shrout P, et al. Prevalence of mental illness in immigrant and non-immigrant U.S. Latino groups. *Am J Psychiatry* 2008;165:359–369.
4. Takeuchi DT, Alegria M, Jackson JS, et al. Immigration and mental health: Diverse findings in Asian, Black, and Latino populations. *Am J Public Health* 2007;97(1):11.
5. Breslau J, Aguilar-Gaxiola S, Kendler KS, et al. Specifying race-ethnic differences in risk for psychiatric disorder in a USA national sample. *Psychol Med* 2006;36(1):57.
6. Williams D, Gonzalez H, Neighbors H, et al. Prevalence and distribution of major depressive disorder in African Americans, Caribbean blacks, and non-Hispanic whites. *Arch Gen Psychiatry* 2007;64:305–315.
7. Broman CL, Neighbors HW, Delva J, et al. Prevalence of substance use disorders among African Americans and Caribbean Blacks in the National Survey of American Life. *Am J Public Health* 2008;98(6):1107–1114.
8. Alegria M, Woo M, Cao Z, et al. Prevalence and correlates of eating disorders in Latinos in the United States. *Int J Eating Disord* 2007;40(S3):S15–S21.
9. Taylor JY, Caldwell CH, Baser RE, et al. Prevalence of eating disorders among Blacks in the National Survey of American Life. *Int J Eating Disord* 2007;40:10–14.
10. Fortuna L, Perez DJ, Canino G, et al. Prevalence and correlates of lifetime suicidal ideation and suicide attempts among Latino subgroups in the United States. *J Clin Psychiatry* 2007; 68(4):572–581.
11. Joe S, Baser RE, Breeden G, et al. Prevalence of and risk factors for lifetime suicide attempts among Blacks in the United States. *JAMA* 2006;297(17):2112–2123.
12. Alegria M, Canino G, Rios R, et al. Inequalities in use of specialty mental health services among Latinos, African Americans, and non-Latino whites. *Psychiatr Serv* 2002;53(12): 1547–1555.
13. Stockdale S, Tang L, Zhang L, et al. The effects of health sector market factors and vulnerable group membership on access to alcohol, drug, and mental health care. *Health Serv Res* 2007;42(3):1020–1041.

14. Alegría M, Cao Z, McGuire T, et al. Health insurance coverage for vulnerable populations: Contrasting Asian Americans and Latinos in the U.S. *Inquiry* 2006;43:231–254.

15. Alegría M, Mulvaney-Day N, Woo M, et al. Correlates of twelve-month mental health service use among Latinos: Results from the National Latino and Asian American Study (NLAAS). *Am J Public Health* 2007;97:76–83.

16. Wang PS, Lane M, Olfson M, et al. Twelve-month use of mental health services in the United States: Results from the National Comorbidity Survey Replication. *Arch Gen Psychiatry* 2005;62(6):629–640.

17. Abe-Kim J, Takeuchi DT, Hong S, et al. Use of mental health-related services among immigrant and US-born Asian Americans: Results from the National Latino and Asian American Study. *Am J Public Health* 2007;97(1):91.

18. Jackson JS, Neighbors HW, Torres M, et al. Use of mental health services and subjective satisfaction with treatment among Black Caribbean immigrants: Results from the National Survey of American Life. *Am J Public Health* 2007;97(1):60–67.

19. Cook B, McGuire T, Miranda J. Measuring trends in mental health care disparities, 2000–2004. *Psychiatr Serv* 2007;58(12):1533–1539.

20. Gee GC, Spencer M, Chen J, et al. The association between self-reported racial discrimination and 12-month DSM-IV mental disorders among Asian Americans nationwide. *Soc Sci Med* 2007;64(10):1984–1996.

21. Chae DH, Takeuchi DT, Barbeau EM, et al. Unfair treatment, racial/ethnic discrimination, ethnic identification, and smoking among Asian Americans in the National Latino and Asian American Study. *Am J Public Health* 2008;98(3):485.

22. Lincoln KD, Chatters LM, Taylor RJ, et al. Profiles of depressive symptoms among African Americans and Caribbean blacks. *Soc Sci Med* 2007;65(2):200–213.

23. Cook BL, Lin J, Guo J, et al. Pathways and correlates connecting exposure to the U.S. and Latinos' Mental Health. *Am J Public Health* (in press).

24. Cho Y, Park G-S, Echevarria-Cruz S. Perceived neighborhood characteristics and the health of adult Koreans. *Soc Sci Med* 2005;60(6):1285–1297.

25. Alegría M, Takeuchi D, Canino G, et al. Considering context, place and culture: The National Latino and Asian American Study. *Int J Methods Psychiatr Res* 2004;13(4):208–220.

26. Lewis-Fernandez R, Kleinman A. Culture, personality, and psychopathology. *J Abnorm Psychol* 1994;103(1):67–71.

27. Vega WA, Alegría M. Latino mental health and treatment in the United States. In: Aguirre-Molina M, Molina C, Zambrana R, eds. *Health Issues in the Latino Community*. San Francisco: Jossey-Bass Publishers, 2001:179–208.

28. Geller JD. Racial bias in the evaluation of patients for psychotherapy. In: Comas-Diaz DL, Griffith EH, eds. *Clinical Guidelines in Cross-Cultural Mental Health*. New York: Wiley, 1988:112–134.

29. Borowsky SJ, Rubenstein LV, Meredith LS, et al. Who is at risk of nondetection of mental health problems in primary care? *J Gen Intern Med* 2000;15(6):381–388.

30. Alegria M, Nakash O, Lapatin S, et al. How missing information in diagnosis can lead to disparities in the clinical encounter. *J Public Health Manag Pract* 2008;14 Suppl:S26–35.

31 The Role of Parity

Robert C. Bransfield and Douglas R. Bransfield

INTRODUCTION

Access to mental healthcare protects the greatest resource—our mental capacities. An intact mind has great potential for productivity; conversely mental illness has significant potential to harm both the individual and society. Although everyone agrees mental health has value, there is often a resistance and cost-shifting of the financial responsibility to pay what is required to achieve mental health and concerns regarding the cost-effectiveness of mental healthcare. Mental health parity is an equalization of mental heath benefits and is an ethical commitment to enhancing humane values, while lack of parity is an exploitation of human vulnerability that erodes our stature as a compassionate society with humanitarian priorities. Ninety-eight percent of Americans have healthcare insurance with lesser coverage for mental healthcare, causing false security and discouraging budgeting and saving for these expenses. This underinsurance is a failure of the insurance and healthcare payment systems and results in greatly reduced access to the advances that exist with our current mental healthcare technology and compromises the infrastructure that could provide this care. Although some with adequate financial resources are able to access care outside the insurance and public assistance systems, many, particularly the more severe and chronically mentally ill that are the most needy, have impairments from their illness that also limits their earning capacity and further obstructs access to care. Most commonly, lack of mental health parity is synonymous with lack of access to mental healthcare which further increases mental health disparities between those who are healthier or can afford care and those who are mentally ill that need but cannot afford to access medically necessary care. This lack of access fuels to a vicious spiral of decline in mental and physical health, functional capacities, socially appropriate behavior and socioeconomic status which increases the numbers of disenfranchised individuals and detracts from our social stability.

To understand this issue more thoroughly, it is necessary to first understand the total burden and financial cost of mental illness then review the current technical capability and cost effectiveness for prevention and treatment and compare this to the burden and cost incurred from reduced access from lack of mental health parity.

THE BURDEN OF MENTAL ILLNESS

Mental illness, including alcohol and substance abuse disorders, affects 50 million American adults, and almost 50% of the population meets one of *The Fourth Diagnostic and Statistical Manual of Mental Health* (DSM-IV) criterion for mental

319

illness in their lifetime. Many illnesses primarily affecting the body cause impairment and disability late in life; however, many mental illnesses can begin early in life (50% by age 14 and 75% by age 24). Failure to access care early in life and early in the course of the disease when these conditions are more readily treated can and does lead to a lifetime of impairment and chronic and costly burden of diseases that could have been avoided.

Neuropsychiatric disorders are the second leading cause of premature death and also one of the leading causes of preventable death caused by suicide. For every two murders in the United States, there are three suicides, with 90% of suicides attributable to mental illness. There are 1000 suicide attempts per month among veterans at Veterans Administration (VA) facilities and approximately 6600 suicides per year among veterans, with an average of about 126 suicides per week. In addition, 300,000 U.S. troops who served in the wars in Afghanistan and Iraq are suffering from major depression or post traumatic stress and 320,000 received brain injuries.

The leading cause of disability and disability payments among developed nations is depression, even though it is readily treated. At 27.3% mental illness is the leading cause of the burden of disease by daily adjusted life-years in high income countries in year 2002. A 2006 George Washington University report found 59% of Medicare beneficiaries with disabilities have a mental disease, only half of which are receiving mental health treatment. The causes of disability in the United States, Canada, and Western Europe in year 2000 are mental illnesses, 24.0%; alcohol and drug use disorders, 12.0% and Alzheimer's disease and dementias, 7.9% (1). Mental illnesses can be as debilitating as serious heart condition; more disabling than other chronic physical illnesses such as lung or gastrointestinal problems, angina, hypertension and even diabetes; persist for a longer duration and inadequately treated depression with diabetes or heart disease increases mortality.

Patients with a diagnosable mental disorder generally visit their primary care physician twice as often as a person without a mental illness. Mental illness is associated with lack of exercise, poor eating habits, insomnia, smoking, and poor compliance with medical treatment and patients are at increased risks for cardiovascular disease, HIV/AIDS, diabetes, upper respiratory infections, asthma, herpes viral infections, autoimmune diseases, and decreased wound healing. Mental disorders, substance abuse, degenerative diseases of the central nervous system (CNS), and psychiatric components of general medical illnesses increase the severity of many general medical illnesses, cause psychosomatic illness, and increase the need for many diagnostic procedures and contribute to a massive burden of disease.

Inadequately treated metal illness can also contribute to burden of crime. Between 5% and 10% of seriously mentally ill persons living in the community will commit a violent act each year, almost all because they are not receiving treatment. Such individual are responsible for at least 5% of all homicides. A study of 81 American cities demonstrates a significant statistical correlation between the lack of public psychiatric beds in that city and the prevalence of violent crimes (murder, robbery, assault, and rape) (2). There are multiple reports of murders as a result of inadequate access to hospital care. Half of the males and 40% of females arrested before age 21 had been diagnosed with a prior mental disorder (3). Youths in the correctional system are far more likely to be mentally ill. Sixty percent to 70% of youths in juvenile justice facilities have been found to have diagnosable psychiatric disorders (4). Twenty percent are afflicted with a serious mental disorder, such as bipolar disorder, major depression, or schizophrenia; up to 39% have a primary or co-occurring substance abuse disorder and one fifth are suicidal. Restricted access to psychiatric treatment facilities has resulted in trans-institutionalization from the mental healthcare system into the prison system. The Los Angeles County jail is now the largest mental health provider in the nation with 3000 mentally ill inmates. "Prisons and jails have become the nation's primary mental health facilities for those with serious illnesses. In 1999 the Department of Justice estimated 283,800 inmates were mentally ill and more than 700,000 mentally ill Americans are processed through either jails or prison each year."

Serious mental disorders also have a social effect that can have tragic consequences, such as family disruption, loss of employment, and housing issues. In any given week, an estimated 842,000 homeless adults and children will sleep on the streets, with that number ballooning to 3.5 million during a yearly peak. Sixty-six percent of homeless people report substance abuse and/or mental health problems, with 20% to 25% meeting the criteria for serious mental illness.

FINANCIAL COSTS OF MENTAL ILLNESS

Diseases and disorders of the central nervous system CNS cause more direct (health-care costs) and indirect costs (e.g., preabsenteeism, absenteeism, premature retirement, lost productivity, and caretaker burden) than any other disease category. Mental disorders, substance abuse, degenerative diseases of the CNS, and psychiatric components to behavioral disorders and general medical illnesses are all contributors to this massive burden.

Depression costs U.S. business at least $44 billion a year in absenteeism, lost productivity, and direct treatment costs, according to Mental Health America. Experts at Harvard Medical School, put that figure closer to $50 billion. About half of this cost is attributable to lost productivity in the workplace. Workers with depression averaged 5.6 hours per week of lost productivity because of health problems, compared with 1.5 hours per week from nondepressed workers (5). For any 30-day period, 8 million people experience depression that leads to absenteeism and lost productivity, with annual productivity losses ranging from $10 billion to $31 billion (5) and Kessler calculated a total cost of $193 billion in lost productivity for all mental illnesses.

In 2007, I reviewed some of the statistics associated with the yearly cost of mental illness. Some statistics on the costs of mental illness are missing and some are more than 15 years old and vastly underestimate current costs. The costs in billions of dollars include alcoholism, 279 (1998); drug abuse, 172 (1995); Alzheimer's disease, 100, (2003); insomnia, 108 (1994); depression, 83 (2000); attention deficit/hyperactivity disorder, 77 (2004); schizophrenia, 62.7 (2002); brain injury, 48; bipolar disorders, 45 (1990); anxiety disorders, 42 (1990) and developmental disabilities, 30. The total of these costs of mental illness alone are $1.047 trillion per year. The costs in billions of dollars of other conditions that often have a psychiatric component include violence, 425 (1998); work-related accidents, 145 (2001); obesity, 102 (1999); pain 100; cigarette smoking 73 (1998); work related violence, 35 (1995) and $2.2 trillion for total medical costs (2007), which is a total of $3 trillion. If we estimate these conditions as having a 25% psychiatric component, the psychiatric component of these costs would be $750 billion per year. When this is added to $1.047 trillion plus $193 billion in lost productivity, this equals $2 trillion as the total cost of mental illness per year.

Societal and government costs include costs associated with emergency services, law enforcement, legal, correctional systems, special education, housing, bankruptcy, welfare, cost-shifting to state budgets and charity fund, direct care, Medicaid, Medicare, health insurance other government subsidized programs, and associated tax burdens.

THE CURRENT TECHNICAL CAPABILITY OF MENTAL HEALTHCARE

Mental illnesses were mostly untreatable in the middle of the last century, but now treatment is quite effective for most patients. Many of the conditions that do not fully respond to treatment may still demonstrate significant functional improvement that results in higher levels of functioning. Brain imaging and other studies demonstrate early effective treatment protects the integrity of the brain, improves brain functioning, and prevents the progression of disease that would otherwise occur if there had been inadequate treatment. This finding has been demonstrated in several conditions including bipolar illness, schizophrenia, posttraumatic stress disorder, attention deficit/hyperactivity disorder, anorexia nervosa, depression, anxiety disorders, obsessive compulsive disorder, and Alzheimer's disease. Early effective treatment helps to prevent the more expensive costs to individuals and society associated with the consequences of late stage disease with higher levels of impairment. Conversely, treatment delays are associated with increasing impairments and increasing treatment resistance and costs.

THE VALUE AND COST-EFFECTIVENESS OF MENTAL HEALTHCARE

American society cannot afford to view mental health as separate and unequal to general health, but mental health must be part of the mainstream of health. With our current capability, most mental illnesses are often effectively treated and many of the consequences of mental illness can be avoided. Most deaths and disability from mental illness are treatable and have a higher treatment success rate than other branches of medicine and other major leading causes of death, such as heart disease. In addition, psychiatric help can prevent some violent activity before it starts and save the public from the effects of an impaired person's antisocial behavior.

Higher levels of mental fitness and resilience correlate not only with happiness, but with creativity and productivity as well, which provides security in the highly competitive global economy. Conversely, inadequately treated mental illness correlates with diminished productivity, increased physical illness, increased risk of substance abuse, greater social discord, and pain and suffering. The goal is to prevent and treat whenever possible to alleviate suffering and promote sustained full recovery with resumption of normal productive functioning. Every person experiencing psychiatric symptoms needs access to an adequate medical/psychiatric assessment, an individually appropriate treatment plan, and medically indicated treatment. Mental hygiene should be viewed as a form of primary preventative healthcare along with fundamental hygiene, nutrition, sanitation, vaccinations and healthy habits of daily living. Mental health and physical health are assets that need to be maintained and protected by fostering viable mental heath and healthcare systems. Increased utilization of mental healthcare services directly and indirectly reduce many burdens and costs.

Prior developments have been quite cost-effective. For example, the development of antipsychotic drugs allowed 400,000 patients to be discharged from state mental hospitals and the development of the newer agents have allowed a further reduction of the census of state, community and private mental hospitals. One facet of treatment is psychiatric medications which help avoid the disability and death caused by disease, lower overall treatment costs, increase productivity, enable people to live more comfortably and reduce costs by eliminating the need for other, more costly medical services. Early detection and preventive treatment of mental illness and six other chronic diseases could save $1.1 trillion in the year 2023. For every dollar spent on substance abuse treatment taxpayers save 7 dollars in future costs.

Whenever mental health parity is implemented, access to care is improved quality of life is improved, many indirect costs are reduced and mental healthcare costs are only modestly increased and offset by other reduced total costs. For example, improved parity for federal employees resulted in less hospital care and reduced out of pocket expenses which resulted in only a 1.6% increase in fee-for-service plans and a 0.3% increase for Health Maintenance Organization (HMO) plans at a direct cost of $2.04 a month for parity. PricewaterhouseCoopers, L.L.P. determined the cost of parity in New Jersey would be $0.55 per member per month or a 0.24% increase in premiums based on an actuarial analysis of full parity and substance abuse benefits. The United States spends $20 billion in agricultural subsidies that economists argue only produces a vicious downward spiral of overproduction, artificially reduced prices, and subsidy reliance. Subsidizing mental health treatment is a better investment.

Medicaid patients hospitalized for physical ailments and provided mental health interventions realized average cumulative savings of $1500 over a subsequent 2.5 year period, which completely offset the cost of the mental health intervention. Medicaid "patients hospitalized without physical ailments who received mental health treatment" realized a reduction in costs that ranged from $296 to $392 with cost reductions correlating to the severity of the diagnosis. Private insurers have also benefited by covering mental health treatment. A 3-year study of more than 10,000 Aetna beneficiaries found after Aetna plans covered mental health treatment, beneficiary medical costs dropped from $242 for the first year to $162 for the 2 years following the inclusion of mental health coverage. This demonstrates that providing coverage for mental health services reduces total costs. When a large HMO in New Mexico made access to Selective Serotonin Reuptake Inhibitors (SSRIs) unrestricted and followed 2000 depressed patients, costs for mental health visits and psychotropic medications increased, but total healthcare costs were substantially reduced.

Business interests have benefited from parity. Two examples are Pitney Bowes and Merrill Lynch. Pitney Bowes reported that investing in employee mental health assessment and treatment programs reduced absence, increased productivity, and helped address overall healthcare and disability costs. Merrill Lynch reported that by removing restrictions on mental health and psychotropic medications, the firm's total healthcare costs after adjusting for inflation was reduced by 25% per employee.

The V.A. has benefited from improved access. An economic assessment during a time of open access to atypical antipsychotic medications showed an 8% increase in the number of mentally ill patients treated and a total cost reduction of 8% reduction in average length of stay and a 33% reduction in psychiatric hospitalization. In another veterans study, researchers found abbreviated mental health treatment reduced outpatient visits by 36%. However, the veterans in the study who did not receive mental health treatment increased outpatient medical utilization.

Mental health and substance abuse treatment spending has grown at a slower rate than other healthcare spending in spite of increased numbers being treated. In 2003 this was only 7.5% of healthcare spending ($121 billion). The single greatest category was prescription medications at 23%, an increase from 7% in 1986 (6). However much of the increased pharmaceutical costs associated with the new generation drugs were attributed to the "woodwork effect" where patients would come out, seek and stay on medications that were more tolerable. In spite of increased drug utilization, there was an associated reduction in overall healthcare costs. The cost of antipsychotic agents was $10.5 billion in 2005. Antidepressants are the most prescribed family of drugs in America with 30 million (10% of Americans) being treated with 233 million prescriptions of antidepressants in 2007 at a cost of $11.9 billion, which is a reduction from $12.5 billion in 2005. The cost of drugs to treat alcohol and drug abuse was less than a billion; the cost of alcoholic beverages was $94.5 billion in 1997 and the social cost of alcohol abuse was estimated at more than $184 billion in 1998, the social cost of drug abuse was $110 billion in 1995 and the money spent on illegal drugs was $62.4 billion in 2000. The cost of drugs to treat cigarette smoking was less than a billion: the total cost of caring for people with health problems caused by cigarette smoking was about $72.7 billion per year in 1998. The cost of Alzheimer's disease drugs was $1.2 billion in 2004, but the cost of Alzheimer's disease was at least $100 billion in 2003. The cost of insomnia medications was $2.76 billion in 2005, but the cost of insomnia was $107.5 billion in 1994. The cost of attention deficit/ hyperactivity disorder medications was $3.1 billion in 2004, but the cost of attention deficit/hyperactivity disorders was $77 billion. Many of these figures on the costs if illnesses need to be adjusted to current costs and these costs are proportionately small when considering the burden and costs of the conditions they treat.

THE CONSEQUENCES AND COSTS OF NOT HAVING MENTAL HEALTH PARITY

Although diseases and disorders of the CNS cause more direct and indirect costs than any other disease category and highly effective and cost-effective treatments now exist, the treatment of these diseases receive less resources than other conditions. Many policies regarding mental health insurance coverage have been highly restrictive and were established at a time when mental health treatment capabilities were very limited. These policies have continued unchanged or have become more restrictive in spite of the improvements in treatments in recent years. In addition stigma, third-party intrusions, misguided cost containment, some realistic cost limitations and fragmentation of the healthcare system have further restricted access to quality mental healthcare for many at a time when insurance companies and their executives make record profits and incomes.

Unlike other medical conditions mental health benefits are subjected to intensive "management" from carve-out management companies, excessive limitations of benefits, inefficient bureaucracy, phantom provider networks, denial of coverage for out of network physicians, 2-year limitations on disability, reduced coverage by Medicare, inadequate coverage for veterans, low reimbursement rates, excessively restrictive psychotropic formularies, and restricted access to psychiatrists and other more highly trained professionals. Phantom networks exist in many managed mental health plans. For example, only 18.6% of listed Magellan Behavioral Health Providers in New Jersey and 13.8% in southeastern Pennsylvania were willing to accept new Magellan patients (7).

Access to mental health coverage is impeded by the insurance industry by altering the definition of words and phrases such as *psychiatric illness, medically necessary psychiatric care, standard of care, standard of practice, experimental or investigational, qualified healthcare practitioner, healthcare insurance, customary and reasonable fees, psychiatric care, evidence based medicine, experts consensus, qualified provider, medically necessary and reasonable care, adequate provider network, adequate and quality care, guidelines, criteria, psychotherapy, appropriate dose and quantity, therapeutic equivalents, class of drugs, generic equivalents, pharmacy benefit management, hospital care, quality assurance criteria, pay for performance criteria, physician quality ranking program criteria, disease management, appeal processes, healthcare, clinical necessity, treatment necessity, behavioral health, generally accepted mental health practice* and *other contractual definitions.* Other techniques that impede access to care include *closed formularies, preferred formularies, managed formularies, tiered formularies, tiered co-pays, therapeutic class substitutions, dispensing or prescribing limits, prior authorization requirements, step therapy, fail first policies, prospective utilization review, concomitant utilization review, retrospective utilization review, physician incentives and disincentives, pharmacist incentives,* and *prescription compliance monitoring.*

Under current Medicare rules, Medicare pays 80% of the cost of a doctor treating a physical ailment and patients pay 20%. But mental health patients must pay half the cost for therapy treatments out of pocket because Medicare only covers 50%. Parity for mental healthcare is also lacking for returning veterans and their families.

It is easy to curtail mental healthcare from vulnerable individuals who are the neediest. Lack of mental health parity is best conceptualized as an unethical experiment on vulnerable individuals that would never acquire approval from an institutional review board. When mental illness is not properly treated, it does not disappear; instead it leads to some other burden to society. In our currently restricted system, less than 50% of all Americans in need of mental healthcare receive it and only one-third of those receive minimally adequate care (8). Families USA and the Institute of Medicine calculate thousands die each year from inadequate insurance. The underinsured and uninsured are more likely to delay or not receive healthcare and less likely to pay for and receive recommended treatments, including prescription medications. In addition they are less likely to receive preventive care, more likely to utilize emergency rooms and are more likely to be hospitalized for preventable health problems. A Commonwealth Fund study in 2006 found 59% of uninsured people with chronic conditions either skipped a dose of their medicine or went without it because it was too expensive. One-third of that group visited an emergency room or stayed in a hospital overnight or did both, compared with 15% of their counterparts with access through insurance. Inadequate access to psychiatric medications in Medicare D resulted in 53% of patient having at least one problem with medication access, 22% discontinuing or temporarily stopping medication, 31% not able to access medication refills, and 20% could not access new medications. Most commonly, these problems were with antipsychotics followed by antidepressants (9). More recent data demonstrated that 48% had access problem and 26% discontinued medication. Thirty-three percent of psychiatrists and nurse practitioners to a Maine survey linked the use of a substitute drug as mandated by Maine care's process to a Medicaid patient's suicide attempt within the prior 6 months. The American Psychiatric Association recently testified before Congress that it has received hundreds of calls from doctors and individuals reporting the denial of essential medications.

Lack of parity with associated failure to access mental healthcare are also associated with higher risks for child abuse and neglect, more risk to innocent bystanders, more debt, more problems with credit rating, and more claims for workers' compensation and welfare and social instability.

Critical to the decision about limiting mental health parity is information about the effect on total healthcare costs. If mental healthcare is limited, do inpatient hospital costs increase? If decision-makers are focused only on one facet of cost reductions, then they miss the larger picture. The "silo effect," in which each decision-maker is concerned that his costs are reduced in his area of responsibility and unconcerned that the cost of healthcare in another "silo" is increasing as a result of his decision (i.e., hospitalizations, both psychiatric and medical, increase use of emergency rooms). Aggressive tactics implemented by managed care have created financial barriers to accessing mental healthcare and have greatly reduced the utilization of mental health services. There have been many objective studies demonstrating increased total costs as a result of obstructing access to mental healthcare (10–12). Although a few studies have demonstrated that lack of parity reduce a few direct costs, no study has ever demonstrated it has reduced total direct and indirect costs. A New Hampshire study found that placing limits on psychotropic medications reduced psychotropic medication costs but increased overall healthcare costs by a factor of 17. While pharmaceutical costs decreased, overall costs increased because of increases in emergency mental health services and partial hospitalizations. A different study with 20,000 of the Columbia Medical Plan's enrollees showed cost savings for treating mentally ill enrollees as compared with not treating mentally ill enrollees. The study found that untreated mentally ill people had a 61% increase in medical utilization compared with mentally ill people who received mental health treatment and increased medical expenditures by only 11%. A controlled study involving 23,000 patients found that fail first policies for atypical antipsychotics cost the state more than $2500 per patient in a 6-month period (13). Medi-Cal formularies for psychotropics in California are typically made up of numerous HMO's each with its own restrictive formulary that leads to confusion, numerous denials, delays and disruption of treatment. Patients from an HMO with a single preferred SSRI were 80% less likely to complete treatment than patients in an HMO with two SSRIs on the formulary (14).

THE COST OF COST CONTAINMENT

There are avoidable and unavoidable costs. Immediate direct costs are very clear but long term benefit is complex and far reaching. The cost of cost containment is often greater than the cost of providing care. The most rapidly increasing costs are the hidden costs of healthcare middlemen and the administrative costs of the dealing with them.

A Boston University study demonstrated only half of healthcare spent on healthcare and the other half is wasted on unnecessary spending, and in particular administrative costs and profit in the insurance company and a 2003 Harvard Medical School study demonstrating that $400 billion is wasted on bureaucratic inefficiency. PricewaterhouseCoopers, L.L.P. puts the value of the waste in the healthcare system at $1.2 trillion a year, and "more than half the $2.2 trillion spent on healthcare in this country" is "wasteful spending." Areas of waste include the "ineffective use of information technology ($81 to $88 billion), claims processing ($21 to $210 billion), and defensive medicine ($210 billion)." Based on this research, $1 trillion, rather than $2.2 trillion is actually being spent on healthcare, a modest figure for an industrialized society. The problem is wasted money, not the money spent on actual mental health or healthcare. In spite of greatly improved technology, the healthcare system appears to be in a declining spiral with increasing management costs, waste, excessive profits, and conflict within the system and decreasing expenditures on actual healthcare.

CONCLUSION

Insurance inequality for the mentally ill is similar to other forms of discrimination based on race, religion, sex and ethnic background. Discrimination against diseases of the brain and those afflicted by brain diseases is unethical and a violation of fundamental human rights. This discrimination is implemented and concealed by the use of managed care, pharmacy benefit management plans, carve-out programs and phantom provider networks. Although employer mandated health insurance coverage is unfair, it is also unfair to use bad faith insurance practices that are inappropriately shielded by ERISA. We cannot allow excessive insurance company profits and cost shifting to government programs by permitting stigma and discrimination with unequal benefits for the mentally ill that are ethically, economically, and scientifically unsound. Those patients unable to physically protect themselves must be protected from the predators in our society. It is a return to the Middle Ages, when the mentally ill roamed the streets and little boys threw rocks at them (15). Throughout history, most civilizations have declined from internal failures rather than external threats. The global perception of our country as a world leader is compromised when the mentally ill, handicapped and disabled veterans wander in our streets and fill our jails and we allow others to benefit at the expense of vulnerable groups. America is the world leader and the major exporter of healthcare technology, but access to mental healthcare is currently challenging. Parity for mental healthcare is an opportunity for us to also be a leader for access to humane care.

Parity is the only ethical and economically sound approach to correct this serious failure in our healthcare system. Our mental health and someone else's mental health have value. Lack of parity must be replaced by an ethical science based, cost-effective, structure with foresight for the greater good and coordinated management of chronic illness through care that is sensitive to patient preferences and supported by adequate infrastructure and is clearly understandable, transparent, responsible and accountable. "Management" of mental health benefits should be the same as the "management" of any other benefit. Accepting parity in return for excessive or deceptive "management" techniques would be phantom parity. Implementation of parity will improve the overall quality of life, save hundreds of billions in many indirect healthcare and other costs, enhance productivity, foster the development of a larger tax base, increase our nation's competitiveness in the global market, reduce the number of inmates of prisons who are mentally disturbed by treating these convicts before they commit a crime and reduce costs to our justice system. As David Sacher, MD, former U.S. Surgeon General stated, "There is no health without mental health."

References

1. Insel TR, Fenton WS. Psychiatric epidemiology. *Arch Gen Psychiatry* 2005;62:590–592.
2. Markowitz FE. Psychiatric hospital capacity, homelessness, and crime and arrest rates. *Criminology* 2006;44:45–72.
3. Copeland WE, Miller-Johnson S, Keeler G, et al. Childhood psychiatric disorders and young adult crime: A prospective, population-based study. *Am J Psychiatry* 2007;164(11): 1668–1675.
4. Teplin LA, Abram KM, McClelland GM, et al. Detecting mental disorder in juvenile detainees: Who receives services. *Am J Public Health* 2005;95(10):1773–1780.
5. Stewart WF. Cost of lost production work time among U.S. workers with depression. *JAMA* 2003;28:3135–3140.

6. Leavitt MO, Gerberding JL, Sondik EJ. *Health, United States, 2007.* DHSS Publication No. 2007–1232, 2007.

7. Markov DM, Goldman M, Kunkel EJS, et al. Lack of parity in mental health care coverage affects physicians in all specialties. *N J Psychiatrist* 2006;40:6.

8. Kessler RC, Berglund P, Demler O, et al. Lifetime prevalence and age of onset distributions of DSM-IV disorders in the national comorbidity survey replication. *Arch Gen Psychiatry* 2005;62:593–602.

9. West JC, Wilk JE, Muszynski IL, et al. Medication access and continuity: the experiences of dual-eligible psychiatric patients during the first 4 months of the Medicare prescription drug benefit. *Am J Psychiatry* 2007;164(5):789–796.

10. Bartels SJ, Horn S, Sharkey P, et al. Treatment of depression in older primary care patients in health maintenance organizations. *Int J Psychiatry Med* 1997;27:215–231.

11. Tennison C. Responding to restrictive formularies. *Psychiatr Ann* 2004;34(2):139–148.

12. Yanos PT, Lu W, Minsky S, et al. Correlates of health insurance among persons with schizophrenia in a statewide behavioral health care system. *Psychiatr Serv* 2004;55(1):79–82.

13. Del Paggio D, Finley PR, Cavano JM, et al. Clinical and economic outcomes associated with olanzipine for the treatment of psychiatric symptoms in a county mental health population. *Clin Ther* 2002;24:803–817.

14. Mitchell J, Greenburg J, Finck K, et al. Effectiveness and economic impact of antidepressant medication: A review. *Am J Managed Care* 1997;3:323–330.

15. Reich R. Care of the chronically mentally ill: A national disgrace. *Am J Psychiatry* 1973; 130:912.

32 | Global Perspectives

Mario Maj and David Baron

"Despite the great attention Western countries pay to the mind and human consciousness in philosophy and the arts, disturbances of mental health remain not only neglected but also deeply stigmatized across our societies."
— Dr. Richard Horton, Editor, The Lancet, 2008.

On September 3, 2007, *The Lancet* launched a series of eleven commentaries and six review articles on global mental disorders in primarily low- and middle-income countries.

This work was produced by 39 international experts, convened as the Lancet Global Mental Health Group. The Group articulated five main goals: (i) placing mental health on the public health priority agenda; (ii) improving organization of mental health services; (iii) integrating the availability of mental health in general healthcare; (iv) developing human resources for mental health; and (v) strengthening public mental health leadership. Each of these goals addresses critical issues related to the current disparities in psychiatric care (1).

Professor Vikram Patel, one of the lead authors, concluded that, "while most persons with mental disorders live in low or middle income countries, most mental health resources are found in high-income countries, reflecting a vast treatment gap" (2). This chapter will explore disparities in psychiatric care from a global perspective.

Mental disorders are highly prevalent in all regions of the world and represent a major source of disability and social burden worldwide. Treatments for all these disorders are currently available and have been found to be effective in both developed and developing countries. However, mental disorders are remarkably undertreated worldwide, especially in low-income countries. National mental health policies are lacking in several countries, especially low-income ones. Resources for mental healthcare are scarce and unequally distributed.

PREVALENCE AND BURDEN OF MENTAL DISORDERS WORLDWIDE

The World Health Organization (WHO) estimates that more than 25% of individuals worldwide develop one or more mental disorders during their lifetime (3). This estimate has been recently supported by a series of face-to-face community surveys conducted in 17 countries in Africa, Asia, the Americas, Europe, and the Middle East, with a total number of 85,052 respondents (4,5). In these surveys, the lifetime prevalence of any mental disorder has been found to be higher than 25% in 11 out of 17 countries, and higher than 15% in all countries but two (China and Nigeria), where prevalence rates were likely to be downwardly biased because of respondent reluctance to admit mental health problems. Anxiety disorders were the most prevalent in 10 out of 17 countries, and mood disorders in six (Table 32.1). Lifetime co-occurrence of two or more mental disorders was quite common, so that the sum of the prevalence rates across the various disorder types was between 30% and 50% higher than the proportion of people having at least one mental disorder. Survival analysis showed that the odds ratios for anxiety, mood, and substance use disorders were higher in younger compared with older cohorts.

To quantify the burden of the various diseases and injuries, the WHO, in collaboration with the Harvard School of Public Health and the World Bank, introduced in 1993 a new measure, called disability-adjusted life year (DALY). DALYs for a given disease or injury are the sum of the years of life lost caused by premature mortality plus the years lost caused by disability for incident cases of that disease or injury in the general population.

In low-income countries, the disability caused by mental and neurological disorders was estimated to be comparatively lower, because of the impact of infectious,

TABLE 32.1	Lifetime Prevalence of DSM-IV Mental Disorders in the World Mental Health Surveys			
	Any Mental Disorder, % (SE)	**Any Anxiety Disorder, % (SE)**	**Any Mood Disorder, % (SE)**	**Any Substance Use Disorder, % (SE)**
The Americas				
Colombia	39.1 (1.3)	25.3 (1.4)	14.6 (0.7)	9.6 (0.6)
Mexico	26.1 (1.4)	14.3 (0.9)	9.2 (0.5)	7.8 (0.5)
United States	47.4 (1.1)	31.0 (1.0)	21.4 (0.6)	14.6 (0.6)
Europe				
Belgium	29.1 (2.3)	13.1 (1.9)	14.1 (1.0)	8.3 (0.9)
France	37.9 (1.7)	22.3 (1.4)	21.0 (1.1)	7.1 (0.5)
Germany	25.2 (1.9)	14.6 (1.5)	9.9 (0.6)	6.5 (0.6)
Italy	18.1 (1.1)	11.0 (0.9)	9.9 (0.5)	1.3 (0.2)
Netherlands	31.7 (2.0)	15.9 (1.1)	17.9 (1.0)	8.9 (0.9)
Spain	19.4 (1.4)	9.9 (1.1)	10.6 (0.5)	3.6 (0.4)
Ukraine	36.1 (1.5)	10.9 (0.8)	15.8 (0.8)	15.0 (1.3)
Africa and Middle East				
Israel	17.6 (0.6)	5.2 (0.3)	10.7 (0.5)	5.3 (0.3)
Lebanon	25.8 (1.9)	16.7 (1.6)	12.6 (0.9)	2.2 (0.8)
Nigeria	12.0 (1.0)	6.5 (0.9)	3.3 (0.3)	3.7 (0.4)
South Africa	30.3 (1.1)	15.8 (0.8)	9.8 (0.7)	13.3 (0.9)
Asia and the Pacific				
Japan	18.0 (1.1)	6.9 (0.6)	7.6 (0.5)	4.8 (0.5)
China	13.2 (1.3)	4.8 (0.7)	3.6 (0.4)	4.9 (0.7)
Oceania				
New Zealand	39.3 (0.9)	24.6 (0.7)	20.4 (0.5)	12.4 (0.4)

From Kessler RC, Angermeyer M, Anthony JC, et al. Lifetime prevalence and age-of-onset distributions of mental disorders in the World Health Organization's World Mental Health Surveys. *World Psychiatry* 2007;6(3):168–176.

TABLE 32.2	Leading Causes of Disability-Adjusted Life-Year (DALYs) Worldwide as Estimated for the Year 2030

Disease or injury	% Total
1. HIV/AIDS	12.1
2. Unipolar depressive disorders	5.7
3. Ischemic heart disease	4.7
4. Road traffic accidents	4.2
5. Perinatal conditions	4.0
6. Cerebrovascular disease	3.9
7. Chronic obstructive pulmonary disease	3.1
8. Lower respiratory infections	3.0
9. Hearing loss, adult onset	2.5
10. Cataracts	2.5

From Mathers CD, Loncar D. Projections of global mortality and burden of disease from 2002 to 2030. *PLoS Med* 2006;3:2011.

perinatal, and nutritional conditions. However, mental and neurological disorders accounted for 17.6% of all DALYs in Africa in the year 2000 (3).

In the estimates for the year 2005 (6), mental and neurological disorders accounted for 13.5% of all DALYs in the world (27.4% in high-income countries, 17.7% in middle-income countries, and 9.1% in low-income countries), being the main contributor to burden among noncommunicable diseases (27.5%, versus 22% for cardiovascular diseases and 11% for cancer).

According to the updated estimates for the year 2030 (6), mental and neurological disorders will account for 14.4% of all DALYs in the world and 25.4% of those caused by noncommunicable diseases. Depression will rank second in the percent of total DALYs in that year (5.7%), following HIV/AIDS and preceding ischemic heart disease (Table 32.2). It will be first in high-income countries (9.8%), second in middle-income countries (6.7%) and third in low-income countries (4.7%) (Table 32.3). Community surveys carried out in low- and high-income countries, focusing on children/adolescents between 1 and 15 years of age, have reported prevalence rates of mental disorders between 12% and 22% (3). This presents a significant challenge globally. There are simply not enough trained child psychiatrists to diagnose and treatment psychopathology in the young. The problem is more acute in low-income countries compared with high income countries. Virtually all low-income countries have only a few child psychiatrists, and they tend to be restricted to large urban areas, leaving rural areas devoid of child/adolescent psychiatric services.

TREATMENT GAP AND PROJECTED POPULATION-LEVEL TREATMENT EFFECTIVENESS WORLDWIDE

The efficacy of pharmacological and psychosocial treatments for mood, anxiety, psychotic, and substance-related disorders is now convincingly proved by clinical trials carried out in low- and middle-income, as well as in high-income countries. However, the treatment gap is substantial for all mental disorders worldwide, in particular in low-income countries.

TABLE 32.3	Leading Causes of Disability-Adjusted Life Years (DALYs) in High-, Middle-, and Low-Income Countries, as Estimated for the Year 2030

Disease or Injury	% Total
High-income countries	
1. Unipolar depressive disorders	9.8
2. Ischemic heart disease	5.9
3. Alzheimer's and other dementias	5.8
4. Alcohol use disorders	4.7
5. Diabetes mellitus	4.5
6. Cerebrovascular disease	4.5
7. Hearing loss, adult onset	4.1
8. Trachea, bronchus, lung cancers	3.0
9. Osteoarthritis	2.9
10. Chronic obstructive pulmonary disease	2.5
Middle-income countries	
1. HIV/AIDS	9.8
2. Unipolar depressive disorders	6.7
3. Cerebrovascular disease	6.0
4. Ischemic heart disease	4.7
5. Chronic obstructive pulmonary disease	4.7
6. Road traffic accidents	4.0
7. Violence	2.9
8. Vision disorders, age-related	2.9
9. Hearing loss, adult onset	2.9
10. Diabetes mellitus	2.6
Low-income countries	
1. HIV/AIDS	14.6
2. Perinatal conditions	5.8
3. Unipolar depressive disorders	4.7
4. Road traffic accidents	4.6
5. Ischemic heart disease	4.5
6. Lower respiratory infections	4.4
7. Diarrheal diseases	2.8
8. Cerebrovascular disease	2.8
9. Cataracts	2.8
10. Malaria	2.5

From Mathers CD, Loncar D. Projections of global mortality and burden of disease from 2002 to 2030. *PLoS Med* 2006;3:2011.

In the World Mental Health Surveys, carried out in representative community samples in 17 countries in Africa, the Americas, Asia, Europe, and the Middle East, the proportion of lifetime cases of anxiety disorders making treatment contact in the year of disorder onset ranged from 0.8% in Nigeria to 36.4% in Israel. The proportion of cases making treatment contact by 50 years ranged from 15.2% in Nigeria to 95.0% in Germany. The median delay to treatment among cases eventually making contact ranged from 3 years in Israel to 30 years in Mexico (5) (Table 32.4). The proportion of lifetime cases of mood disorders making treatment contact in the year of disorder

TABLE 32.4	Treatment Delay for Anxiety Disorders in the World Mental Health Surveys		
	Making Treatment Contact in Year of Onset, % (SE)	**Making Treatment Contact by 50 Years, % (SE)**	**Median Duration of Delay in Years (SE)**
The Americas			
Colombia	2.9 (0.6)	41.6 (3.9)	26.0 (1.5)
Mexico	3.6 (1.1)	53.2 (18.2)	30.0 (5.1)
United States	11.3 (0.7)	87.0 (2.4)	23.0 (0.6)
Europe			
Belgium	19.8 (2.8)	84.5 (4.9)	16.0 (3.5)
France	16.1 (1.8)	93.3 (1.9)	18.0 (1.8)
Germany	13.7 (1.8)	95.0 (2.3)	23.0 (2.3)
Italy	17.1 (2.1)	87.3 (8.5)	28.0 (2.2)
Netherlands	28.0 (3.7)	91.1 (2.8)	10.0 (1.6)
Spain	23.2 (2.0)	86.6 (5.2)	17.0 (3.2)
Africa and Middle East			
Israel	36.4 (0.9)	90.7 (1.3)	3.0 (0.1)
Lebanon	3.2 (1.1)	37.3 (11.5)	28.0 (3.9)
Nigeria	0.8 (0.5)	15.2 (2.6)	16.0 (4.2)
Asia and the Pacific			
Japan	11.2 (2.4)	63.1 (6.2)	20.0 (2.4)
China	4.2 (2.0)	44.7 (7.2)	21.0 (3.1)
Oceania			
New Zealand	12.5 (0.8)	84.2 (2.5)	21.0 (0.8)

From Wang PS, Angermeyer M, Borges G, et al. Delay and failure in treatment seeking after first onset of mental disorders in the World Health Organization's World Mental Health Survey Initiative. *World Psychiatry* 2007;6(3):177–185.

onset ranged from 6% in Nigeria and China to 52.1% in the Netherlands. The proportion of cases making treatment contact by 50 years ranged from 7.9% in China to 98.6% in France. The median delay to treatment among cases eventually making contact ranged from one year in Belgium, the Netherlands, Spain, and Japan to 14 years in Mexico (5) (Table 32.5).

The proportion of lifetime cases of substance use disorders making treatment contact in the year of disorder onset ranged from 0.9% in Mexico to 18.6% in Spain. The proportion of cases making treatment contact by 50 years ranged from 19.8% in Nigeria to 86.1% in Germany. The median delay to treatment among cases eventually making contact ranged from 6 years in Spain to 18 years in Belgium (5) (Table 32.6).

In the World Mental Health Surveys, failure and delays in treatment seeking were generally greater in low-income countries, older cohorts, men, and cases with earlier ages of onset. The earlier treatment contact of people with mood disorders may be due at least in part to the fact that these disorders have been targeted in some countries by educational campaigns and primary care quality improvement programs. These government sponsored programs offer the added benefit of decreasing the stigma of mental illness, a significant factor in seeking treatment.

TABLE 32.5	Treatment Delay for Mood Disorders in the World Mental Health Surveys		
	Making Treatment Contact in Year of Onset, % (SE)	**Making Treatment Contact by 50 Years, % (SE)**	**Median Duration of Delay in Years (SE)**
The Americas			
Colombia	18.7 (2.7)	66.6 (3.7)	9.0 (1.6)
Mexico	16.0 (2.2)	69.9 (8.5)	14.0 (3.1)
United States	35.4 (1.2)	94.8 (2.5)	4.0 (0.2)
Europe			
Belgium	47.8 (2.7)	93.7 (2.5)	1.0 (0.3)
France	42.7 (2.1)	98.6 (1.4)	3.0 (0.3)
Germany	40.4 (3.8)	89.1 (5.0)	2.0 (0.4)
Italy	28.8 (3.0)	63.5 (5.9)	2.0 (0.5)
Netherlands	52.1 (2.9)	96.9 (1.7)	1.0 (0.3)
Spain	48.5 (2.3)	96.4 (3.1)	1.0 (0.3)
Africa and Middle East			
Israel	31.9 (0.8)	92.7 (0.5)	6.0 (0.3)
Lebanon	12.3 (2.0)	49.2 (5.2)	6.0 (2.1)
Nigeria	6.0 (1.7)	33.3 (7.2)	6.0 (3.3)
Asia and the Pacific			
Japan	29.6 (4.0)	56.8 (7.3)	1.0 (0.7)
China	6.0 (2.2)	7.9 (2.6)	1.0 (2.0)
Oceania			
New Zealand	41.4 (1.3)	97.5 (1.0)	3.0 (0.2)

From Wang PS, Angermeyer M, Borges G, et al. Delay and failure in treatment seeking after first onset of mental disorders in the World Health Organization's World Mental Health Survey Initiative. *World Psychiatry* 2007;6(3):177–185.

The Disease Control Priorities Project Report (7) estimated the cost of a mental healthcare package consisting of outpatient-based treatment of schizophrenia and bipolar disorder with first-generation antipsychotics or mood stabilizers and adjuvant psychosocial interventions, and treatment of depression and panic disorder in primary care with generic selective serotonin reuptake inhibitors. The cost per capita of the package was projected to be $3 to $4 USD in sub-Saharan Africa and South Asia, and $7 to $9 USD in Latin America and the Caribbean. The addition of brief interventions by primary care physicians for high-risk alcohol users was projected to cost a further $0.04 USD per capita in sub-Saharan Africa and South Asia and up to $0.36 USD per capita in central Asia and Latina America.

RESOURCES FOR MENTAL HEALTHCARE WORLDWIDE

According to the Mental Health Atlas 2005 (8), only 62.1% of countries worldwide, accounting for 68.3% of the world population, have a mental health policy (i.e., a document of the government or ministry of health specifying the goals for improving the

TABLE 32.6	Treatment Delay for Substance Use Disorders in the World Mental Health Surveys		
	Making Treatment Contact in Year of Onset, % (SE)	**Making Treatment Contact by 50 Years, % (SE)**	**Median Duration of Delay in Years (SE)**
The Americas			
Colombia	3.6 (0.8)77	23.1 (7.1)	11.0 (5.0)
Mexico	0.9 (0.5)	22.1 (4.8)	10.0 (3.3)
United States	10.0 (0.8)	75.5 (3.8)	13.0 (1.2)
Europe			
Belgium	12.8 (4.8)	61.2 (17.7)	18.0 (5.8)
France	15.7 (5.4)	66.5 (14.1)	13.0 (3.7)
Germany	13.2 (5.7)	86.1 (8.6)	9.0 (3.9)
Netherlands	15.5 (5.4)	66.6 (7.9)	9.0 (3.1)
Spain	18.6 (7.6)	40.1 (14.1)	6.0 (4.9)
Africa and Middle East			
Israel	2.0 (0.5)	48.0 (2.4)	12.0 (0.5)
Nigeria	2.8 (1.7)	19.8 (7.2)	8.0 (1.8)
Asia and the Pacific			
Japan	9.2 (5.1)	31.0 (7.8)	8.0 (4.6)
China	2.8 (1.8)	25.7 (9.0)	17.0 (3.7)
Oceania			
New Zealand	6.3 (0.8)	84.8 (15.4)	17.0 (1.3)

From Wang PS, Angermeyer M, Borges G, et al. Delay and failure in treatment seeking after first onset of mental disorders in the World Health Organization's World Mental Health Survey Initiative. *World Psychiatry* 2007;6(3):177–185.

mental health situation of the country, the priorities among those goals and the main directions for attaining them). A mental health policy is present in 58.8% of low-income and 70.5% of high-income countries. In Africa, only 50% of countries have a mental health policy. In South-East Asia, only 54.5% of countries have a mental health policy, and 76.4% of the population is not covered by such a policy (Table 32.7).

TABLE 32.7	Presence of a Mental Health Policy in the Countries of Each Region of the World Health Organization	
WHO Region	**% Countries**	**% Population Coverage**
Africa	50.0	69.4
Americas	72.7	64.2
Eastern Mediterranean	72.7	93.8
Europe	70.6	89.1
South-East Asia	54.5	23.6
Western Pacific	48.1	93.8

From World Health Organization. *Mental Health Atlas 2005.* Geneva: World Health Organization; 2005.

Community care facilities exist in only 68.1% of the countries (51.7% of low-income and 93% of high-income countries). In South-East Asia, they are present in 50% of the countries, and in Africa in 56.5% of the countries. Only 60.9% of the countries report to provide treatment facilities for severe mental disorders at the primary care level (55.2% of low-income and 79.5% of high-income countries). About a quarter of low-income countries do not provide even basic antidepressant medications in primary care settings. In many others, the supply does not extend to all regions of the country or is very irregular. Since medicines are often not available in healthcare facilities, patients and families are forced to pay for them out of pocket.

While more than 61.5% of European countries spend more than 5% of their health budget in mental healthcare, 70% of countries in Africa and 50% of countries in South-East Asia spend less than 1%. Out-of-pocket payment is the most important method of financing mental healthcare in 38.6% of countries in Africa and 30% of countries in South-East Asia, whereas it is not the primary method of financing mental healthcare in any European country (Table 32.8). All countries with out-of-pocket payment as the dominant method of financing mental healthcare belong to low-income or lower middle-income categories, while almost all countries with social insurance as the dominant method of financing belong to high-income or upper middle-income categories (9).

The median of psychiatric beds per 10,000 population ranges from 0.33 in South-East Asia and 0.34 in Africa to 8 in Europe. Globally, 72% of psychiatric beds are located in mental hospitals and the rest in other settings, including psychiatric units in general hospitals and community services. The percentage of psychiatric beds located in mental hospitals is 74% in low-income and 83% in middle-income countries, compared with 64% in high-income countries. The lower figures for high-income countries reflect the trend toward deinstitutionalization in those countries. Of the psychiatric beds available in Europe, more than 80% are located in mental hospitals in low- and middle-income countries of Central and Eastern Europe (10).

The median number of psychiatrists per 100,000 population ranges from 0.04 in Africa and 0.2 in South-East Asia to 9.8 in Europe. It is 0.1 in low-income countries compared with 9.2 in high-income countries. Two thirds of low-income countries have less than one psychiatrist per 100,000 population. Chad, Eritrea, and Liberia (with populations of 9, 4.2, and 3.5 million, respectively) have just one psychiatrist

TABLE 32.8	Countries in Which Out-of-Pocket Payment Is the Most Common Method of Financing Mental Healthcare in Each Region of the World Health Organization

WHO Region	**% Countries**
Africa	38.6
Americas	12.9
Eastern Mediterranean	15.8
Europe	0
South-East Asia	30.0
Western Pacific	18.5

From World Health Organization. *Mental Health Atlas 2005.* Geneva: World Health Organization; 2005.

each. Afghanistan, Rwanda, and Togo (with populations of 25, 8.5, and 5 million, respectively) have just two psychiatrists each. Large-scale migration of psychiatrists from low- and middle-income countries to high-income countries, as part of the larger picture of migration of health professionals in general ("brain drain"), has been consistently documented (10). India and some sub-Saharan African countries are the most important contributors to the mental health workforce in the United Kingdom, although this country has around 40 psychiatrists per million population, while India has 4 per million and sub-Saharan Africa less than one per million (11).

The median number of psychiatric nurses per 100,000 population ranges from 0.1 in South East Asia and 0.2 in Africa to 24.8 in Europe. Nearly 47% of low-income countries have less than one psychiatric nurse per 100,000 population. The median number of psychologists working in mental healthcare per 100,000 population ranges from 0.03 in South-East Asia and 0.05 in Africa to 3.1 in Europe. Approximately 69% of low-income countries have less than one psychologist per 100,000 population (Table 32.9).

From the above figures, it is clear that resources for mental healthcare are grossly inadequate in comparison to the needs, and that inequalities across countries are large, especially between low-income and high-income countries (9). Moreover, resources tend to be concentrated in urban areas, especially in low-income countries, leaving vast regions without any form of mental healthcare.

Even worse is the situation concerning child and adolescent mental healthcare. According to the WHO (11), only 7% of countries worldwide have a specific child and adolescent mental health policy. In less than one third of all countries it is possible to identify an institution or a governmental entity with an overall responsibility for child mental health. School-based services are almost exclusively present in high-income countries, and even in Europe only 17% of countries have a sufficient number of these services. There are no pediatric beds for mental health identified in low-income countries, while such beds are identified in 50% of high-income countries. In all African countries outside South Africa, fewer than 10 psychiatrists could be identified who were trained to work with children. In European countries, the number of child psychiatrists ranges from one per 5300 to one per 51,800. In more than 70% of countries worldwide, there is no list of essential psychotropic medications for children. In 45% of countries worldwide, psychostimulants are either prohibited or unavailable for use in children with attention-deficit/hyperactivity disorder.

TABLE 32.9	Median Number of Mental Health Professionals per 100,000 Population in Each Region of the World Health Organization		
WHO Region	**Psychiatrists**	**Psychiatric Nurses**	**Psychologists Working in Mental Health**
Africa	0.04	0.20	0.05
Americas	2.00	2.60	2.80
Eastern Mediterranean	0.95	1.25	0.60
Europe	9.80	24.80	3.10
South-East Asia	0.20	0.10	0.03
Western Pacific	0.32	0.50	0.03

From World Health Organization. *Mental Health Atlas 2005.* Geneva: World Health Organization; 2005.

CURRENT TRENDS IN MENTAL HEALTHCARE AND BARRIERS TO CHANGE WORLDWIDE

The current trends in mental healthcare worldwide have been summarized by the WHO in its recommendations issued in 2001 (3). They include (a) providing treatment in primary care; (b) making psychotropic medications available; (c) giving care in the community; (d) educating the public; (e) involving communities, families, and consumers; (f) establishing national policies, programs, and legislations; (g) developing human resources; (h) linking with other relevant sectors; (i) monitoring community mental health; (j) supporting more research.

Providing treatment in primary care involves the inclusion of recognition and treatment of common mental disorders in training curricula of all health personnel, the provision of refresher training to primary care physicians, and the improvement of referral patterns in primary healthcare. Making psychotropic medications available includes ensuring the availability of essential drugs in all healthcare settings and, in high-income countries, providing easier access to newer psychotropic drugs under public or private treatment plans. Giving care in the community implies moving people with mental disorders out of prisons, downsizing mental hospitals and improving care within them, developing general hospital psychiatric units, and providing community care facilities.

Educating the public includes promoting public campaigns against stigma and discrimination; using the mass media to promote mental health, foster positive attitudes, and help prevent mental disorders; and, in high-income countries, launching public campaigns for the recognition and treatment of common mental disorders. Involving communities, families, and consumers includes supporting the formation of self-help groups; ensuring the representation of communities, families, and consumers in services and policy-making; and foster advocacy initiatives.

Establishing national policies, programs and legislations includes revising legislations on the basis of current knowledge and human rights considerations, formulating mental health programs and policies, and increasing the budget for mental healthcare. Developing human resources involves training psychiatrists and psychiatric nurses, and, in middle- and high-income countries, creating national training centres for psychiatrists, psychiatric nurses, psychologists, and psychiatric social workers. Linking with other relevant sectors involves initiating school and workplace mental health programs, encouraging the activities of nongovernmental organizations in these areas, and, in high-income countries, initiating evidence-based mental health promotion programs in collaboration with other appropriate sectors.

Monitoring community mental health involves including mental disorders in basic health information systems, surveying high-risk population groups, instituting surveillance for specific disorders in the community, and, in high-income countries, monitoring effectiveness of preventive programs. Supporting more research includes conducting studies in primary healthcare settings on the prevalence, course, outcome and impact of mental disorders in the community; instituting effectiveness and cost-effectiveness studies for management of common mental disorders in primary healthcare; and, in high-income countries, carrying out research on the risk factors for mental disorders and on service delivery, and investigating evidence on the prevention of mental disorders (3).

The main interventions proposed for the prevention of suicide worldwide include: (a) reduction of access to means of suicide (e.g., pesticides, firearms); (b) treatment of people with mental disorders; (c) improvement of media portrayal of suicide; (d) training of primary healthcare personnel; (e) school-based programs; (f) availability of hot lines and crisis centres (11). The most significant barriers to the implementation of the above principles worldwide, according to the WHO (12), include the following: (a) some stakeholders may be resistant to the changes; (b) health authorities may not believe in the effectiveness of mental health interventions; (c) there may be no consensus among the country's stakeholders about how to formulate or implement the new policy; (d) financial and human resources may be scarce; (e) other basic health priorities may compete with mental healthcare for funding; (f) primary care teams may feel overburdened by their workload and refuse to accept the introduction of the new policy; (g) many mental health specialists may not want to work in community facilities or with primary care teams, preferring to remain in hospitals. The solutions which are suggested include: (a) adopting an "all-winners approach," ensuring that the needs of all stakeholders are taken into account; (b) developing pilot projects and evaluating their impact on health and consumer satisfaction; (c) asking for technical reports from international experts; (d) focusing the implementation of the mental health policy on a demonstration area and performing cost-effectiveness studies; (e) linking mental health programs to other health priorities; (f) showing primary care practitioners that people with mental disorders are already a hidden part of their burden, and that this burden will decrease if these disorders are identified and treated (12).

STIGMATIZING ATTITUDES TOWARD PEOPLE WITH MENTAL DISORDERS RESULTING IN DISPARITY OF CARE

Stigmatizing attitudes toward people with mental disorders have been reported to be widespread in the general public and even among mental health professionals. Although it has been suggested that stigma may be less severe in Asian and African countries, a study carried out in India within the Stigma Programme of the World Psychiatric Association (WPA), in which 463 persons with schizophrenia and 651 family members were interviewed in four cities, reported that two thirds of the respondents had suffered discrimination (13). Women and people living in urban areas were more stigmatized. Males experienced greater discrimination in the job area, whereas women experienced more problems in the family and social area. In the family area, subtle discrimination in the form of decreased love, avoidance, rejection, distance and excessive caution was frequently reported. In Ethiopia, among relatives of people with a diagnosis of schizophrenia or mood disorders, 75% reported they had experienced stigma caused by the presence of mental illness in the family, and 37% wanted to conceal the fact that a relative was ill (14). In a large survey carried out in China among people with schizophrenia and their family members, one half of the respondents reported they had felt significantly stigmatized, and levels of stigma were found to be higher in urban areas (15). Stigmatization of people with mental disorders has been reported to be rare in Islamic countries (16).

Unlike people with physical disabilities, those with mental disorders are often perceived by the public to be in control of their disabilities and responsible for causing them (16). The view that "weakness," "laziness," or "lack of willpower" contribute toward the development of mental disorders has been observed in several countries, including Turkey, Mongolia, and South Africa (10). The stigmatization of people with mental disorders may result in public avoidance, systematic discrimination and reduced help-seeking behavior. In a survey carried out in 1996 in a probability sample of 1444 adults in the United States, more than one half of the respondents reported to be unwilling to spend an evening socializing, work next to, or have a family member marry a person with mental illness (17). While most countries in the world have some provision for disability benefits, mental ill people are often specifically excluded from such entitlements. Moreover, mental disorders are frequently not considered in social and private insurance schemes for healthcare. Shame is reported to be one of the main barriers from seeking help for mental disorders in both developed and developing countries (10).

Strategies for addressing stigmatization of people with mental disorders have been subdivided into three groups: protest, education, and contact (16). There is some evidence that protest campaigns may be effective in reducing stigmatizing behaviors against people with mental disorders. Education may promote a better understanding of mental illness, and educated people may be less likely to endorse stigma and discrimination. An inverse relationship between having contact with a person with mental illness and endorsing stigmatizing behaviors has been documented.

The access of people with mental illness to physical healthcare is reduced with respect to the general population. In the above-mentioned study conducted in Australia (18), the SMR for ischemic heart disease was found to be 1.78 in men with schizophrenia. However, hospital admission for that disease was remarkably less common in both males and females with schizophrenia compared with the general population. Moreover, both men and women with schizophrenia were more than threefold less likely to receive revascularization procedures than the general population.

The quality of physical healthcare received by patients with severe mental illness is often worse than the general population. A study conducted in the United States (19) found that adverse events during medical and surgical hospitalizations were significantly more frequent in patients with schizophrenia than in the other people, including infections caused by medical care, postoperative respiratory failure, postoperative deep venous thrombosis or pulmonary embolism, and postoperative sepsis. All these adverse events were associated with significantly increased odds of admission to an intensive care unit and of death.

The decreased access of people with mental disorders to medical services has been related to several factors concerning the healthcare system. Well documented is the impact of lack of insurance and cost of care. In a study carried out in the United States (20), people with mental disorders were twice as likely than those without mental disorders to have been denied insurance because of a pre-existing condition (odds ratio = 2.18). Having a mental disorder conferred a greater risk of having delayed seeking care because of cost (odds ratio = 1.76) and of having been unable to obtain needed medical care (odds ratio = 2.30).

Even when people with mental illness are seen by a doctor, their physical diseases often remain undiagnosed. Primary care providers may misperceive the medical complaints of people with mental disorders as "psychosomatic," be unskilled or feel uncomfortable in dealing with this population. An underlying stigmatization may be involved. Moreover, during hospitalizations in medical and surgical wards, healthcare professionals may not be experienced in dealing with the special needs of patients with schizophrenia, may minimize or misinterpret their somatic symptoms, and may make an inappropriate use of restraints or sedative drugs, or fail to consider possible interactions of psychotropic drugs with other medications (19). On the other hand, many psychiatrists are unable or unwilling to perform physical and even neurological examinations or are not up-to-date on the management of even common physical diseases.

To address this situation, the first step is raising awareness of the problem among mental healthcare professionals, primary care providers, patients with schizophrenia and their families. Available research information about the increased morbidity and mortality caused by physical illness in people with schizophrenia should be appropriately disseminated.

Education and training of mental health professionals and primary care providers is a further essential step. Mental health professionals should be trained to perform at least basic medical tasks. They should be educated about the importance of recognizing physical illness in people with severe mental disorders, and encouraged to familiarize themselves with the most common reasons for under diagnosis or misdiagnosis of physical illness in these people. On the other hand, primary care providers should overcome their reluctance to treat people with severe mental illness, and learn effective ways to interact and communicate with them: it is not only an issue of knowledge and skills, but most of all one of attitudes.

This final point cannot be overstated. Any meaningful change in the current global disparity in psychiatric care must start with a change in the attitude and perception of mental illness. As advances in neuroscience continue to document the physiologic abnormalities associated with psychopathology, more medical students will choose to become psychiatrists, government and public health officials will better fund mental health treatment facilities and the general population will view psychiatric disease and its treatment, in parity with other medical disorders. This is our goal and hope for the future.

FUTURE PERSPECTIVES

Among the strategies proposed to place mental health on the public health priority agenda are the development and use of uniform and clearly understandable messages for mental health advocacy, and the education of decision-makers within governments and donor agencies on the evidence concerning the public health significance of mental disorders and the cost-effectiveness of mental healthcare. Strategies suggested to improve the organization of mental health services include, among the others, the provision of incentive arrangements to overcome vested interests blocking change, and the organization of international technical support to learn from countries that have experienced successful mental health reform. To integrate the availability of mental health in general healthcare, it is proposed to appoint and train mental health professionals specifically for supporting and supervising primary healthcare staff. To promote the development of human resources for mental health, it is suggested to increase and diversify the professional and specialist workforce, and to improve the quality of mental health training, ensuring that it is practical and occurs in community or primary care settings. Government ministries are asked to identify and scale-up a priority package of service interventions and to increase mental health budget allocations, with a view to attain a minimum level of investment within 10 years of $2 USD per capita in low-income countries and $3 to $4 USD per capita in lower middle-income countries. International donors and governments of high-income countries, in particular those which are beneficiaries of the brain drain, are asked to place mental health on their priority agenda for health assistance to low- and middle-income countries. Finally, several outcome indicators are proposed to monitor progress worldwide.

References

1. Patel V. Global mental health: A call to action. *WPA News Third Quarter* 2007;4.
2. Levin A. "Vast treatment gap" plagues mental illness around globe. *Psych News* 2008; 43:11.
3. World Health Organization. *The World Health Report 2001. Mental Health: New Understanding, New Hope.* Geneva: World Health Organization, 2001.
4. Kessler RC, Angermeyer M, Anthony JC, et al. Lifetime prevalence and age-of-onset distributions of mental disorders in the World Health Organization's World Mental Health Surveys. *World Psychiatry* 2007;6(3):168–176.
5. Wang PS, Angermeyer M, Borges G, et al. Delay and failure in treatment seeking after first onset of mental disorders in the World Health Organization's World Mental Health Survey Initiative. *World Psychiatry* 2007;6(3):177–185.
6. Mathers CD, Loncar D. Projection of global mortality and burden of disease from 2002 to 2030. *PLoS Med* 2006;3:2001.
7. World Health Organization. *Disease Control Priorities Related to Mental, Neurological, Developmental and Substance Abuse Disorders.* Geneva: World Health Organization, 2006.
8. World Health Organization. *Mental Health Atlas 2005.* Geneva: World Health Organization, 2005.
9. Saxena S, Sharan P, Garrido Cumbrera M, et al. World Health Organization's Mental Health Atlas 2005: Implications for policy development. *World Psychiatry* 2006;5:179.
10. Saxena S, Thornicroft G, Knapp M, et al. Scarcity, inequity and inefficiency of resources: The three major barriers to better mental health. *Lancet* (in press).
11. Patel V, Boardman J, Prince M, et al. Returning the debt: How rich countries can invest in mental health capacity in developing countries. *World Psychiatry* 2006;5:67.
12. World Health Organization. *Atlas: Child and Adolescent Mental Health Resources.* Geneva: World Health Organization, 2005.
13. World Health Organization. *Mental Health Policy, Plans and Programmes.* Geneva: World Health Organization, 2005.
14. Corrigan PW, Watson AC. Understanding the impact of stigma on people with mental illness. *World Psychiatry* 2002;1:16.
15. Murthy RS. Stigma is universal but experiences are local. *World Psychiatry* 2002;1:28.
16. Bertolote JM. Suicide prevention: At what level does it work? *World Psychiatry* 2004; 3:147.
17. Shibre T, Negash A, Kullgre G, et al. Perception of stigma among family members of individuals with schizophrenia and major affective disorders in rural Ethiopia. *Soc Psychiatry Psychiatr Epidemiol* 2001;36:299.
18. Brown S, Inskip H, Barraclough B. Causes of the excess mortality of schizophrenia. *Br J Psychiatry* 2000;177:212.
19. Filik R, Sipos A, Kehoe PG, et al. The cardiovascular and respiratory health of people with schizophrenia. *Acta Psychiatr Scand* 2006;113:298.
20. de Leon J, Diaz FJ. A meta-analysis of worldwide studies demonstrates an association between schizophrenia and tobacco smoking behaviors. *Schizophr Res* 2005;76:135.

33 | The Need for Universal Access to Care

Pedro Ruiz and Annelle B. Primm

INTRODUCTION

The current crisis in the delivery of psychiatric and mental health services is not unique to the United States; this crisis is also observed in all regions of the world as well. The prevalence and burden of psychiatric disorders and mental conditions is well known to be a worldwide phenomenon. For instance, the World Health Organization (WHO) estimates that over 25% of persons across the world will suffer from mental illness and conditions during their lifetime. Comorbidity conditions, with more than one mental condition being present in the same individual, are quite commonly observed these days worldwide.

The effectiveness of biological and psychological approaches in the treatment of mental illness has always been well demonstrated worldwide. Unfortunately, however, major gaps exist in the access, parity, and distribution of care across the world. Ethnic minority populations are well known to be negatively affected in this regard among developed nations, especially in the United States. Among low-income countries or evolving countries these gaps are definitely more pronounced. In this regard, only 62% of countries across the world had in 2005 well-established mental health policies. Among industrialized nations, about 70% have mental health policies; however, this number lowers to about 59% among low-income nations (1). Among these lines, the lack of appropriate mental health manpower is quite significant in poorest countries, and among poor populations in developed/industrialized countries, particularly among ethnic minority populations. This situation sometimes reaches major crisis among children and the elderly population. Stigma, of course, is a contributing factor in the current neglect that persons with mental illness are exposed to worldwide.

THE CASE OF THE UNITED STATES

As previously discussed, the current ills of the mental healthcare systems are quite widespread across the world. What is unique, however, in the United States, is that economically and scientifically the United States is the most powerful country in the world. Unfortunately, however, the mental health system in this country has deteriorated significantly in the last several decades. As a result of this, the United States does

343

not have any longer the pre-eminence status that it used to have a couple of decades ago. Today, many nations have a much better mental health system, as well as a better healthcare system than the United States; actually, the United States is considered to be the 35th nation insofar as its healthcare status is concerned.

Today, there are approximately 47 millions of Americans without any type of access to health/mental healthcare (2). Additionally, several millions do have medical coverage but this coverage is insufficient and minimal. Besides, the lack of psychiatric parity of care, forces persons with mental illness to pay more for their care than persons suffering from medical illness. For instance, in accordance to current Medicare regulations, Medicare pays 80% of the physician's costs for medical illnesses; however, Medicare only pays 50% of the physician (psychiatrists) costs for psychiatric illnesses. This current lack of psychiatric parity leads to the unfortunate situation that less than 50% of all Americans in need of mental healthcare receive such care, and one third of those who receive care only receive minimal adequate care.

This unfortunate situation also leads to deleterious impact in the mental health system that currently prevails in the United States; for instance, depression cost businesses about $44 billion per year in the United States because of absenteeism, lack of productivity, and treatment cost; other psychiatric disorders also lead to similar situations. Many mental healthcare providers in the United States are currently refusing to see psychiatric patients under these highly discriminatory psychiatric parity policies that are very detrimental to the persons who suffer from mental illnesses in the United States, and, thus, add a high financial burden to the government, industry, and the U.S. population at large.

FOCUSING ON THE MENTAL HEALTH NEEDS OF THE MINORITY POPULATION IN THE UNITED STATES

The issues previously addressed with respect to access to care, comprehensive parity of psychiatric care and humane care are also quite unjust, detrimental, and discriminatory vis-à-vis the minority populations of the United States; that is, the ethnic minorities, gender/sexual minorities, and age-group minorities.

With respect to the ethnic minority populations who reside in the United States, the disparities in their psychiatric care approaches are already well demonstrated. For instance, it has recently been well documented that there are significant differences between ethnic groups insofar as demographic characteristics, geographic location, zone of residence, insurance status, income, wealth, and use of mental health services in this country. Clearly, poor Latinos/Hispanics with family income of less than $15,000 per year have lower access to specialty mental healthcare than poor non-Latino/Hispanic whites; additionally, African Americans who were not classified as poor were less likely to receive specialty mental healthcare than their white counterparts, even after adjusting for demographic characteristics, medical insurance status, and psychiatric comorbidity (3). Hispanics who reside in the United States also have the unique distinction of being the ethnic minority group with the highest percentage of uninsured persons (33.4%); the Caucasian population has an uninsured rate of 11% (4). In this respect, it is of interest to note that in the United States, native/U.S.-born citizens have an uninsurance rate of 14.2%, while the naturalized U.S. population has an uninsurance rate of 18.2%, the U.S. foreign-born alien population has an uninsurance rate of 34.2%, and the U.S. illegal alien population has an uninsurance rate of 43.6%. Obviously, in the United States, being foreign or non-native leads to discrimination and rejection in this regard (4). Along these lines, among the 32.3 million Americans living in poverty in the United States, 10.4 million (32.3%) are uninsured; of this number, 33.4% are Hispanics. This unfortunate situation leads to the fact that annually, 40% of Mexican Americans, 40% of Cuban Americans, and 33% of mainland Puerto Ricans have not had any physician annual visits (4). From a professional man-power point of view, in the United States, only 2% of medical students, 5.4% of physicians, 4.6% of psychiatrists, and 3% of nurses are Hispanics (4).

With respect to gender/sexual aspects, it has already been shown that the rates of reperfusion therapy, coronary angiography, and in-hospital death after myocardial infraction, but not the use of aspirin and β-blockers, vary according to race and sex; similar patterns are also being observed with respect to psychiatric care (5).

Age differences also play a roll in the delivery of mental healthcare in the United States. Mental healthcare disparities are also observed in different age groups; for instance, it is well known that eligibility and enrollment into Medicaid and State Children's Health Insurance Program (SCHIP) are hindered by financial, nonfinancial, and social policy barriers. Disparities in insurance and access indicators shows that lack of parental employment-linked benefits, procedural barriers to enrollment, and lack of clarification on eligibility for children of noncitizen parents are associated with low levels of insurance coverage among Latino children (6). Female-headed households in the United States shows a rate of 42.4% among African American families and about 40% for Puerto Rican families who reside in the United States mainland; this situation definitely leads to stress, poverty, and poor social support; eventually, it also leads to depression posttraumatic stress disorder, sexual use/abuse, prostitution, increased level of HIV infection and AIDS, increased levels of criminal activities, and the like. Definitely and unfortunately, society discriminates and/or ignores the unique mental health needs of these women and children (4).

It is also interesting to note that the existence of mental health disparities in this country also extends to the care of patients suffering from substance use/abuse, as well as alcoholism. We should also emphasize that the factors that influence mental health disparities, particularly access to mental healthcare, are multifactorial; among them, cultural differences, language barriers, lack of sufficient ethnic minority professional manpower, low education and socioeconomic levels among patients who suffer from mental illness, the high number of uninsured populations among the ethnic minority groups, ethnic and racial prejudices, and racial/ethnic discrimination (8).

THE ROLE OF MANAGED CARE

In addressing such an important topic, it is important to review what role, if any, managed care has vis-à-vis mental health disparities. In this regard, a study was conducted in Harris County (Houston) with patients admitted at the Harris County Psychiatric Center (HCPC), between the ages of 18 and 65 years, and during the years of 1994 and 1998 (9). The focus of this study was to measure the impact of managed care in the public-sector population of Texas. In 1994, 3245 patients were studied and in 1998, 3469 patients were also studied. The outcome of this study demonstrated that after the implementation of the Medicaid managed care program in Harris County (Houston), the bed utilization at HCPC decreased by 32%, and the readmission rate increased by 21%; concomitantly, the length of stay decreased from 16.5 days to 9.3 days. Additionally, African American and Hispanic American patients were more negatively affected than Caucasian patients. Undoubtedly, the implementation of the Medicaid managed care system in Texas has led to untoward effects in the quality of care provided to one of the most disadvantaged populations of this State (9).

Another study focusing on the role of managed care can also provide light in this regard (10). In this study, the experiences of low-income, nonelderly Hispanics, African Americans, and whites in managed care are compared with their racial/ethnic counterparts enrolled in the fee-for-service health plans. This study took place in three states: Florida, Tennessee, and Texas. The outcome of this study shows that patients/enrollees do not differ substantially on most access and satisfaction measures, except for a few notable exceptions. However, when compared with their fee-for-service counterparts, African Americans enrollees are twice as likely to report problems in obtaining needed care, and Hispanic enrollees are nearly twice as likely to rate the extent to which their providers care about them as "fair" to "poor." In contrast, however, whites in managed care are less likely to be without a regular provider than their fee-for-services counterparts, but they report greater dissatisfaction with the extent to which providers care about them (10).

In a third study (11), the authors investigate whether managed care ameliorates or aggravates ethnic and racial healthcare disparities in Medicare. In this study a disparity was defined, as proposed by the Institute of Medicine in 2002, as any difference in the use of health services after adjusting for preferences and healthcare needs. In this context, income or insurance may be mediators of disparities in healthcare. This study focused on the impact of managed care on healthcare disparities in two ways (a) whether aged minorities are more or less likely than whites to choose a managed care plan versus a regular indemnity plan when offered the same choices; and (b) comparison of selected measures of health services access and use by Medicare enrollees across racial groups and types of plans. The outcome of this study shows that minorities as a group are at least as well off in Medicare managed care as whites. Additionally, the impact of managed care on the use of services is at least as positives for Hispanics as for whites. Blacks, however, showed smaller gains and some losses in access relative to whites and Hispanics, but the differences are very small in magnitude and in significance. Also, minorities benefit more than whites from managed care's lower out-of-pocket costs.

On a report produced by the Committee on Managed Care of the American Psychiatric Association in 2002, entitled "Alternatives to Managed Care: A Resource Document" the negative impact of managed care on people suffering from mental illness is strongly emphasized. In this report, it clearly says that access to mental healthcare has been limited and drastically restricted. Patients have to call several physician/psychiatrists to find out who is in their plans, and they often have to wait for weeks before they are seen. Also frequently, the managers of Managed Care Organizations erroneously rule that the psychiatric care is not necessary, thus denying needed psychiatric services to patients.

Overall, the benefits of the managed care model in improving access to care, in achieving parity between psychiatry and medical services and in providing a more humane care approach leaves much to be desired, or has miserably failed.

EXPLORING SOLUTIONS

The previous discussions held in this chapter clearly depicts that the current health/mental healthcare system that prevails in this country is not only in a state of chaos, but is also negatively impacting in the health and mental healthcare outcomes of the population residing in the United States, especially the minority populations. Therefore, it is imperative that alternative models of care be sought, studied, and implemented as soon as possible in the United States. To continue in this deficient and chaotic health/mental health system is not only improper, but is also rapidly becoming an unethical position. How can we remain silent any longer or sustain a system that is causing the death of hundreds of persons weekly and perpetuating the complete lack or inferior provision of health/mental healthcare to millions of Americans on an annual basis. It is obviously time to say "enough is enough" and to find a humane solution and fair solution to the health/mental healthcare crisis of this nation. This country is the most powerful nation on earth in every respect; thus, it is imperative that health/mental healthcare be accessible to all persons living in this country, under a symbol of fairness and parity, and under the principles of humane care. Certainly, health/mental healthcare must be a right of all persons residing in this country rather than the privilege of the rich and wealthy.

Several models should be explored and discussed. For instance, the Canadian health/mental healthcare system has been already in existence for several years. In general, Canadian psychiatrists express satisfaction with their government run health insurance program; however, some physicians/psychiatrists are not too happy with the government's control over hospitals and the medical education system. Decisions about type of care or length of care are not a problem for psychiatrists in Canada. Psychoanalysis, for instance, is easily prescribed and delivered to patients in Canada. In Canada, managed care exclusions or precertification requirements are nonexisting. Ability to pay for health/mental health services is not an issue in Canada. In Canada, a single payer, the government, and universal access to care have been two major improvements in the Canadian health/mental healthcare system. Two issues that are often heard from psychiatrists in Canada are that only one payer decides the level of payment (the government) and that the current health/mental health system costs taxpayers in Canada a lot of money. Another issue raised at times is the lack of hospital beds in Canada to meet the current medical needs of the Canadian population. Control of medications can also potentially be a problem. In any case, when we compare the current health/mental healthcare system that prevail in Canada with ours in the United States, it looks to us that the Canadian is definitely better. Therefore, it makes sense to us to adapt the Canadian system in the United States until such a time that we are able to design a better system than the one in Canada.

It is, however, fair that we note the pitfalls of a potential "single-payer" health/mental healthcare system. For instance, lack of access because lack of available beds, possible rationing, potential for high overhead/administrative costs, assurance of "quality" care, viability of research efforts, overuse of the system, etc. Well, after taking into consideration all of these potential pitfalls, the current health/mental healthcare system in the United States if far worse.

With respect to the ethnic disparities, the major problem that we have in this country is the fact that although the government and policy-makers in the health/mental healthcare system are fully aware of its existence, little agreement has been reached regarding what type of intervention should be implemented to eliminate them (12). In this context, it has already been proven that if Hispanics and African Americans were provided medical insurance with levels comparable to the medical insurance of whites, many of the current minority disparities would be reduced if not eliminated (12).

The American Psychiatric Association has also addressed the issue of health/mental healthcare disparities among the minority groups of this country, and has made suggestions to resolve them (13).

It should also be emphasized in this context that policies addressing the poor socioeconomic conditions of the minority groups who reside in this country could clearly help to improve or eliminate the rate of health/mental health disparities that currently exist in the United States; for instance, housing, education, and income (14). Along these lines, it has also been demonstrated that lack of health insurance is a key factor in white and Hispanic mental healthcare differences and also in white and African American mental healthcare differences. When one has health insurance, one is likely to seek health/mental healthcare for unmet medical and psychiatric needs and is more likely to see the same doctor over time and less likely to let a year go by without a medical check-up (15). It should also be mention here that the cost to provide full health insurance to all persons in the United States, although costly, is not necessarily exaggerated. Based on 1996 to 1998 insurance coverage data with persons with private and public insurance among persons with lower or middle-income levels will cost from about $34 million to about $69 million based on 2001 dollar value. This amount will increase healthcare spending by 3% to 6% and will raise the healthcare's share of the Gross Domestic Product (GDP) by less than one percent point (16).

There are also other options and/or models that need to be taken into consideration when attempting to find solutions for a health/mental healthcare system that is currently shameful. For instance, it is estimated that if a National Health Insurance (NHI) program were to be created in this country, similar to the current Medicare program or conceptualized as an expansion of the current Medicare program, based on a universal and single payer program, it will save $200 billion annual, which is enough to provide health insurance coverage to every one who lacks it in this country (17). It is obvious that this country must do something to resolve the current health/mental healthcare chaos that prevail in this nation. To remain with the status quo is rather unethical.

CONCLUSION

In this chapter, we first described the current delivery of mental healthcare system that prevails at a worldwide level, especially in poverty-stricken regions. Next, we focused on the current crisis that exists in the health/mental healthcare system of the United States. Subsequently, we discussed the unmet mental health needs of the minority populations of the United States. Afterward, we addressed the potential role of managed care vis-à-vis the disparities that currently exist in the health/mental healthcare system of this country. Later, we examine the options and models that should be considered as possible solutions to the problems that prevail in the health/mental healthcare system of this nation.

What is clear to us is that the status quo is no longer viable. The current health/mental healthcare system of this country borders on being unethical. Solutions must be found and implemented as soon as possible. In this context a series of principles must be kept in mind. They are as follows:

- Health insurance coverage must be a right rather than a privilege.
- All persons living in the United States must be provided health insurance.
- Every person living in this country must have full access to health and mental health insurance at all times.

- Parity of care between medical/surgical and psychiatric conditions must be implemented. Not to provide this parity is unethical.
- Quality of care, level of care, and comprehensiveness of health/mental healthcare must be identical for all persons in this country.
- All current health/mental health disparities (racial, ethnic, cultural, gender, etc.) must be fully eliminated from the health/mental healthcare system of this country.
- Issues pertaining to health/mental health manpower needs must be addressed and resolved in this country.
- No discrimination should be permitted in the health/mental healthcare system of this country based on racial, ethnic, gender, age, religious, or cultural differences.
- Confidentially must prevail at all times in the health/mental healthcare system of this country.
- Health/mental health coverage in this country needs to be universal, continuous, affordable, and sustainable for all persons living in this country.
- The health insurance program in this country must be well-being oriented and must enhance health.
- Research and education should be integral components of the health/mental healthcare system of this country.
- Evidence-based should be an integral component of the health/mental healthcare system of this country.
- Cultural competence should be an integral component of the health/mental healthcare system of this country.

References

1. May M. World aspects of psychiatry. In: Sadock BJ, Sadock VA, Ruiz P, eds. *Kaplan & Sadock's Comprehensive Textbook of Psychiatry*, 9th ed. Philadelphia, PA: Lippincott Williams & Wilkins (in press).
2. Ruiz P. Presidential address: Addressing patient needs: Access, parity and humane care. *Am J Psychiatry* 2007;16(10):1507–1509.
3. Alegria M, Canino G, Rios R, et al. Inequalities in use of specialty mental health services among Latino, African Americans, and Non-Latino whites. *Psychiatric Serv* 2002;53(12): 1547–1555.
4. Ruiz P. Hispanics' mental health plight. *Behav Health Management* 2005;11:17–19.
5. Vaccarino V, Rathore SS, Wenger N, et al. Sex and racial differences in the management of acute myocardial infarction, 1994–2002. *N Engl J Med* 2005;353:671–682.
6. Zambrana RE, Carter-Pokras O. Improving health insurance coverage for Latino children: A review of barriers, challenges and state strategies. *J Natl Med Assoc* 2004;19(14):508–523.
7. Ruiz P, Venegas Samuels K, Alarcon RD. The economics of pain: mental healthcare cost among minorities. *Psychiatr Clin North Am* 1995,18(3).659 670.
8. Ruiz P. Hispanic access to health/mental health services. *Psychiatr Q* 2002;73(2):85–91.
9. Averill P, Ruiz P, Small DR, et al. Outcome assessment of the medicaid managed care program in Harris County (Houston). *Psychiatr Q* 2003;74(2):103–114.
10. Leigh WA, Lillie-Blanton M, Martinez RM, et al Managed care in three states: Experiences of low-income African Americans and Hispanics. *Managed Care* 1999;36: 318–331.
11. Balsa AI, Cao Z, McGuire TG. Does managed healthcare reduce healthcare disparities between minorities and whites? *J Health Economics* 2007;26(1):101–121.
12. Lillie-Blanton M, Hoffman C. The role of health insurance coverage in reducing racial/ethnic disparities in healthcare. *Health Affairs* 2005;24(2):398–408.
13. Ruiz P, Primm A. APA's efforts to eliminate disparities. *Psychiatr Serv* 2005;56(12): 1603–1605.

14. Alegría M, Perez DJ, Williams S. The role of public policies in reducing mental health status disparities for people of color. *Health Affairs* 2003;22(5):51–64.

15. Hargraves JL, Hadley J. The contribution of insurance coverage and community resources to reducing racial/ethnic disparities in access to care. *Health Serv Res* 2003;38(3): 809–829.

16. Hadley J, Holahan J. Covering the uninsured: How much would it cost? *Data Watch* 2003;4:W3-250–W3-265.

17. The Physician's Working Group for Single-Payer National Health Insurance. *JAMA* 2003;290(6):798–805.

INDEX

Note: Page numbers followed by an *f* indicate figures; those followed by a *t* indicate tables